Library of Congress Cataloging-in-Publication Data

Exercise gas exchange in heart disease / editor, Karlman Wasserman.
     p.   cm.
  Includes bibliographical references and index.
  ISBN 0-87993-629-0
  1. Heart function tests.   2. Pulmonary function tests.   3. Pulmonary gas exchange—Evaluation.   4. Heart failure—
Pathophysiology.   I. Wasserman, Karlman.
  [DNLM: 1. Heart Diseases—diagnosis.   2. Heart Diseases—
physiopathology.   3. Pulmonary Gas Exchange.   4. Exertion—
physiology.   5. Exercise Test.   WG 210 E96 1995]
RC683.5.H4E95   1995
616.1′20754—dc20
DNLM/DLC
for Library of Congress   95-38676
                                                                  CIP

Copyright © 1996

Published by
Futura Publishing Company, Inc.
135 Bedford Road
Armonk, New York 10504

LC#: 95-38676
ISBN#: 0-87993-629-0

Every effort has been made to ensure that the information in this book
is up to date and accurate at the time of publication. However, due to
the constant developments in medicine, neither the authors, nor the editor, nor the publisher can accept any legal or any other responsibility
for any errors or omissions that may occur.

Printed in the United States of America.

Printed on acid-free paper.

EXERCISE GAS EXCHAN
IN HEART DISEASE

Editor:

Karlman Wasserman, MD, PhD

Professor of Medicine
Division of Respiratory and Critical Care Physiology
Medicine
Department of Medicine
Harbor-UCLA Medical Center
University of California, Los Angeles
Torrance, CA

**Futura Publishing
Company, Inc.**
Armonk, NY

Contributors

Gert Baumann, MD   Professor of Medicine, Director, I. Med. Klinik und Poliklinik, Zentrum fur Innere Medizine, Charite, Universitat Zu Berlin, Berlin, Germany

Gianni Carini, MD   Cattedra di Cardiologia, Universita di Torino, Torino, Italy

Frederick R. Cobb, MD   Veterans Affairs Medical Center, Durham, North Carolina

Alain Cohen-Solal, MD   Service de Cardiologie, Hospital Beaujon, Clichy, France

Jay N. Cohn, MD   Professor of Medicine, Head of Cardiovascular Division, University of Minnesota Medical School, Minneapolis, Minnesota

Robert J. Cody, MD   Division of Cardiology, Ohio State University, Columbus, Ohio

Livio Dei Cas, MD   Universita de Brescia, Brescia, Italy

Brian D. Duscha, MS   Exercise Physiologist, Center for Living, Duke University Medical Center, Durham, North Carolina

Adrian Hall, MB, BS, FANZCA   Deputy Director ICU, Western Hospital, Victoria, Australia

William R. Hiatt, MD   Professor of Medicine, University of Colorado Health Sciences Center, Section of Vascular Medicine, Denver, Colorado

Michael B. Higgenbotham, MD   Associate Professor of Medicine, Duke University Medical Center, Heart Failure Service, Durham, North Carolina

Michiaki Hiroe, MD   Second Department of Internal Medicine, Tokyo Medical and Dental University, Tokyo, Japan

Haruki Itoh, MD   Director of Internal Medicine, The Cardiovascular Institute, Tokyo, Japan

Gary Johnson, MS   Veterans Affairs Medical Center, West Haven, Connecticut

Kazuzo Kato, MD   President, The Cardiovascular Institute, Tokyo, Japan

Franz X. Kleber, MD   Professor of Medicine, I. Med. Klinik und Poliklinik, Zentrum fur Innere Medizin, Charite, Med. Fakultat der Humboldt, Universitat zu Berlin, Berlin, Germany

Toshio Kobayashi, MD   Associate Professor, Health Science Center, Tokyo University of Mercantile Marine, Tokyo, Japan

Kazuzo Kato, MD   President, The Cardiovascular Institute, Tokyo, Japan

Akira Koike, MD   Second Department of Internal Medicine, Tokyo Medical and Dental University, Tokyo, Japan

Mark D. Kraemer, MD   Cardiology Fellow, University of Minnesota, Cardiovascular Division, Minneapolis, Minnesota

Fumiaki Marumo, MD   Second Department of Internal Medicine, Tokyo Medical and Dental University, Tokyo, Japan

Marco Metra, MD   Cattedra di Cardiologia, Universita de Brescia, Brescia, Italy

Savina Nodari, MD   Universita de Brescia, Brescia, Italy

Paul Older, MB, BS, FRCA, FANZCA, FFIANZCA   Director ICU and Head CPX Laboratory, Western Hospital, Victoria, Autralia

Fulvio Orzan, MD   Cattedra di Cardiologia, Universita di Torino, Torino, Italy

Antimo Papa, MD   Fondazione Clinica del Lavoro, Centro di Raibilitazione, Campoli, Italy

Phillip A. Poole-Wilson, MD, FRCP, FESC, FACC   Professor of Cardiology, National Heart and Lung Institute, London, England

D. Domencia Raccagni, MD   Cattedra di Cardiologia, Universita de Brescia, Brescia, Italy

Judith G. Regensteiner, PhD   Associate Professor of Medicine, University of Colorado Health Sciences Center, Section of Vascular Medicine, Denver, Colorado

Irmingard Reindt, MD   I. Med. Klinik und Poliklinik, Zentrum fur Innere Medizin, Charite, Med. Fakultat der Humboldt, Universitate zu Berlin, Berlin, Germany

Kathy E. Sietsema, MD   Associate Professor of Medicine, Division of Respiratory and Critical Care Physiology and Medicine, Harbor-UCLA Medical Center, Torrance, California

Cris A. Slentz, PhD   Exercise Physiologist, Veterans Administration Medical Center, Durham, North Carolina

Lynne Warner Stevenson, MD   Associate Professor of Medicine, Medical Director, Cardiomyopathy and Transplant Program, Brigham and Women's Hospital, Harvard Medical School, Boston, Massachusetts

William W. Stringer, MD   Assistant Professor of Medicine, Division of Respiratory and Critical Care Physiology and Medicine, Harbor-UCLA Medical Center, Torrance, California

Darryl Y. Sue, MD   Professor of Medicine, Division of Respiratory and Critical Care Physiology and Medicine, Harbor-UCLA Medical Center, Torrance, California

Martin J. Sullivan, MD   Associate Professor of Medicine, Division of Cardiology, Duke University Medical Center, Durham, North Carolina

Karlman Wasserman, MD, PhD   Professor of Medicine and Chief, Division of Respiratory and Critical Care Physiology and Medicine, Harbor-UCLA Medical Center, Torrance, California

Karl T. Weber, MD   Professor of Medicine and Chairman, Department of Internal Medicine, University of Missouri-Columbia, Columbia, Missouri

Klaus D. Wernecke, Dr. Institut für Biomathematik, Med. Fakultat der Humboldt, Universitat zu Berlin, Berlin, Germany

Eugene E. Wolfel, MD Associate Professor of Medicine, Division of Cardiology, University of Colorado Health Sciences Center, Denver, Colorado

Hiroshi Yamabe, MD First Department of Internal Medicine, Kobe University School of Medicine, Kobe, Japan

Mitsuhiro Yokoyama, MD First Department of Internal Medicine, Kobe University School of Medicine, Kobe, Japan

Susan Zeische, RN Veterans Affairs Medical Center, Minneapolis, Minnesota

Preface

Adolf Fick published his principle for measuring cardiac output in the University of Wurzburg Press (Wurzburg, Germany) in 1870. He recognized that pulmonary blood flow, and therefore cardiac output, were inextricably linked to oxygen uptake and arteriovenous oxygen difference through the law of conservation of mass. Since then, the Fick Principle has been the "gold standard" for measuring cardiac output.

Application of the Fick Principle to clinical medicine had to await the development of cardiac catheterization. However, in the third decade of this century, with the development of methods for measuring oxygen and carbon dioxide in the expired air, physiologically-oriented cardiologists, notably Tinsley R. Harrison, used gas exchange measurements to study heart failure. They recognized that heart failure resulted in a low oxygen consumption and a high carbon dioxide production to perform exercise compared to normal subjects; however, technology was too cumbersome to exploit these early findings and it was not pursued for the next 30 years.

In the middle of this century, academic cardiologists stopped defining heart failure by its backward signs (e.g., pulmonary edema, increased vascular pressures) and recognized that the primary role of the heart is to supply oxygen to the tissues to support cellular respiration. Thus, heart failure could logically be defined by respiratory gas analysis as had already been shown. Because the measurement of oxygen and carbon dioxide in the expired air and minute ventilation required special referral laboratory skills, this information was not readily available to most physicians treating patients with heart failure. Consequently, gas exchange methods to evaluate patients for heart disease and effectiveness of therapy could not be used in the routine care of patients with heart disease.

However, in the 1950s and 1960s, electronic gas analyzers for carbon dioxide, nitrogen, and oxygen were developed so that expired and inspired gas composition could be easily and accurately measured breath-by-breath. With the further development of digital computers in the late 1960s and early 1970s, followed by the availability of relatively cheap personal computers, it was possible to return to measuring gas exchange during exercise for studying heart failure and all types of cardiovascular diseases. Furthermore, it became possible to make the measurements dynamically, to track the transient cardiovascular responses to exercise stimuli. The recent development of accurate and automated analyses of gas exchange during exercise makes this technology one of the lowest cost and potentially one of the most widely applied approaches for evaluating cardiovascular function during exercise.

Recognizing the rapid development of new research in this area leading directly to applications relevant to patient care, a monograph describing many of these advances seems timely. The chapters in this monograph are written by experienced authorities from around the world who have used the new technology of cardiopulmonary exercise testing with gas exchange measurements to address important questions in cardiology.

To address the advances in gas exchange measurements in cardiopulmonary exercise testing in a systematic way, this monograph is divided into four sections preceded by an introductory chapter on exercise physiology. The latter establishes the motivation for using gas exchange measurements during exercise to uncover pathophysiology. Following this introductory chapter, the first section describes gas exchange measurements which can be used to evaluate cardiac function. The next section focuses on the abnormal ventilatory responses to exercise, and the possible mechanisms of the abnormality and their relationship to the severity of heart failure. The third section examines peripheral factors affecting the reduced exercise capacity in cardiovascular diseases. The final section describes clinical applications to which exercise gas exchange testing is currently applied. It is anticipated that the information in this monograph will provide the basis for new research as well as serve as a guide for established and new applications of cardiopulmonary exercise testing in patients with cardiovascular diseases.

Karlman Wasserman, MD, PhD
Editor

Contents

Contributors   iii

Preface   vii

Section 1   Introduction

Chapter 1   **Cardiovascular Coupling of External
to Cellular Respiration**
Karlman Wasserman, MD; Darryl Y. Sue, MD   1

Section 2   Central Circulation-Cardiac Function and
Exercise Gas Exchange

Chapter 2   **Cardiopulmonary Exercise Testing
in Chronic Heart Failure**
Alain Cohen-Solal, MD   17

Chapter 3   **Diastolic Dysfunction and Exercise Gas
Exchange**
Michael B. Higgenbotham, MD   39

Chapter 4   **Cardiopulmonary Exercise Testing and the
Evaluation of Systolic Dysfunction**
Karl T. Weber, MD   55

Chapter 5   **Gas Exchange During Recovery from
Exercise in Patients with Heart Failure**
Mark D. Kraemer, MD   63

Chapter 6   **Analysis of Gas Exchange Dynamics
in Patients with Cardiovascular Disease**
Kathy E. Sietsema, MD   71

Section 3   The Ventilatory Response to Exercise in Patients
               with Heart Disease

Chapter 7   **The Relation Between Muscle Function
               and Increased Ventilation in Heart Failure**
               Phillip A. Poole-Wilson, MD   83

Chapter 8   **Dyspnea in Heart Failure**
               Franz X. Kleber, MD; Irmingard Reindl, MD
               Klaus D. Wernecke, MD; Gert Baumann, MD   95

Chapter 9   **Increased Ventilatory Response to
               Exercise as Related to Functional Capacity**
               Akira Koike, MD; Michiaki Hiroe, MD
               Fumiaki Marumo, MD   109

Chapter 10   **Ventilatory and Arterial Blood Gas Changes
               During Exercise in Heart Failure**
               Marco Metra, MD; Domenica Raccagni, MD
               Gianni Carini, MD; Fulvio Orzan, MD
               Antimo Papa, MD; Savina Nodari, MD
               Robert J. Cody, MD; Livio Dei Cas, MD   125

Chapter 11   **The Role of Increased Dead Space in the
               Augmented Ventilation of Cardiac Patients**
               Toshio Kobayashi, MD; Haruki Itoh, MD
               Kazuzo Kato, MD   145

Section 4   Peripheral Mechanisms Determining
               Exercise Capacity

Chapter 12   **Critical Capillary PO$_2$, Net Lactate
               Production, and Oxyhemoglobin
               Dissociation: Effects on Exercise
               Gas Exchange**
               Karlman Wasserman, MD, PhD
               William W. Stringer, MD   157

Chapter 13   **Peripheral and Central Oxygen Extraction
               in Chronic Heart Failure**
               Hiroshi Yamabe, MD; Mitsuhiro Yokoyama, MD   183

Contents · xi

Chapter 14 **Peripheral Arterial Disease: Pathophysiology, Exercise Performance, and Effect of Exercise Training on Gas Exchange and Muscle Metabolism**
William R. Hiatt, MD; Eugene E. Wolfel, MD
Judith G. Regensteiner, PhD   197

Chapter 15 **Peripheral Determinants of Exercise Intolerance in Patients with Chronic Heart Failure**
Martin J.Sullivan, MD; Brian D. Duscha, MS
Cris A. Slentz, PhD   209

Section 5   Clinical Applications

Chapter 16 **Short-Term Exercise Training After Cardiac Surgery**
Haruki Itoh, MD; Kazuzo Kato, MD   229

Chapter 17 **Use of Exercise Gas Exchange Measurements in Multicenter Drug Studies**
Jay N. Cohn, MD; Susan Ziesche, RN
Gary Johnson, MS; Frederick R. Cobb, MD   245

Chapter 18 **Exercise Gas Exchange to Evaluate Cardiac Pacemaker Function**
Norbert Treese, MD   257

Chapter 19 **Role of Exercise Testing in the Evaluation of Candidates for Cardiac Transplantation**
Lynne Warner Stevenson, MD   271

Chapter 20 **The Role of Cardiopulmonary Exercise Testing for the Preoperative Evaluation of the Elderly**
Paul Older, MB; Adrian Hall, MB   287

Index   299

Section 1

Introduction

1

Cardiovascular Coupling of External to Cellular Respiration

Karlman Wasserman, MD, PhD
Darryl Y. Sue, MD

Elementary Considerations of Muscle Bioenergetics

The energy for muscle contraction during exercise is provided by the splitting of the terminal phosphate of adenosine triphosphate. Adenosine triphosphate (ATP) undergoes hydrolysis, releasing energy in the cytosol at the site of the myofibril where the conformational change in actin and myosin takes place (Figure 1).[1] The majority of ATP is generated in the mitochondria from adenosine diphosphate (ADP) and inorganic phosphate, as a result of energy derived in the process of proton transport along the electron transport chain to oxygen. These reactions result in the consumption of oxygen and the formation of water.

Phosphocreatine (Cr~P) serves both as a shuttle for the transfer of high energy phosphate (~P) from mitochondrial ATP, the site of ~P generation, and the cytosolic ATP, the site of its consumption (Figure 1). It also serves as a buffer source of ~P for the rapid resynthesis of cytosolic ATP as it is consumed during muscle contraction.[2] The ~P stores in the form of Cr~P are limited in the muscle (approximately 16 to 35 mmol/L of muscle water),[3] and Cr~P concentration changes very rapidly at the onset of exercise with similar dynamics to that of oxygen uptake ($\dot{V}O_2$).[4] Thus, the net contribution of Cr~P to muscle bioenergetics is complete by the time $\dot{V}O_2$ reaches a steady state

From Wasserman, K (ed): *Exercise Gas Exchange in Heart Disease*. Armonk, NY: Futura Publishing Company, Inc., © 1996.

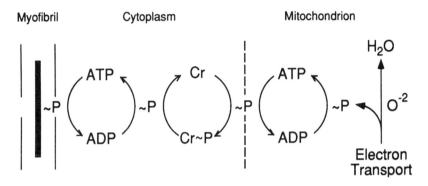

Figure 1. Scheme by which phosphocreatine (Cr~P) shuttles high energy phosphate (~P) between adenosine triphosphate (ATP) in the mitochondrion and the cytosol of the myocyte. Phosphocreatine also serves as a buffer source of ~P for the immediate availability of cytosolic ATP for contraction of the myofibril. In the mitochondrion, the regeneration of 3 ATP during electron transport consumes one atom of oxygen.

(<3 minutes for moderate intensity exercise). Similarly, the oxygen stores in the blood are largely depleted by the third minute of exercise. Therefore, to sustain exercise, the ATP must be regenerated primarily aerobically, and the source of oxygen for these reactions must be the atmosphere. The aerobic regeneration of ATP is reflected in the increase in $\dot{V}O_2$ in response to exercise. The delivery of the atmospheric oxygen to the myocyte required for ATP regeneration is totally dependent on the ability of the circulation to transport the oxygen at the rate required by the active muscles (Figure 2).

$\dot{V}O_2$ as a Function of Increasing Work Rate

The number of molecules of ATP regenerated from each molecule of oxygen consumed is well established (approximately 6 ATP:1 O_2). The amount of oxygen required to perform a given amount of work totally aerobically is also well characterized, approximately 10 mL/min/W (Figure 3), regardless of the degree of fitness, age, or gender of the subject.[5,6] Thus, failure of the circulation to deliver oxygen at the required rate to sustain exercise will slow the rate of aerobic regeneration of ATP by the muscles. This slowing should be reflected in a slowed rate of $\dot{V}O_2$ at the airway, and the stimulation of anaerobic ATP regeneration in the cell. The latter is accompanied by lactic acidosis and increased carbon dioxide output ($\dot{V}CO_2$) over that predicted from aerobic metabolism alone (Figure 4). Thus, we might predict that the

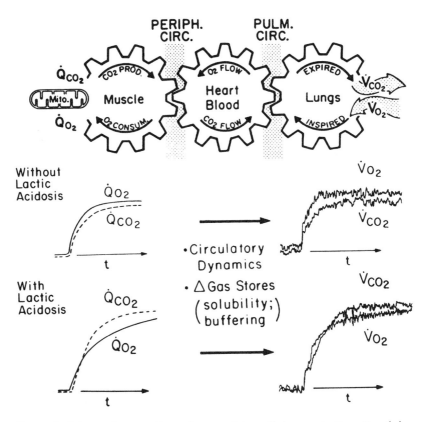

Figure 2. Scheme for coupling of external to cellular respiration. Breath-by-breath data (**right**), interpolated second-by-second for 6 minutes of 2 constant work-rate exercise tests, 1 above and 1 below that at which a lactic acidosis occurs. Each study on the right is an overlay of 4 repetitions to reduce random noise in the data and enhance the physiological events. The factors that modulate the relationship between cellular respiration and external respiration are shown in the center of the diagram. For work rates without a lactic acidosis, $\dot{V}O_2$ reaches a steady state by 3 minutes and $\dot{V}CO_2$ by 4 minutes (**upper right**). For work rates with a lactic acidosis, $\dot{V}O_2$ kinetics are slowed and may not reach a steady state. In contrast, $\dot{V}CO_2$ increases in magnitude over without an apparent slow-rising component (**lower right**). (Reproduced from Reference 7.)

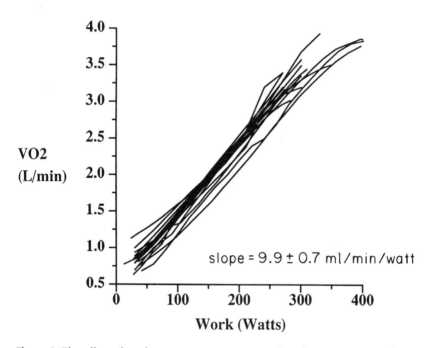

Figure 3. The effect of work rate on oxygen consumption during progressively increasing work-rate cycle ergometer exercise for 17 normal subjects. The oxygen consumption response in normal subjects is predictable for cycle ergometer work regardless of age, gender, or training. The average regression slope is given in the figure. The slope is consistent among subjects, but is displaced upward depending on the body weight. The displacement upward is 5.8 mL/min/kg body weight.[5,6]

slope of the relationship between $\dot{V}O_2$ and work rate during progressively increasing work-rate exercise might become more shallow in patients with cardiovascular dysfunction as has been previously described.[6]

Peripheral Blood Flow Requirements During Exercise

The oxygen flow to the exercising muscles depends on the blood flow, hemoglobin concentration, and the partial pressure of oxygen (PO_2) in the patient's arterial blood.[7] Each liter of arterial blood con-

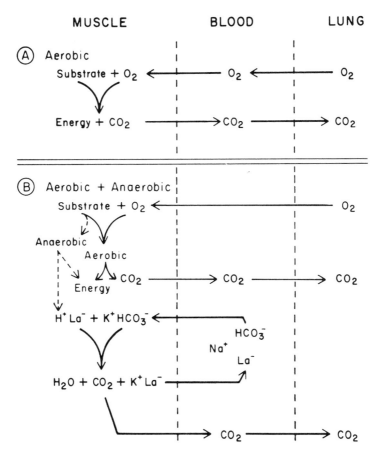

Figure 4. Gas exchange during aerobic (**A**) and aerobic-plus-anaerobic (**B**) exercise. The acid-base consequence of the latter is a net increase in cellular lactic acid production. The buffering of the accumulating lactic acid takes place in the cell at the site of formation, predominantly by bicarbonate. The latter mechanism increases the CO_2 production of the cell by approximately 22.3 mL/mmol of bicarbonate buffering lactic acid. The increase in cell lactate and decrease in cell bicarbonate results in chemical concentration gradients causing lactate to be transported out of and bicarbonate to be transported into the cell. (From Reference 21.)

taining 15 g hemoglobin/dL at normal sea level PO_2 contains about 200 mL of O_2. To perform a relatively fast walk (3 mph), the average size adult's lower extremity muscles consume O_2 at a rate of about 1 L/min. Because not all of the O_2 can be extracted from the capillary blood, the maximal extraction being about 85%, the blood flow to the legs must be at least 6 L/min to perform this walk totally aerobically. The requirement for increased lower extremity blood flow is even higher in patients with anemia, carboxyhemoglobinemia, or a hemoglobinopathy with a left shifted oxyhemoglobin dissociation curve.

If the blood supply is inadequate to maintain the critical capillary PO_2 required to perform exercise totally aerobically, anaerobic metabolism will be stimulated with the accumulation of lactic acid,[8] buffering of the H^+ by HCO_3^-, and increased CO_2 production (Figure 4). Since lactic acid is highly dissociated (>99.9%) at the pH of cell water, the H^+ must be immediately buffered in the cell as it is formed. Because HCO_3^- is the primary buffer of the increased cellular H^+, H_2CO_3 is formed at the same rate that lactate accumulates. The H_2CO_3 formed dissociates to CO_2 and H_2O, resulting in an increased CO_2 production by the cell over that predicted from the rate of aerobic metabolism alone (Figure 4). Arterial blood lactate and HCO_3^- change reciprocally and approximately stoichiometrically in response to exercise above the subject's lactic acidosis threshold (*LAT*) (heavy intensity exercise).[9-13] Also, the increase in $\dot{V}CO_2$ over that predicted from aerobic metabolism has been shown to occur simultaneously with the development of lactic acidosis (Figure 5). Consequently, the excess $\dot{V}CO_2$ has been used to quantify the metabolic rate at which lactic acidosis develops[14] and the magnitude of the lactic acidosis. Therefore, the failure of the circulation to provide oxygen at the required rate to support the aerobic regeneration of ATP should be reflected in a disproportionately increased $\dot{V}CO_2$ relative to the $\dot{V}O_2$ (Figures 2 and 5). An inadequate cardiovascular response to exercise should also cause $\dot{V}O_2$ kinetics to be relatively slow[16-18] and $\dot{V}CO_2$ at the lungs to be increased, reflecting the anaerobic contribution to the bioenergetics of exercise.[7,19]

Exercise Lactic Acidosis, Fitness, and Heart Disease

Failure of the circulation to deliver oxygen at the rate needed to sustain exercise limits the rate of aerobic regeneration of ATP and $\dot{V}O_2$ by the muscles. When ATP is generated anaerobically, lactic acidosis develops because of a net increase in lactate production. Arterial lactate measurement is one of the more sensitive ways of determining the

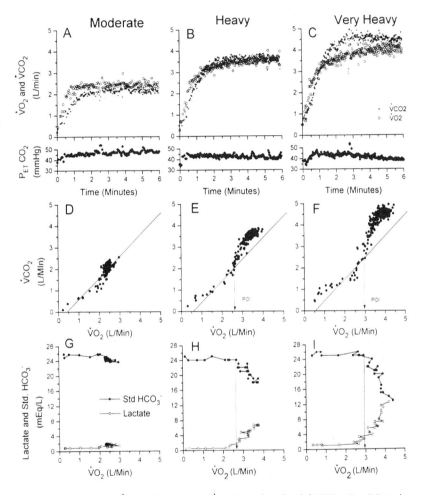

Figure 5. O_2 uptake ($\dot{V}O_2$), CO_2 output ($\dot{V}CO_2$), and end-tidal PCO_2 ($P_{ET}CO_2$) plotted as a function of time (**panels A, B** and **C**), and $\dot{V}CO_2$ arterial lactate, and standard (Std) HCO_3^- plotted as a function of $\dot{V}O_2$ (**panels D** to **I**) for constant work-rate tests of moderate, heavy, and very heavy work intensity. Steepening of $\dot{V}CO_2$ relative to $\dot{V}O_2$ (arrow in **panels E** and **F**) occurs simultaneously with the increase in lactate and the decrease in standard HCO_3^- (arrow in **panels H** and **I**), reflecting the buffering of the lactic acid by HCO_3^-. The diagonal lines in panels D, E & F have a slope of "1." (From Reference 21.)

fitness of the subject to perform aerobic work (Figure 6). The more fit the subject, the higher the $\dot{V}O_2$ before the arterial lactate starts to increase. Once the arterial lactate starts to increase, it increases progressively and more steeply rather than linearly as $\dot{V}O_2$ increases (Figure 6). Patients with heart disease resulting in exercise limitation may begin to increase arterial lactate concentration at extremely low $\dot{V}O_2$ levels (Figure 6). This reflects their inability to supply the active myocytes with the oxygen flow necessary to sustain ATP regeneration, aerobically. However, the arterial lactate concentration versus $\dot{V}O_2$ relationship of patients with mild heart disease, or patients with coronary artery disease who manifest myocardial ischemia at work levels above their predicted *LAT*, may overlap with that of normal sedentary subjects.

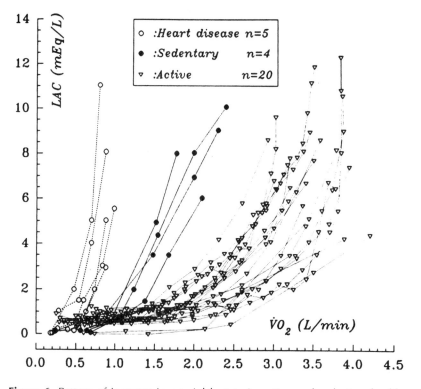

Figure 6. Pattern of increase in arterial lactate in active and sedentary healthy subjects and in patients with chronic heart failure, secondary to mitral valve disease, as related to increasing exercise oxygen uptake ($\dot{V}O_2$). Arterial lactate (LAC) concentration increased from approximately the same resting value to approximately the same concentration at maximal exercise in each of the three groups. The fitter the subject for aerobic work, the higher the $\dot{V}O_2$ before lactate started to increase significantly above resting levels. (Reproduced from Reference 7.)

$\dot{V}O_2$ and $\dot{V}CO_2$ Kinetics Below and Above the Lactic Acidosis Threshold

Figure 2 shows the typical responses of $\dot{V}O_2$ and $\dot{V}CO_2$ for moderate intensity exercise, i.e., exercise that does not engender lactic acidosis, and heavy intensity exercise, i.e., exercise that results in lactic acidosis. These data were obtained from a normal subject,[20] but the same patterns are observed in patients with heart disease.[16,21] The pattern of gas exchange has been shown to differ between the work-rate domains associated with and without lactic acidosis.[7,22] Thus, in the absence of lactic acidosis, $\dot{V}O_2$ reaches a steady state by 3 minutes, while $\dot{V}CO_2$ increases slightly more slowly, reaching a steady state by 4 minutes at a somewhat lower value than $\dot{V}O_2$. The $\dot{V}CO_2$ is slightly lower than $\dot{V}O_2$ (Figure 2) because the metabolic substrate respiratory quotient is less than 1.0.

For exercise performed above the *LAT*, $\dot{V}O_2$ dynamics are slow compared to exercise performed below the *LAT*, and a steady state in $\dot{V}O_2$ is often not reached before the subject fatigues (Figure 7). In contrast to $\dot{V}O_2$ dynamics, $\dot{V}CO_2$ dynamics do not change appreciably during above *LAT* exercise (Figure 7),[22] and usually after 1 minute of such exercise, $\dot{V}CO_2$ exceeds $\dot{V}O_2$ (Figures 5 and 7), the magnitude depending on the rate of lactate increase.[15] The extra CO_2 can be accounted for by the CO_2 produced as HCO_3^- buffers the H^+ from lactic acid produced during heavy intensity exercise (Figure 5).

Sites of Cardiovascular Dysfunction and the Pattern of Coupling of External to Cellular Respiration

From the Fick equation for measuring cardiac output (cardiac output = $\dot{V}O_2$/arteriovenous O_2 difference), it is evident that $\dot{V}O_2$ is a measure of cardiac function. Studies have demonstrated that changing the ventilatory response to exercise does not affect $\dot{V}O_2$ kinetics,[23] but changing the circulatory response to exercise does affect $\dot{V}O_2$ kinetics.[24] Accordingly, $\dot{V}O_2$ is our best global marker of the rate of aerobic regeneration of ATP, and, thereby, $\dot{V}O_2$ becomes a sensitive indicator of the adequacy of the cardiovascular response to exercise stress.

To demonstrate how disease can impair the coupling of external to cellular respiration, examples of gas exchange abnormalities found at three different anatomic sites of cardiovascular function are described. While the gas exchange measurements are abnormal in all three types of dysfunction, there are specific findings in each type. Importantly, recognizing these abnormal patterns of the gas exchange re-

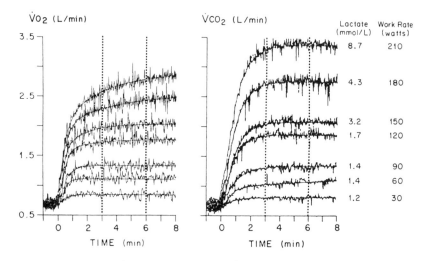

Figure 7. O_2 uptake ($\dot{V}O_2$) and CO_2 output ($\dot{V}CO_2$) as related to time at seven different levels of work for a healthy subject. On the right side of each study is the work rate performed and the forearm vein lactate measured 1 minute after the end of exercise. The 3 lowest work rates were below the subject's lactic acidosis threshold (*LAT*), whereas the 4 highest work rates were above it. The $\dot{V}O_2$ continued to increase during the 4 work rates above the *LAT*, the rate of increase being more marked the higher the work rate. In contrast, the $\dot{V}CO_2$ kinetics are not appreciably different, reaching a constant level by 3 to 4 minutes in all 7 tests. (Modified from Reference 22.)

sponses may enable the investigator to distinguish one disorder from the other when it is desirable to make a distinction. Only the graphical display of gas exchange abnormalities in myocardial ischemia are illustrated here (Figure 8, Patient B) and contrasted with a study of a patient with a similar predicted maximum oxygen uptake ($\dot{V}O_2$max), but who had a normal exercise response (Figure 8, Patient A). (Refer to Chapter 8, Reference 6 for similar graphical displays of the other disorders described.)

Myocardial Ischemia

$\Delta\dot{V}O_2/\Delta WR$. When perfusion of a region of the myocardium is inadequate to supply oxygen at the rate needed to regenerate ATP to sustain contraction, that region of the myocardial muscle cannot contract and contribute to the force required to effect a normal stroke volume. Simultaneously, myocardial work increases as heart rate and blood pressure increase, creating a further imbalance between myocardial oxygen supply and demand. During a progressively increasing work-

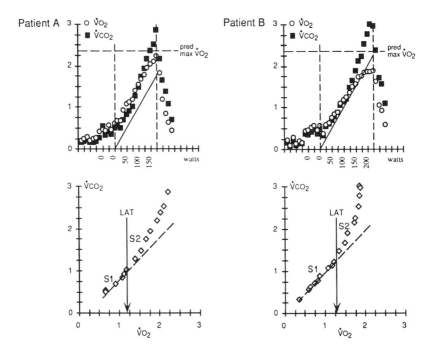

Figure 8. $\dot{V}CO_2$ and $\dot{V}O_2$ (L/min, STPD) as related to work rate for a 1-minute incremental (25 W/min) cycle ergometer exercise test for a normal 37-year-old man, 157 cm tall (**Patient A**) and a 47-year-old man, 175 cm tall (**Patient B**). In the **upper panels,** the diagonal solid line is drawn with a slope of 10 mL/min/W, the normal O_2 cost of cycle ergometer work (Figure 3), in order to detect, visually, if $\dot{V}O_2$ fails to increase appropriately for the increasing work rate performed. The start of the work-rate increment is indicated by the left vertical dashed line and the end of the exercise is indicated by the right vertical dashed line. The 47-year-old man (Patient B) had significant ST segment depression in the left precordial leads of the electrocardiogram, but without angina at 150 watts of work, whereas the 37-year-old man (Patient A) had a normal electrocardiogram and gas exchange response to exercise. Both subjects stopped exercise because of leg fatigue. The peak $\dot{V}O_2$ for Patient A was 95% of predicted (normal) whereas it was 80% of predicted (abnormal) for Patient B. Patient A had a normal pattern for $\dot{V}O_2$ increase, being almost linear to the maximum tolerated work rate with a slope of 10 mL/min/W (i.e., parallel to the diagonal solid line on the upper panel). In contrast, $\dot{V}O_2$ abruptly stopped increasing at the work rate at which the electrocardiogram became abnormal in Patient B, suggesting myocardial ischemia. The failure of $\dot{V}O_2$ to increase, despite increasing work rate and heart rate, indicates that the product of cardiac output and arteriovenous O_2 difference is no longer increasing due to a decreasing stroke volume. This abrupt decrease in the $\Delta\dot{V}O_2/\Delta$work-rate relationship is commonly seen during exercise testing in patients with coronary artery disease in response to increasing work-rate exercise. $\dot{V}CO_2$ increased steeply despite the flattening of the $\dot{V}O_2$ response, eliciting an increased difference between $\dot{V}O_2$ and $\dot{V}CO_2$. The V-slope plots for the two patients are shown on the **lower panels.** The diagonal dashed line has a slope of "1." The vertical arrow extending from the intersection of S1 and S2 (the breakpoint) to the x-axis identifies the lactic acidosis threshold (*LAT*). Coronary angiography confirmed the presence of coronary artery disease in Patient B.

rate exercise test, the $\dot{V}O_2$ might abruptly change from its normal rate of rise (10 mL/min/W), illustrated by the solid diagonal line in the upper panels of Figure 8, to a more shallow slope as work rate increases to the level at which myocardial ischemia develops (Figure 8, Patient B).[21] In such instances, $\dot{V}O_2$ plotted against work rate shows a flattening of $\dot{V}O_2$ increase, simultaneously with electrocardiographic changes reflecting myocardial ischemia, and a reduced $\dot{V}O_2$max. In contrast, $\dot{V}CO_2$ continues to rise steeply because the anaerobic production of carbon dioxide from buffering the increasing rate of lactic acid accumulation offsets the slowed rate of carbon dioxide production from aerobic metabolism (Figure 8, upper panels). To date, there has been no systematic study of the altered $\Delta\dot{V}O_2/\Delta$ work-rate relationship in patients with coronary artery disease. An exercise test that could determine the level of cardiac work at which the myocardium becomes sufficiently ischemic to impair cardiac output could be a valuable diagnostic aid.

Lactic Acidosis (Anaerobic) Threshold.   To determine the $\dot{V}O_2$ at which lactic acidosis develops (*LAT*), Beaver et al[25] plotted moles of $\dot{V}CO_2$ against moles of $\dot{V}O_2$ by the lungs, breath-by-breath, on equal scales. Because the units were left in volumes per unit of time, this method for determining the *LAT* was called the V-slope method. This method had advantages over that of other methods of determining the anaerobic or lactic acidosis threshold because it was insensitive to ventilation noise since ventilation was on both the *x* and *y* axes. These plots are shown on the lower panels of Figure 8. The *LAT* is selected as the $\dot{V}O_2$ at which the slope of the $\dot{V}CO_2$ versus $\dot{V}O_2$ changes from 1 (S1, diagonal dashed line) or slightly less than 1 to a slope which is steeper than 1 (S2). The intersection of S1 and S2 is the $\dot{V}O_2$ above which the increased $\dot{V}CO_2$ can only be explained by a metabolic acidosis. The theory was confirmed by arterial blood lactate, blood gas, and pH measure- . ments (e.g.,[21,25]). Sue et al,[26] noting that S1 had a slope of approximately 1 in almost every subject, determined the threshold with a 45° right triangle placed over or next to the data points (diagonal dashed line in lower panels of Figure 8). Thus, when $\dot{V}CO_2$ increased faster than $\dot{V}O_2$ during a progressively increasing work-rate test, the slope was steeper than 45°, visually measured by the edge of the 45° angle. This made possible an objective selection of the $\dot{V}O_2$ above which lactic acidosis becomes evident by gas exchange during an increasing work-rate test. The resolution of the threshold selection depends on scaling and the ability to read the breakpoint on the $\dot{V}CO_2$ versus $\dot{V}O_2$ plot after placement of the 45° angle on the data points of S1.

Peripheral Vascular Disease

Occlusive disease of the conducting vessels would also pre-dictably limit the muscle utilization of oxygen. This would manifest a smaller than expected increase in $\dot{V}O_2$ as work rate is increased during a progressive exercise test. This again has not been systematically studied, but the finding of a significantly reduced $\Delta\dot{V}O_2/\Delta$work-rate slope below the normal value of approximately 10 mL/min/W has been observed[21] in patients with peripheral vascular disease. In con-trast to coronary artery disease, however, this defect does not appear to show an abrupt change in the slope of $\dot{V}O_2$ versus work rate as shown in the right upper panel of Figure 8. Rather a shallower than normal slope throughout the exercise test is observed. The ability to detect this defect is largely dependent on the investigator's under-standing of the oxygen requirement of the muscles to perform the work aerobically, i.e., the normal $\Delta\dot{V}O_2/\Delta$work-rate slope for the type of work performed.

Pulmonary Vascular Disease

Pulmonary vascular occlusive disease limits the ability of the right ventricle to return the venous blood through the lungs to the left side of the heart to meet the increased oxygen requirement of exercise. Thus, the $\dot{V}O_2$ again increases more slowly than that required to per-form the exercise aerobically,[6,21] and the rate of increase becomes pro-gressively more shallow as work rate increases. As with the other causes of failure of the cardiovascular system to meet the oxygen re-quirement for aerobic ATP regeneration, $\dot{V}CO_2$ is disproportionately increased,[21] reflecting the buffering of the lactic acid from the in-creased anaerobic metabolism. The abnormality in the coupling of ex-ternal to cellular respiration in pulmonary vascular disease is further distinguished from those mentioned above because the decreased per-fusion of ventilated airspaces increases physiological dead space and, therefore, the ventilatory requirement for a given $\dot{V}CO_2$.

The three anatomically distinct sites of interruption of the normal coupling of external to cellular respiration described above have a common physiological feature, namely the inability of the cardiovas-cular system to maintain the high flow of oxygen needed to support the energetic requirement of the exercising muscles. However, there are differences in the pattern of the gas exchange and ventilatory re-sponses that make it possible for them to be distinguished. The mea-surement of gas exchange to evaluate cardiovascular performance has advantages over many other techniques in that it is quantitative, noninvasive, reproducible, and repeatable for purposes of studying the clinical course and effectiveness of therapy.

Summary

The delivery of atmospheric oxygen to the muscle to sustain regeneration of ATP needed for muscle contraction is totally dependent on the ability of the circulation to transport the oxygen at the rate required by the muscles. Failure of the circulation to deliver oxygen at the rate needed to sustain exercise will slow the rate of aerobic regeneration of ATP and oxygen consumption by the muscles. This will invoke anaerobic ATP regeneration and result in lactic acidosis. Lactic acid is buffered by HCO_3^-, resulting in an increased rate of $\dot{V}CO_2$ over that predicted from aerobic metabolism alone. Thus, the patterns of $\dot{V}O_2$ and $\dot{V}CO_2$ during exercise differ, depending on whether the work is, or is not, accompanied by lactic acidosis. For work rates which engender a lactic acidosis, $\dot{V}O_2$ kinetics are slowed and may not reach a steady state while $\dot{V}CO_2$ exceeds $\dot{V}O_2$. Different types of cardiovascular dysfunction may elicit different patterns of gas exchange abnormality. Measurement of gas exchange to evaluate cardiovascular function has advantages over many other technologies because it is quantitative, noninvasive, reproducible, and repeatable for purposes of studying the clinical course of patients and effectiveness of therapy.

References

1. Engelhardt VA, Lyubimova MN: Myosin and adenosine triphosphatase. *Nature* 144:668, 1939.
2. Meyer RA, Sweeney HL, Kushmerick MJ: A simple analysis of the phosphocreatine shuttle. *Am J Physiol* 248:C365–C377, 1984.
3. Meyer RA, Brown TR, Kushmerick MD: Phosphorus nuclear magnetic resonance and fast- and slow-twitch muscle. *Am J Physiol* 248:279–287, 1985.
4. Barstow TJ, Buchthal S, Zanconato S, Cooper DM: Muscle energetics and pulmonary oxygen uptake kinetics during moderate exercise. *J Appl Physiol* 74:1742–1749, 1994.
5. Wasserman K, Whipp BJ: Exercise physiology in health and disease (State of the Art). *Am Rev Respir Dis* 112:219–249, 1975.
6. Hansen JE, Sue DY, Oren A, Wasserman K: Relation of oxygen uptake to work rate in normal men and men with circulatory disorders. *Am J Cardiol* 59:669–674, 1987.
7. Wasserman K: Coupling of external to cellular respiration during exercise: the wisdom of the body revisited. *Am J Physiol* 266:E519–E539, 1994.
8. Koike A, Wasserman K, Taniguchi K, Hiroe M: Critical capillary oxygen partial pressure and lactate threshold in patients with cardiovascular disease. *J Am Coll Cardiol* 23:1644–1650, 1994.
9. Osnes J-B, Hermansen L: Acid-base balance after maximal exercise of short duration. *J Appl Physiol* 32:59–63, 1972.

10. Bouyhus A, Pool J, Binkhorst RA, Van Leeuwen P: Metabolic acidosis of exercise in healthy males. *J Appl Physiol* 21:1040–1046, 1966.
11. Wasserman K, Van Kessel A, Burton GG: Interaction of physiological mechanisms during exercise. *J Appl Physiol* 22:71–85, 1967.
12. Beaver WL, Wasserman K, Whipp BJ: Bicarbonate buffering of lactic acid generated during exercise. *J Appl Physiol* 60:472–478, 1986.
13. Stringer W, Casaburi R, Wasserman K: Acid-base regulation during exercise and recovery in man. *J Appl Physiol* 72:954–961, 1992.
14. Beaver WL, Wasserman K, Whipp BJ: Improved detection of the lactate threshold during exercise using a log-log transformation. *J Appl Physiol* 59:1936–1940, 1985.
15. Zhang YY, Sietsema KE, Sullivan C, Wasserman K: A method for estimating bicarbonate buffering of lactic acid during constant work rate exercise. *Eur J Appl Physiol* 69:309–315, 1994.
16. Zhang Y-Y, Wasserman K, Sietsema KE, Barstow TJ, Mizumoto G, Sullivan CS: O_2 uptake kinetics in response to exercise: measure of tissue anaerobiosis in heart failure. *Chest* 103:735–741, 1993.
17. Auchincloss JH, Ashutosh K, Rana S, Peppi D, Johnson LW, Gilbert R: Effect of cardiac, pulmonary, and vascular disease on one-minute oxygen uptake. *Chest* 70:486–493, 1976.
18. Nery LE, Wasserman K, Andrews JD, Huntsman DJ, Hansen JE, Whipp BJ: Ventilatory and gas exchange kinetics during exercise in chronic airways obstruction. *J Appl Physiol* 56:1594–1602, 1982.
19. Harrison TR, Pilcher C: Studies in congestive heart failure. II. The respiratory exchange during and after exercise. *J Clin Invest* 8:291–315, 1929.
20. Sietsema KE, Cooper DM, Rosove MA, et al: Dynamics of oxygen uptake during exercise in adults with cyanotic congenital heart disease. *Circulation* 73:1137–1144, 1986.
21. Wasserman K, Hansen JE, Sue DY, Whipp BJ, Casaburi R: *Principles of Exercise Testing and Interpretation.* 2nd ed. Lee & Febiger, 1994.
22. Casaburi R, Barstow TJ, Robinson T, Wasserman K: Influence of work rate on ventilatory and gas exchange kinetics. *J Appl Physiol* 67:547–555, 1989.
23. Casaburi R, Weissman ML, Huntsman D, Whipp BJ, Wasserman, K: Determinants of gas exchange kinetics during exercise in the dog. *J Appl Physiol* 46:1054–1060, 1979.
24. Casaburi R, Spitzer S, Haskell R, Wasserman, K: Effect of altering heart rate on oxygen uptake at exercise onset. *Chest* 95:6–12, 1988.
25. Beaver WL, Wasserman K, Whipp BJ: A new method for detecting the anaerobic threshold by gas exchange. *J Appl Physiol* 60:2020–2027, 1986.
26. Sue DY, Wasserman K, Moricca RB, Casaburi, R: Metabolic acidosis during exercise in patients with chronic obstructive pulmonary disease. *Chest* 94:931–938, 1988.

Section 2

Central Circulation — Cardiac Function and Exercise Gas Exchange

---

2

Cardiopulmonary Exercise Testing in Chronic Heart Failure

Alain Cohen-Solal, MD

Heart failure can be defined as an inability of the heart to deliver an output sufficient to meet the demands of the peripheral tissues. This definition underlines the importance of assessing the coupling between the heart and the periphery to define heart failure, and therefore the importance of using any kind of dynamic test (exercise, volume loading, etc.) to demonstrate the inability of cardiac output to follow the increase of the energy requirements of the body. Once the exclusive province of research physiologists, cardiopulmonary exercise testing has gained increasing popularity in cardiology over the last 15 years. Evolving technological advances and the ready availability of computerized systems have both greatly simplified and increased the amount of information obtained from patients with stable chronic heart failure (CHF); cardiopulmonary exercise testing is now widely used to study the pathophysiology of heart failure, assess the severity of the disease, evaluate the response to therapy, distinguish dyspnea from cardiac or respiratory origin, and assess the prognosis.

Rationale for Performing an Exercise Test in Chronic Heart Failure

It has long been considered that in CHF, symptoms and exercise capacity closely correlate with hemodynamics parameters. However,

From Wasserman, K (ed): *Exercise Gas Exchange in Heart Disease.* Armonk, NY: Futura Publishing Company, Inc., © 1996.

numerous studies performed in the last 15 years have clearly shown that this was not the case (Figure 1).[1–5] To understand that, one has to consider the multiple systems in the chain that deliver oxygen (O_2) from the outside to the muscles and remove carbon dioxide (CO_2) in the reverse direction during exercise. It can be depicted as a succession of resistances, serially arranged. At least in normally trained subjects, the heart, via its ability to increase cardiac output, is the limiting factor. In heart failure, all the elements of this chain, besides the heart, may alter the oxygen transport and limit exercise tolerance (Figure 2). Among those factors, the impairment of the peripheral circulation, incorrectly distributing the oxygen transported, and the metabolic abnormalities of the peripheral muscles, impairing normal utilization of oxygen, seem to play an important role. The mechanisms leading to exertional fatigue and/or dyspnea appear to be more complex than previously believed. Not only increase in capillary wedge pressure, but an increase in lung physiological dead space,[6] peripheral muscle underperfusion,[7] bronchial hyperreactivity,[8] and perhaps respiratory muscle fatigue[9] are suspected as possible participants in the sensation of dyspnea. Fatigue probably results from abnormalities of muscle me-

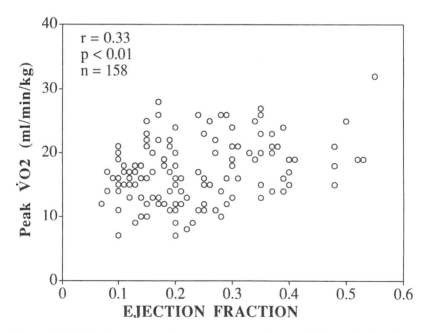

Figure 1. Relation between peak oxygen consumption and left ventricular ejection fraction in 158 patients with chronic heart failure. There was a weak significant correlation.

The O2/CO2 transport chain

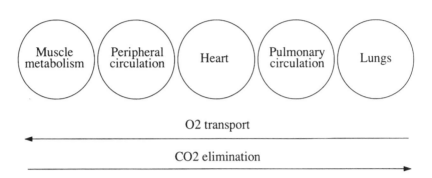

Figure 2. The chain of transport of oxygen in normal subjects. It can be depicted as a succession of conductances. In normal subjects, the heart is generally the limiting factor of exercise capacity.

tabolism as well as reduced nutritive muscle blood flow.[10,11] Moreover, there may be an exercise cardiac reserve[3,12,13] that cannot be predicted from resting hemodynamic measurements. Training-induced peripheral changes can compensate for a reduced exercise cardiac response. Often, structural and functional changes at the arterial or muscular level aggravate the consequences of reduced oxygen transport by altering the distribution and utilization of oxygen. These mechanisms explain the discrepancies observed between exercise capacity and resting cardiac hemodynamics.

General Methodology

Modern analyzers and computers allow measuring, on-line, ventilatory variables (breathing rate, minute ventilation, tidal volume, inspired and expired fractions of O_2 and CO_2) without significantly increasing the duration of the test. Oxygen uptake ($\dot{V}O_2$), carbon dioxide output ($\dot{V}CO_2$), and other useful measurements can be derived which permit an objective, reliable, and reproducible assessment of the exercise response. Various systems are now commercialized. They still require knowledge of the exercise physiology as well as of technology of gas analyzers. Although systems using a mixing chamber are often sufficient to measure peak $\dot{V}O_2$, the trend in recent years has been to use breath-by-breath technology mandatory to assess dynamic gas exchange during unsteady states. Patients breathe through a mouthpiece with a nose clip or a face mask. The first is preferable whenever possible, but the face mask may be better tolerated by patients; however, the risk of leaks is constant and the physiological dead space is increased. It is very important to carefully calibrate the system with gas of known concentration before each test; this quality control should ideally be given with every report. It is also important to familiarize the patient with the system before making the first measurements. Graded maximal exercise tests are generally used. Treadmill exercise is generally the way of testing in the United States and Great Britain, whereas bicycle exercise is preferred in continental Europe. Treadmill exercise mimics walking exercise, but peak $\dot{V}O_2$ kg is highly dependent on body weight and on the way of walking on the treadmill; holding on handrails decreases the metabolic requirements of treadmill exercise at a given walking grade or speed. Linearity of the increase in $\dot{V}O_2$ during treadmill exercise is not as good as with the bicycle.[14] The Bruce protocol, which produces the highest values of peak $\dot{V}O_2$, uses work-rate steps which are too abrupt for the more disabled patients. The modified Naughton treadmill protocol has been the most frequently used in patients with CHF during recent years because work-rate increments are smaller. However, duration of exercise with this protocol appears longer than generally recommended.[15]

Bicycle exercise tests yield fewer artifacts on the ECG than treadmill tests. Exercise is generally limited by lower limb fatigue even in patients complaining of exercising dyspnea during daily activities. Bicycle exercise uses a smaller muscle mass than treadmill and, therefore, peak $\dot{V}O_2$ has been generally found to be about 10% less than for treadmill exercise (Figure 3).[14,16,17] Jondeau et al[18] recently reported that exercising with both upper and lower limbs increases peak $\dot{V}O_2$ in patients with CHF. Because patients with severe heart failure often have peripheral muscle atrophy, abnormal distribution of blood flow and extraction of oxygen within the muscle, and intrinsic abnormalities of muscle metabolism,[19] systemic $\dot{V}O_2$ during exercise is actually smaller than that of normal subjects at the patient's maximal work rate. Engaging additional muscle mass in exercise (upper limbs, for example) may increase $\dot{V}O_2$ at peak exercise when patients' peak $\dot{V}O_2$ are lower than 15 mL/min/kg.[18]

Before breath-by-breath gas exchange techniques were available, exercise protocols with large steps in work rate of relative long duration were used for testing.[20,21] Because patients with severe heart failure have a slow hemodynamic and therefore $\dot{V}O_2$ response to exercise,[22] use of long stages in order to try to achieve a hypothetical steady state has no physiological merit, nor is a higher peak $\dot{V}O_2$ achieved. Exercise tests of longer than 15 minutes duration may lead to boredom in normal sub-

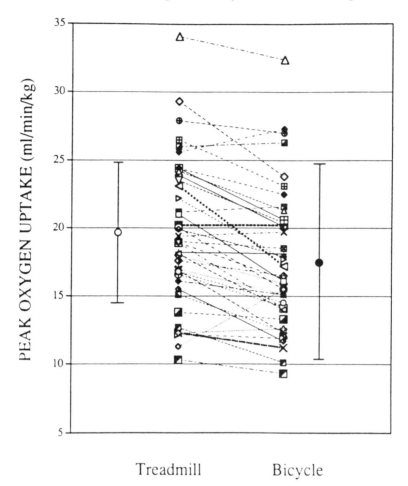

Figure 3. Comparison of peak oxygen uptake ($\dot{V}O_2$) during exercise on treadmill (modified Naughton protocol) and on bicycle (10 W/min protocol) in 40 patients with chronic heart failure. (Reproduced with permission from Reference 14.)

jects.[15] Ramp protocols with small increases in work rate (10 W/min, for example) appear to be better tolerated by the patient and yield fewer ventilatory or ECG artifacts than longer protocols.

The slope of the increase of $\dot{V}O_2$ to increase in work rate is determined by the biochemical efficiency of exercise. Therefore, for cycle ergometer exercise in which work rate is accurately known, $\dot{V}O_2$ increases at the rate of approximately 10 mL/min/W.[23] However, in patients with severe CHF, the rate of $\dot{V}O_2$ increase is not maintained as work rate increased, reflecting increased anaerobic work (Table 1).[24]

Table 1

Oxygen uptake ($\dot{V}O_2$, mL/min/kg) at various levels of exercise in patients with chronic heart failure (CHF) and in age-matched normal subjects during bicycle exercise test (10W/min).

				$\dot{V}O_2$ (mL/min/kg)				$\Delta \dot{V}O_2/\Delta W$
	Rest	20W	40W	60W	80W	100W	120W	(mL/min/W)
Controls	4.1	9.0	11.4	14.1	17.0	19.8	22.7	11.1±0.4
CHF-A	4.3	9.0	11.2	14.0	17.2	19.3	21.7	11.4±1.5
CHF-B	4.3	8.3	10.4	12.9	15.0*	16.7*	18.2*	10.1±1.6
CHF-CD	3.9	7.4*	9.3*	10.8*	12.2*	13.8*	14.2*	8.8±2.1*
CHF-all	4.2	8.3	10.4*	12.9*	15.5*	18.1*	20.7*	10.2±2.0*

Severity of CHF increases from A to C-D class. *p 0.05 vs. controls
(Modified from Reference 24.)

Therefore, a plot of $\dot{V}O_2$ versus work rate may be useful in quantifying the severity of CHF.

Cardiopulmonary Exercise-Derived Parameters of Exercise Capacity

Various criteria can be used to evaluate exercise tolerance, but unfortunately, we have not found a simple, reliable, and reproducible "gold standard."

Exercise duration or peak work rate attained during a maximal exercise test in which work rate is increased in equal steps is influenced by the patient's motivation and by observer bias. Exercise duration is reproducible during treadmill exercise where patients may increase exercise duration (by learning to walk more "efficiently") without a corresponding increase in peak $\dot{V}O_2$. This is not true on the bicycle provided that patients have been familiarized with the exercise protocol. It is very speculative to estimate $\dot{V}O_2$ without measuring it, particularly on the treadmill. $\dot{V}O_2$, the product of cardiac output and arteriovenous difference for oxygen, should thus be measured during exercise in patients. The maximal aerobic capacity (maximal oxygen uptake, $\dot{V}O_2max$) has thus become the gold standard for assessing patients' exercise capacity. It therefore depends on the maximal capacity of the body to transport oxygen to the exercising muscle, and to use oxygen for a given form of exercise.[25] It has been defined classically by a plateauing in the increase in $\dot{V}O_2$ at the end of exercise despite increasing work rate. $\dot{V}O_2max$ can generally be determined and is very reproducible in trained normal subjects. Because maximal arteriovenous difference for oxygen does not markedly differ among normal subjects, $\dot{V}O_2$max is closely related to maximal cardiac output. Its value generally ranges from 30 to 40 mL/min/kg in untrained middle-aged normal subjects. However, it is greatly affected by sex, obesity, age and fitness: for example, 19 mL/min/kg may represent a normal value for a 70-year-old woman; world-class athletes may reach values close to 90 mL/min/kg. It is therefore better to rely on predicted values indexed to normal body weight, age, and gender than on $\dot{V}O_2$/actual body weight.[23,26]

Unfortunately, patients with CHF virtually never reach a true $\dot{V}O_2$max. A plateau of $\dot{V}O_2$ towards the end of exercise may result from a decrease in the rate of pedalling, or a failure for oxygen transport to increase appropriately (e.g., development of myocardial ischemia or severe mitral regurgitation). The absence of plateau of $\dot{V}O_2$max does not necessarily mean that patient effort was not maximal or near-maximal, provided that other criteria (see below) are present. It is important to encourage the patients,[27] who have long been told to avoid strenuous exercise, to give a maximal effort. In severe CHF, we have observed that peak $\dot{V}O_2$ may be reached 15 to 45 seconds after the cessation of exercise, possibly because of the increased transit time between the peripheral muscles and the mouth.[28,29] Nevertheless, it has been our experience[30] and that of others[2,31,32] that peak $\dot{V}O_2$ is the most reproducible criterion of exercise tolerance in these patients, provided a preliminary exercise test has been performed to familiarize the patient with the testing protocol,[31] and gas analysis is correctly performed. Peak $\dot{V}O_2$, however, is not entirely independent of the exercise protocol (treadmill or bicycle, slow or rapid protocols).[33-35] Its determination necessitates performing an exercise test to exhaustion. However, despite these limitations, peak achieved $\dot{V}O_2$ remains the most satisfactory of all the available measures of exercise capacity.

In order to circumvent the limitations of the determination of peak $\dot{V}O_2$, the anaerobic threshold has been proposed as an index of exercise capacity independent of the patient's motivation (and therefore more objective and reproducible than peak $\dot{V}O_2$), and not requiring maximal effort.[36] It has been defined as the point where lactate increases in plasma during incremental exercise (Figure 4). This lactate threshold has been considered to result from a switch from total aerobic to aerobic plus anaerobic metabolism in the peripheral muscle, due to limitation in oxygen transport. Because the buffering of plasma lactate during exercise leads to an increase in carbon dioxide production, respiratory gas analysis can be used to determine the $\dot{V}O_2$ at which $\dot{V}CO_2$ increases disproportionately to aerobic metabolism (Figure 5).

The mechanism for the increase in blood lactate during an effort is controversial.[37] This controversy will not be addressed here (see

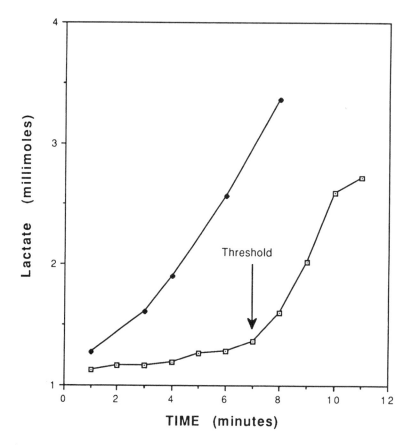

Figure 4. Two examples of blood lactate response during graded bicycle exercise (10 W/min protocol) in patients with CHF. In the **lower curve,** there is a clear-cut lactate threshold; in the second patient (**upper curve**), a progressive increase in lactate from the beginning of exercise prevents any reliable determination of a lactate threshold.

Chapter 12). Nevertheless, despite the controversies about the significance of a lactate threshold, the temporal relationship between the lactate and the ventilatory thresholds, and the interobserver, agreement in the determination of the ventilatory threshold,[38,39] there have been a number of recent studies supporting the concept of a close relationship between the ventilatory threshold and a shift in intracellular metabolism,[40-45] and it is generally accepted that this noninvasive index is an important criterion of exercise capacity in normal subjects.

In patients with CHF, various groups have also emphasized the interest of determining the ventilatory threshold during exercise.[2,46] However, reliability and reproducibility of the ventilatory threshold determination in patients with CHF seem less than in normal subjects

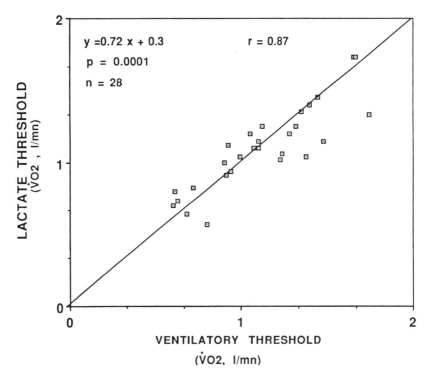

Figure 5. Relationship between the lactate threshold and the ventilatory threshold during exercise in patients with chronic heart failure (CHF). The ventilatory threshold value was calculated as the mean of the values obtained by four methods of detection ($\dot{V}E$, $\dot{V}E/\dot{V}CO_2$, RER, and $\dot{V}CO_2$ methods). (Reproduced with permission from Reference 30.)

(Table 2).[4,30,31,47–58] Also, because of the irregular pattern of breathing of the patients (Figure 6),[54,59,60] a clear-cut threshold is sometimes difficult to detect by ventilation versus $\dot{V}O_2$ and $\dot{V}CO_2$ curves; however, as shown by Wasserman et al,[61] a threshold can be more easily seen in irregularly breathing patients when $\dot{V}CO_2$ is plotted against $\dot{V}O_2$, thereby attenuating the problem of breathing irregularity. In patients with severe CHF or with marked deconditioning, a progressive increase in lactate and in $\dot{V}CO_2$ is often observed from the beginning of exercise (Figure 4); this occurs too early to be explained only by an inadequate blood flow. It is possible that because most of the muscle fibers in these patients are of IIb type ("glycolytic" fibers), lactic acid is produced even if oxygen delivery is adequate. In our studies, we could not determine a ventilatory threshold during exercise in more than about 75% of patients with mild to moderate CHF; this 25% rate of undetermination is a serious limitation to the use of this criterion as an end

---

Table 2

Reproducibility of peak oxygen uptake (peak $\dot{V}O_2$, mL/min/kg)
and the ventilatory threshold (mL/min/kg) during bicycle exercise (10 W/min)
in patients with chronic heart failure (CHF).

	Peak $\dot{V}o_2$ (mL/min/kg)	Ventilatory Threshold (mL/min/kg)
n	29	23
test 1	20.9 ± 6.3	14.3 ± 4.6
test 2	20.9 ± 6.9	15.3 ± 5.1
r	0.93	0.88
coefficient of variation	7.8%	12.7%

The methods used to determine the ventilatory threshold were the $\dot{V}O_2$, V_E, $V_E/\dot{V}O_2$, and RER vs. time graphs. $\dot{V}O_2$max appears to be more reproducible than ventilatory threshold; in 6 patients, it was not possible to determine the ventilatory threshold at one or both of the two exercise tests.

(Reproduced with permission from Reference 30.)

point of exercise capacity, especially in therapeutic trials.[30,62] Moreover, considerable interobserver variability in the way of determining the ventilatory threshold should not be ignored. The commonly employed methods for determining the ventilatory threshold are subjective and suggest that new methods of determination are needed. Currently, we depend on manual calculations from plots of ventilatory responses. The ventilatory equivalent for oxygen (ratio of minute ventilation by $\dot{V}O_2$) appears to be the most reliable of these methods in our experience.[30] Computerized analysis of the $\dot{V}CO_2$ versus $\dot{V}O_2$ relationship (V-slope method)[49,54,63] has been reported to significantly improve the accuracy of the detection of the anaerobic threshold in these patients. Generally, multiple criteria have to be considered and, in the setting of a multicenter trial, it is a good precaution to have a centralized review of the graphical reports (Table 3). The graphs using minute ventilation, or the ventilatory equivalents for O_2 and CO_2 plotted against time, yielded the highest rate of determination (51% and 58% on average respectively), but the crossing point method was, as expected, more simple to use; however, at best, the rate of determination was only 72% (the V-slope method was not used in this study). Finally, reproducibility of the ventilatory threshold is just satisfactory and lower than that of peak $\dot{V}O_2$.[30,62] $\dot{V}O_2$ corresponding to a respiratory exchange ratio equal to 1 during the test may provide a more reproducible index of submaximal performance,[62,64] although it occurs after the actual ventilatory threshold and may vary with the caloric intake of the patient (Figure 7).[65]

Reliability of the detection of the ventilatory response has consid-

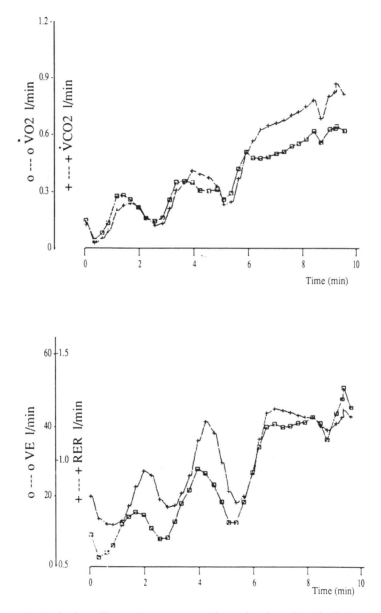

Figure 6. Marked oscillations in oxygen uptake and carbon dioxide during exercise may complicate the detection of a ventilatory threshold, which was found at 520 mL/min of $\dot{V}O_2$.

Table 3

Comparison of the different ways of determining the ventilatory threshold by four committees in a multicenter study involving 85 patients (331 tests).

	Committee 1	Committee 2	Committee 3	Committee 4	Mean
Minute ventilation	44%	65%	56%	40%	51%
$\dot{V}CO_2$	20%	61%	50%	38%	42%
RER	17%	46%	37%	38%	34%
$VE/\dot{V}O_2$	50%	56%	72%	51%	58%
Crossing	64%	76%	73%	74%	72%
Mean	39%	61%	58%	48%	•

Ventilatory threshold was determined by graphical criteria, the $\dot{V}O_2$ vs. $\dot{V}O_2$ curve, minute ventilation vs. time curve, the respiratory exchange ratio (RER) vs. time curve, the ventilatory equivalents vs. time curve ($VE/\dot{V}O_2$), and the crossing of the $\dot{V}O_2$ and $\dot{V}CO_2$ curves.[62,64]
The percentage of all the exercise tests that were possible to determine a ventilatory threshold is reported according to 1) the committee (**column**); 2) the method used to detect the ventilatory threshold (**row**). (The V-slope method was not used in this study.)
(Reproduced with permission from Reference 62.)

erable importance for the interpretation of an exercise test. When peak $\dot{V}O_2$ is low, the ventilatory threshold value is important for determining the cause of exercise intolerance. A low ventilatory threshold reflects reduced oxygen delivery (low cardiac output, decrease in oxygen content in arterial blood), but also an impairment of skeletal muscle oxygen extraction and/or utilization, resulting from deconditioning or mitochondrial abnormalities.[66] The ventilatory threshold can also be used as an index of the patient's motivation; failure to reach the ventilatory threshold strongly suggests poor motivation or a noncardiovascular limitation of exercise tolerance. Assessment of peak $\dot{V}O_2$ alone can be misleading; change in peak $\dot{V}O_2$ without change in the ventilatory threshold suggests change in the patient's motivation rather than in functional capacity (Figure 8). When no ventilatory threshold can be detected, a respiratory exchange ratio higher than 1 or a peak heart rate close to the maximal predicted value are other criteria suggesting a sufficient level of exercise.

Other criteria of functional impairment derived from an incremental test have been proposed, but they have not gained as wide acceptance as the two previous ones.

The oxygen pulse reflects the capacity of the heart to deliver O_2 per beat. It is calculated from the $\dot{V}O_2$ divided by heart rate and is equal to the product of stroke volume and the arterial-mixed venous O_2 difference $C(a-v)O_2$. Peak oxygen pulse is generally low in CHF, de-

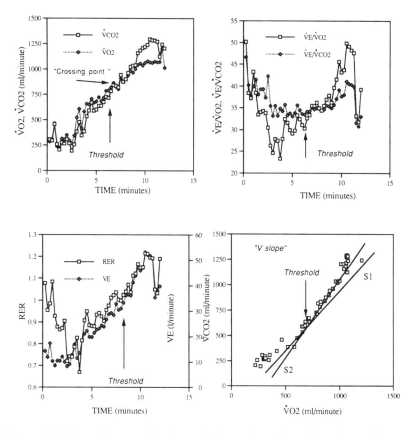

Figure 7. The various graphical methods used to determine the ventilatory threshold during exercise. $\dot{V}O_2$ (oxygen uptake), $\dot{V}CO_2$ (carbon dioxide production) versus time; $\dot{V}E$ (minute ventilation) versus time; RER (respiratory exchange ratio) versus time; $\dot{V}E/\dot{V}O_2$ and $\dot{V}E/\dot{V}CO_2$ (ventilatory equivalents for O_2 and for CO_2) versus time; and the V-slope method ($\dot{V}CO_2$ versus $\dot{V}O_2$); the methods using the end-tidal pressures for O_2 and for CO_2 are not displayed.

pending on the capacity of $C(a-v)O_2$ to widen enough to compensate for a reduced exercise stroke volume. The O_2 pulse response profile also is abnormal in CHF. As stroke volume fails to increase or decreases throughout exercise, the O_2 pulse response is characterized by an early low plateau, or in severe CHF even a decrease at end-exercise; as $C(a-v)O_2$ always increases during exercise, a plateau of O_2 pulse presumably reflects a decreasing stroke volume (Figure 9).

The slope of the $\dot{V}O_2$/time or $\dot{V}O_2$/work-rate response during exercise has appeared as another index of circulatory response during exercise[17,24,50,67]; it reflects the oxygen cost of carrying out work: the more reduced the slope, the more the anaerobic metabolism and severity of

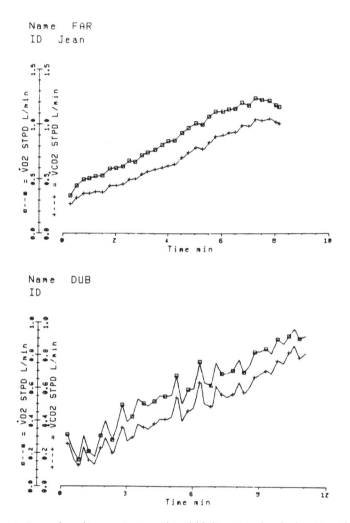

Figure 8. Examples of two patients with mild left ventricular dysfunction (the first on the top due to inferior myocardial infarction, the second at the bottom because of mitral regurgitation) and marked reduction in exercise tolerance. Both stopped exercising before reaching the ventilatory threshold, which suggests that circulatory failure was not the cause of exercise limitation; the first patient actually had severe chronic obstructive pulmonary disease (COPD) and the second one was poorly motivated; the next day, with encouragement, the second patient doubled her exercise time and passed the ventilatory threshold. Without respiratory gas analysis, these patients would probably have been considered having reduced exercise capacity due to severe heart failure.

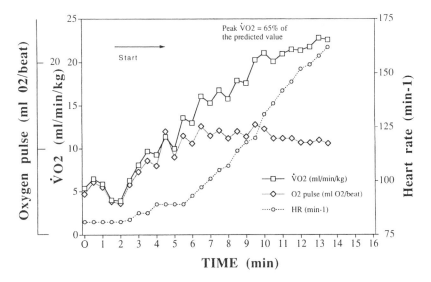

Figure 9. Near normal response of $\dot{V}O_2$ and heart rate in a patient with a markedly enlarged left ventricle (echocardiographic end-diastolic diameter 99 mm, ejection fraction 18%). However, the O_2 pulse response is abnormal, rapidly plateauing, suggesting a decrease in stroke volume during exercise.

the circulatory failure (Table 1). In normal subjects, the $\dot{V}O_2$ work-rate relationship is approximately 10 mL/min/W. It is shifted upward in obesity. This index is best applied with ramp protocols on bicycle, and calculated only after some minutes of zero-workload pedalling. Its main interest is that it can be determined even if exercise is submaximal.

Kinetics of recovery of $\dot{V}O_2$ seems to be another promising parameter[28]; we found the half-time of recovery of $\dot{V}O_2$ to be reduced in parallel with the severity of heart failure and has the advantage over peak $\dot{V}O_2$ of being determinable even if exercise is submaximal. The calculation of the oxygen debt or of the excess post-exercise oxygen consumption[68-70] has also been proposed as a method of cardiovascular assessment.

In summary, cardiopulmonary exercise testing allows for determining various parameters besides exercise duration and peak workload, which provide information about the circulatory, respiratory, and metabolic responses of the whole body during exercise.

Indications for Exercise Testing in Chronic Heart Failure

1) Measures of cardiopulmonary exercise capacity complement the NYHA classification. The NYHA classification is subjective and nonparametric. Discrimination between class II and III is difficult;

most of the patients are in these categories and small, but clinically important changes in functional status may not be detected.[71] Exercise tests permit categorization of patients in a more objective and parametric way than solely by the NYHA classification.[72] Recently, it has been recommended that CHF patients be characterized not only by their NYHA functional class, but also by an objective criterion of their exercise capacity.[73] Franciosa et al,[16] and Weber and Janicki[2] have proposed classifying the functional capacity of patients with CHF by their $\dot{V}O_2$max in four classes: A: $\dot{V}O_2$max > 20 mL/min/kg; B: $\dot{V}O_2$max 16–20 mL/min/kg; C: $\dot{V}O_2$max 10–15 mL/min/kg; D: $\dot{V}O_2$max 10 mL/min/kg. This classification has the advantage over the NYHA one because peak $\dot{V}O_2$ is a continuous variable. However, some limitations should not be ignored: indexation of $\dot{V}O_2$ only by body weight is unsatisfactory. Age, sex, and fitness should be taken into account. The validity of normal values obtained in normal, fit subjects[26] may be questioned when applied to a deconditioned, but otherwise normal population.

2) Exercise testing with respiratory gas analysis is able to differentiate exertional dyspnea of respiratory or cardiac origin (Figure 8).[74-77] Patients with CHF often have alteration in pulmonary function and conversely, patients with pulmonary disease may have a low anaerobic threshold because of deconditioning or alteration in oxygen transport. Cardiopulmonary exercise testing may help distinguish relative importance of heart and lung abnormalities in exercise limitation.[74]

3) Assessing the changes of peak $\dot{V}O_2$ and/or the ventilatory threshold was hoped to be the gold standard for evaluating the effect of treatment in patients with CHF. Indeed, the first applications of respiratory gas analysis in therapeutic trials have shown a clear improvement in peak $\dot{V}O_2$ with some drugs and no improvement with others. However, when patients were familiarized with the exercise protocol and the technique of respiratory gas analysis by at least one preliminary test, it has been much more difficult to demonstate an improvement in peak $\dot{V}O_2$ with drugs in placebo-controlled trials, despite reported improvement in quality of life, especially when patients with mild heart failure are considered or when exercise is performed on bicycle. Recent demonstration that the most marked improvement in $\dot{V}O_2$ is obtained by physical training[78] suggests that improvement of the peripheral abnormalities of CHF translates more rapidly than improvement in cardiac hemodynamics into an increase in peak $\dot{V}O_2$. Moreover, one should not forget that some drugs can have a more effective action on survival than others despite a lesser effect on peak exercise capacity.[79] Finally, as peak $\dot{V}O_2$ remains dependent on the patient's motivation, its superiority over exercise duration may be questionable; one can, however, argue that its reproducibility is higher, and therefore fewer patients are needed to demonstrate an intergroup difference in treatment efficacy in a controlled trial.

4) Currently, peak $\dot{V}O_2$ is a main determinant of the prognosis of patients with CHF.[80] Various studies[3,81-85] have tried to define a cutoff value of peak $\dot{V}O_2$ for predicting survival in patients with CHF, but failed or obtained conflicting results. Mancini et al[86] have shown that patients with a peak $\dot{V}O_2$ lower than 10 mL/min/kg on treadmill had a very poor survival at one year and therefore should be considered for heart transplant, whereas those with a peak $\dot{V}O_2$ higher than 18 mL/min/kg had a 100% survival at one year, and those with a peak $\dot{V}O_2$ higher than 14 mL/min/kg had a 94% one-year survival rate, which represented a clearly better survival than that of the transplants. These results have been confirmed by the V-HeFT study group[84] and Stevenson et al [87] in large populations of patients. Further studies are necessary to determine the relationship between changes in peak $\dot{V}O_2$ during serial exercise testing, and changes in therapy and prognosis.

In conclusion, exercise testing is now the established standard method of functional assessment in patients with CHF. Measurement of gas exchange permits a better understanding of the pathophysiology of the symptoms and provides powerful independent prognostic information.

Summary

Exercise testing is now accepted as the best way of assessing functional capacity in patients with CHF. Coupled with respiratoy gas analysis, cardiopulmonary exercise tests allow assessment of the effects of treatments, distinguishing the cardiac or respiratory origin of exertional dyspnea and more recently assessing the prognosis. In addition to detecting cardiac pump failure, exercise testing has also permitted the development of a better understanding of the complex pathophysiology of the overall oxygen transport during exercise in patients who have skeletal muscle alterations, abnormal vascular dilatation, and pulmonary dysfunction.

References

1. Franciosa JA, Park M, Levine TB: Lack of correlation between exercise capacity and indexes of resting left ventricular performance in heart failure. *Am J Cardiol* 47:33–39, 1981.
2. Weber KT, Kinasewitz GT, Janicki JS, Fishman AP: Oxygen utilization and ventilation during exercise in patients with chronic cardiac failure. *Circulation* 65:1213–1223, 1982.
3. Szlachcic J, Massie BM, Kramer BL, Topic N, Tubau J: Correlates and prognostic implication of exercise capacity in chronic congestive heart failure. *Am J Cardiol* 55:1037–1042, 1985.

4. Metra M, Raddino R, Dei Cas L, Visioli O: Assessment of peak oxygen consumption, lactate and ventilatory thresholds and correlation with resting and exercise hemodynamic data in chronic congestive heart failure. *Am J Cardiol* 65:1127–1133, 1990.
5. Kraemer MK, Kubo SH, Rector ThS, Brunsvold N, Bank AJ: Pulmonary and peripheral vascular factors are important determinants of peak exercise oxygen uptake in patients with heart failure. *J Am Coll Cardiol* 21:641–648, 1993.
6. Sullivan MJ, Higginbotham MB, Cobb FR: Increased exercise ventilation in patients with chronic heart failure: intact ventilatory control despite hemodynamic and pulmonary abnormalities. *Circulation* 77:552–559, 1988.
7. Wilson JR, Ferraro N: Exercise intolerance in patients with chronic left heart failure: relation to oxygen transport and ventilatory abnormalities. *Am J Cardiol* 51:1359–1363, 1983.
8. Cabanes LR, Weber SN, Matran R, Regnard J, Rich MO, Degeorges ME: Bronchial hyperresponsiveness to methacholine in patients with impaired left ventricular function. *N Engl J Med* 320:1317–1322, 1989.
9. Mancini DM, Henson D, LaManca J, Levine S: Respiratory muscle function and dyspnea in patients with chronic congestive heart failure. *Circulation* 86:909–918, 1992.
10. Massie BM, Conway M, Yonge R, et al: Skeletal muscle metabolism in patients with congestive heart failure: relation to clinical severity and blood flow. *Circulation* 76:1009–1019, 1987.
11. Mancini DM, Wilson JR, Bolinger L, et al: In vivo magnetic resonance spectroscopy measurement of deoxymyoglobin during exercise in patients with heart failure. Demonstration of abnormal muscle metabolism despite adequate oxygenation. *Circulation* 90:500–508, 1994.
12. Franciosa JA, Leddy CL, Wilen M, Schwartz DE: Relation between hemodynamic and ventilatory responses in determining exercise capacity in severe congestive heart failure. *Am J Cardiol* 53:127–134, 1984.
13. Sullivan MJ, Knight JD, Higginbotham MB, Cobb FR: Relation between central and peripheral hemodynamics during exercise in patients with chronic heart failure. Muscle blood flow is reduced with maintenance of arterial pressure. *Circulation* 80:769–781, 1989.
14. Page E, Cohen-Solal A, Jondeau G, et al: Comparison of treadmill and bicycle exercise in patients with chronic heart failure. *Chest* 106:1002–1006, 1994.
15. Buchfuhrer MJ, Hansen JE, Robinson TE, Sue DY, Wasserman K, Whipp BJ: Optimizing the exercise protocol for cardiopulmonary assessment. *J Appl Physiol* 55:1558–1564, 1983.
16. Franciosa JA, Ziesche S, Wilen M: Functional capacity of patients with chronic left ventricular failure. *Am J Med* 67:460–466, 1976.
17. Myers J, Buchanan N, Walsh D, et al: A comparison of the ramp versus standard exercise protocols. *J Am Coll Cardiol* 17:339–343, 1991.
18. Jondeau G, Katz SD, Zohman L, et al: Active skeletal muscle mass and cardiopulmonary reserve. Failure to attain peak aerobic capacity during maximal bicycle exercise in patients with severe congestive heart failure. *Circulation* 86:1351–1356, 1992.
19. Mancini DM, Ferraro N, Tuchler M, Chance B, Wilson JR: Detection of abnormal calf muscle metabolism in patients with heart failure using phosphorus-31 nuclear magnetic resonance. *Am J Cardiol* 62:1234–1240, 1988.
20. Franciosa JA: Exercise testing in chronic congestive heart failure. *Am J Cardiol* 54:1447–1450, 1984.

21. Lipkin DP, Canepa-Anson R, Stephens MR, Poole-Wilson PA: Factors determining symptoms in heart failure: comparison of fast and slow exercise tests. *Br Heart J* 55:439–445, 1986.

22. Sietsema KE, Ben-Dov I, Zhang YY, Sullivan C, Wasserman K: Dynamics of oxygen uptake for submaximal exercise and recovery in patients with chronic heart failure. *Chest* 105:1693–1700, 1994.

23. Wasserman K, Hansen JE, Sue DY, Whipp BJ: Normal values. In: Wasserman K, Hansen JE, Sue DY, Whipp BJ, eds. *Principles of Exercise Testing and Interpretation*. Philadelphia: Lea & Febiger, 72–85, 1987.

24. Cohen-Solal A, Chabernaud JM, Gourgon R: Comparison of oxygen uptake during bicycle exercise in patients with chronic heart failure and in normal subjects. *J Am Coll Cardiol* 16:80–85, 1990.

25. Green HJ, Patla AE: Maximal aerobic power: neuromuscular and metabolic considerations. *Med Sci Sports Exerc* 24:38–46, 1992.

26. Jones NL, Makrides L, Hitchcock C, McCartney N: Normal standards for an incremental progressive cycle ergometer test. *Am Rev Respir Dis* 131: 700–708, 1985.

27. Clark AL, Poole-Wilson PA, Coats AJS: Effects of motivation of the patient on indices of exercise capacity in chronic heart failure. *Br Heart J* 71:162–165, 1994.

28. Cohen-Solal A, Laperche Th., Morvan D, Geneves M, Caviezel B, Gourgon R: Kinetics of recovery of ventilation and oxygen uptake after maximal exercise in heart failure. Analysis with gas exchange and NRM spectroscopy? *Circulation* 91:2924–2933, 1995.

29. Daida H, Allison TG, Johnson BD, Nelson SM, Squires RW, Gau GT: Delayed recovery of oxygen consumption after maximal exercise in congestive heart failure. *Circulation* 90 (suppl I):1–15, 1994.

30. Cohen-Solal A, Benessiano J, Himbert D, Paillole C, Gourgon R: Ventilatory threshold during exercise in patients with mild to moderate chronic heart failure: determination, relation with lactate threshold and reproducibility. *Int J Cardiol* 30:321–327, 1991.

31. Elborn JS, Stanford CF, Nicholls DP: Reproducibility of cardiopulmonary parameters during exercise in patients with chronic cardiac failure. *Eur Heart J* 11:75–81, 1990.

32. Dickstein K, Aarsland S, Snapinn S: Reproducibility of cardiopulmonary exercise testing in men following myocardial infarction. *Eur Heart J* 9:948–954, 1988.

33. Froelicher VF, Brammel H, Davis G, Noguera I, Stewart A, Lancaster MC: A comparison of the reproducibility and physiologic response to three maximal treadmill exercise protocols. *Chest* 65:512–517, 1974.

34. Davis JA, Vodak P, Wilmore JH, Vodak J, Kurtz P: Anaerobic threshold and maximal aerobic power for three modes of exercise. *J Appl Physiol* 41:544–550, 1976.

35. Myers J, Buchanan N, Walsh D, et al: Comparison of the ramp versus standard exercise protocols. *J Am Coll Cardiol* 17:1334–1342, 1991.

36. Wasserman K, Whipp BJ, Koyal SN, Beaver WL: Anaerobic threshold and respiratory gas exchange during exercise. *J Appl Physiol* 35:236–243, 1973.

37. Brooks GA: "Anaerobic threshold": review of the concept and direction for future research. *Med Sci Sports Exerc* 17:22–31, 1985.

38. Yeh MP, Gardner RM, Adams TD, Yanowith FG, Crapo RO: Anaerobic threshold: problems of determination and validation. *J Appl Physiol* 55: 1178–1186, 1983.

39. Caiozzo VJ, Davis JA, Ellis JF, et al: A comparison of gas exchange indices used to detect anaerobic threshold. *J Appl Physiol* 53:1184–1189, 1982.
40. Koike A, Weiler-Ravell D, McKenzie DK, Zanconato S, Wasserman K: Evidence that the metabolic acidosis threshold is the anaerobic threshold. *J Appl Physiol* 68:2521–2526, 1990.
41. Systrom DM, Kanarek DJ, Kohler SJ, Kazemi H: 31P nuclear magnetic resonance spectroscopy study of the anaerobic threshold in humans. *J Appl Physiol* 68:2060–2066, 1990.
42. Marsh GD, Paterson DH, Thompson RT, Driedger AA: Coincident thresholds in intracellular phosphorylation potential and pH during progressive exercise. *J Appl Physiol* 71:1076–1081, 1991.
43. Riley M, Nicholls DP, Nugent AM, et al: Respiratory gas exchange and metabolic responses during exercise in McArdle's disease. *J Appl Physiol* 75(2):745–754, 1993.
44. Samaan SA, Icenogle MV, Robergs RA, Hudson TL, Fukushima E, Crawford MH: Onset of regional anaerobic muscle metabolism during exercise does not explain reduced systemic anaerobic threshold in heart failure. *J Am Coll Cardiol* 21 (suppl A):329A, 1993.
45. Koike A, Wasserman K, Taniguchi K, Hiroe M, Marumo F: The critical capillary PO2 and the lactate threshold in patients with cardiovascular disease. *J Am Coll Cardiol* 23:1644–1650, 1994.
46. Matsumura N, Nishijima H, Kojima S, Hashimoto F, Minami M, Yasuda H: Determination of anaerobic threshold for assessment of functional state in patients with chronic heart failure. *Circulation* 68:360–367, 1983.
47. Wilson JR, Fink L, Ferraro N, Dunkman WB, Jones RA: Use of maximal bicycle exercise testing with respiratory gas analysis to assess exercise performance in patients with congestive heart failure secondary to coronary artery disease or to idiopathic dilated cardiomyopathy. *Am J Cardiol* 58:601–606, 1986.
48. Simonton CA, Higginbotham MB, Cobb FR: The ventilatory threshold: quantitative analysis of reproducibility and relation to arterial lactate concentration in normal subjects and in patients with chronic congestive heart failure. *Am J Cardiol* 62:100–107, 1988.
49. Dickstein K, Barvik S, Aarsland T, Snapinn S, Kalsson J: A comparison of methodologies in detection of the anaerobic threshold. *Circulation* 81 (suppl II):II-38—II-46, 1990.
50. Itoh H, Taniguchi K, Koike A, Doi M: Evaluation of the severity of heart failure using ventilatory gas analysis. *Circulation* 81 (suppl II):II-31—II-37, 1990.
51. Shimuza M, Myers J, Buchanan N, et al: The ventilatory threshold: method, protocol, and evaluator agreement. *Am Heart J* 122:509–516, 1991.
52. Katz SD, Berkowitz R, Le Jemtel TH: Anaerobic threshold detection in patients with congestive heart failure. *Am J Cardiol* 69:1565–1569, 1992.
53. Gibelin P, Darmon JP, Mondain JR, Morand Ph: Détermination du seuil anaérobie dans l'insuffisance cardiaque chronique. Intérêts et limites. *Ann Cardiol Angéiol* 41:471–479, 1992.
54. Miyagi K, Asanoi H, Ishizaka S, Kameyama T, Sasayama S: Limited value of anaerobic threshold for assessing functional capacity in patients with heart failure. *Clin Cardiol* 16:133–137, 1993.
55. Katz SD, Bleiberg B, Wexler J, Bhargava K, Steinberg JJ, Le Jemtel TH: Lactate turnover at rest and during submaximal exercise in patients with heart failure. *J Appl Physiol* 75:1974–1979, 1993.

56. Yamabe H, Itoh K, Yasaka Y, Takata T, Yokoyama M: Lactate threshold is not an onset of insufficient oxygen supply to the working muscle in patients with chronic heart failure. *Clin Cardiol* 17:391–394, 1994.
57. Elborn JS, Riley M, Stanford CF, Nicholls DP: Anaerobic threshold in patients with chronic cardiac failure due to ischaemic heart disease. *Presse Med* 23:367–71, 1994.
58. Gitt AK, Winter UJ, Fritsch J, et al: Vergleich der vier verschiedenen Methoden zur respiratorischen Bestimmung der anaeroben Schwelle bei Normalpersonen, Herz- und Lungenkranken. *Z Kardiol* 83 (suppl 1):37–42, 1994.
59. Kremsen CB , O'Toole MF, Leff AR: Oscillatory hyperventilation in severe congestive heart failure secondary to idiopathic dilated cardiomyopathy or to ischemic cardiomyopathy. *Am J Cardiol* 59:900–905, 1987.
60. Yajima T, Koike A, Sugimoto K, Miyahara Y, Marumo F, Hiroe M: Mechanism of periodic breathing in patients with cardiovascular disease. *Chest* 106:142–146, 1994.
61. Wasserman K, Beaver WL, Whipp BJ: Gas exchange theory and the lactic acidosis (anaerobic) threshold. *Circulation* 81 (suppl II):II-14—II-30, 1990.
62. Cohen-Solal A, Zannad F, Guéret P, et al: Multicenter determination of the oxygen uptake and the ventilatory threshold. *Eur Heart J* 12:1055–1063, 1991.
63. Beaver WL, Wasserman K, Whipp BJ: A new method for detecting anaerobic threshold by gas exchange. *J Appl Physiol* 60:2020–2027, 1986.
64. Dickstein K, Aarsland T, Svanes H, Barvik S: A respiratory exchange ratio equal to 1 provides a reproducible index of submaximal cardiopulmonary exercise performance. *Am J Cardiol* 17:1367–1369, 1993.
65. Prusaczyk WK, Cureton KJ, Graham RE, Ray CA: Differential effects of dietary carbohydrate on RPE at the lactate and ventilatory thresholds. *Med Sci Sports Exerc* 24:568–575, 1992.
66. Bogaard JM, Scholte HR, Busch HFM: Anaerobic threshold as detected from ventilatory and metabolic exercise responses in patients with mitochondrial respiratory chain defect. *Adv Cardiol* 35:135–145, 1986.
67. Hansen JE, Sue DY, Oren A, Wasserman K: Relation of oxygen uptake to work rate in normal men and men with circulatory disorders. *Am J Cardiol* 59:669–674, 1987.
68. Pina IL, Madonna DS, Sinnamon EA, Brozena S, Smith AL, Bove AA: Excess post-exercise O2 consumption in class II and III patients with heart failure (abstr). *Circulation* (suppl I) 92:I-399, 1992.
69. Kraemer MD, Kubo SH, Tschumperlin LK, Rector ThS, Bank AJ: Patients with heart failure demonstrate increased oxygen consumption and symptoms following maximal and submaximal exercise. *J Am Coll Cardiol* (suppl A) 23:471A, 1994.
70. Cross AM, Higginbotham MB: Oxygen deficit during exercise testing in heart failure: relation to submaximal exercise tolerance (abstr). *Circulation* 90 (suppl 1):1–15, 1994.
71. Dunselmann PHJM, Kuntze CEE, Van Bruggen A, et al: Value of New York Heart Association classification, radionuclide ventriculography, and cardiopulmonary exercise tests for selection of the patients for congestive heart failure studies. *Am Heart J* 116:1475–1482, 1988.
72. Patterson JA, Naughton J, Pietras RF, Gunnar RM: Treadmill exercise in assessment of functional capacity of patients with cardiac disease. *Am J Cardiol* 30:757–763, 1972.

73. The Criteria Committee of the New York Heart Association: 1994 revision to Classification of functional class and objective assessment of patients with disease of the heart. *Circulation* 92:644–645, 1994.
74. Wasserman K, Hansen JE, Sue DY, Whipp BJ, eds.: *Principles of Exercise Testing and Interpretation.* Philadelphia: Lea & Febiger, 47–57, 1987.
75. Weber K, Janicki JS: Cardiopulmonary exercise testing for evaluation of chronic heart failure. *Am J Cardiol* 55:22A-31A, 1985.
76. Eschenbascher WL, Mannina A: An algorithm for the interpretation of cardiopulmonary exercise tests. *Chest* 97:263–267, 1990.
77. Messner-Pellenc P, Ximenes C, Brasileiro CF, Mercier J, Grolleau R, Prefaut C: Cardiopulmonary exercise testing: determinants of dyspnea due to cardiac or pulmonary limitation. *Chest* 106:354–360, 1994.
78. Coats AJS, Adamopoulos S, Meyer TE, Conway J, Sleight P: Effects of physical training in chronic heart failure. *Lancet* 335:63–66, 1990.
79. Cohn JN, Johnson G, Ziesche S, et al: A comparison of enalapril with hydralazine-isosorbide dinitrate in the treatment of chronic congestive heart failure. *N Engl J Med* 325:303–310, 1991.
80. Mudge GH, Goldstein S, Addonizio LJ, et al: Bethesda Conference: Cardiac Transplantation. *J Am Coll Cardiol* 22:21–31, 1993.
81. Likoff MJ, Chandler SL, Kay HR: Clinical determinants of mortality in chronic congestive heart failure secondary to idiopathic dilated or to ischemic cardiomyopathy. *Am J Cardiol* 59:634–638, 1987.
82. Franciosa JA: Why patients with heart failure die: hemodynamic and functional determinants of survival. *Circulation* (suppl IV) 75:IV-20—IV-27, 1987.
83. Cohn JN, Rector TS: Prognosis of congestive heart failure and predictors of mortality. *Am J Cardiol* 62:25A-30A, 1988.
84. Cohn JN, Johnson G, Shabetai R, et al: Ejection fraction, peak oxygen consumption, cardio-thoracic ratio, ventricular arrhythmias, and plasma norepinephrine as determinants of prognosis in heart failure. *Circulation* 87 (suppl VI):VI-5—VI-16, 1993.
85. van den Broek SAJ, van Veldhuisen DJ, de Graeff PA, Landsman MLJ, Hillege H, Lie KI: Comparison between New York Heart Association classification and peak oxygen consumption in the assessment of functional status and prognosis in patients with mild to moderate chronic congestive heart failure secondary to either ischemic or idiopathic dilated cardiomyopathy. *Am J Cardiol* 70:359–363, 1992.
86. Mancini DM, Eisen H, Kussmaul W, Mull R, Edmunds LH, Wilson JR: Value of peak exercise oxygen consumption for optimal timing of cardiac transplantation in ambulatory patients. *Circulation* 83:778–786, 1991.
87. Stevenson LW, Steimle AE, Chelimsky-Fallick C, et al: Outcomes predicted by peak oxygen consumption during evaluation of 333 patients with advanced heart failure (abstr). *Circulation* 88 (suppl I):I-94, 1993.

3

Diastolic Dysfunction and Exercise Gas Exchange

Michael B. Higginbotham, MB

It is now generally accepted that the ejection fraction, like other measures of left ventricular emptying, correlates poorly with exercise tolerance and peak oxygen uptake ($\dot{V}O_2$) among patients with heart failure.[1,2] Thus, patients with very low ejection fractions can have normal exercise tolerance, while those with well-preserved ejection fractions may be severely limited (Figure 1).

The Fick equation indicates that $\dot{V}O_2$ is the product of cardiac output and arteriovenous oxygen difference, the latter reflecting peripheral mechanisms of blood flow distribution and oxygen extraction. This suggests either that peripheral (or noncardiac) factors may be contributing to exercise limitation, or that the ejection fraction by itself may not be an adequate descriptor of cardiac function. While the first alternative has been emphasized recently by several investigators,[3,4] recent insights concerning abnormalities of ventricular filling and relaxation support the second. Control of cardiac output is complex, relying upon valvular competence and changes in left ventricular stroke volume and heart rate; left ventricular stroke volume, in turn, depends upon preload as well as afterload and contractility (Figure 2). The concept that diastolic dysfunction may limit exercise tolerance has been supported by studies of left ventricular pressure and volume during exercise in several cardiac conditions associated with a normal ejection fraction.

From Wasserman, K (ed): *Exercise Gas Exchange in Heart Disease.* Armonk, NY: Futura Publishing Company, Inc., © 1996.

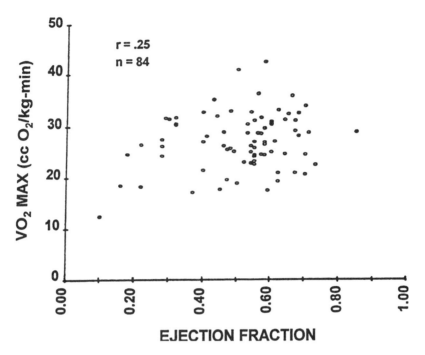

Figure 1. Relationship between ejection fraction and maximal oxygen uptake ($\dot{V}O_{2max}$) in patients with coronary heart disease, but not limited by angina. (Reproduced with permission from Reference 2.)

Cardiac Output = Stroke Volume x Heart Rate

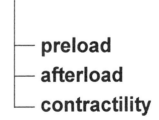

preload
afterload
contractility

Figure 2. Determinants of cardiac output.

Etiology and Hemodynamic Consequences of Diastolic Dysfunction

Left ventricular filling abnormalities are present in a wide variety of cardiac disorders (Figure 3).[5–8] These include:

- **Extrinsic** abnormalities that do not involve the left ventricle itself, such as pericardial constriction, mitral stenosis, primary pulmonary hypertension, and right ventricular failure.
- **Intrinsic** problems with the left ventricle such as hypertrophic cardiomyopathy (idiopathic or hypertensive), restrictive cardiomyopathy, coronary artery disease, and cardiac transplantation. Another important change in left ventricular relaxation—hardly to be regarded as an abnormality—is advanced age.

The hemodynamic consequences of intrinsic left ventricular filling abnormalities can be best illustrated by studying the left ventricular pressure-volume relationship.[7–10] The left ventricular pressure volume loop (Figure 4) clearly separates contraction (phases 1 and 2) from relaxation (phases 3 and 4). When left ventricular filling is abnormal (as in hypertrophic car-

ABNORMAL LV FILLING

EXTRINSIC
Pericardial constriction

Mitral stenosis

Primary pulmonary hypertension

Right heart failure

INTRINSIC
Hypertrophic cardiomyopathy

Restrictive cardiomyopathy

Coronary artery disease

Cardiac transplantation

(Advanced age)

Figure 3. Extrinsic and intrinsic causes of abnormal left ventricular filling.

CARDIOMYOPATHY

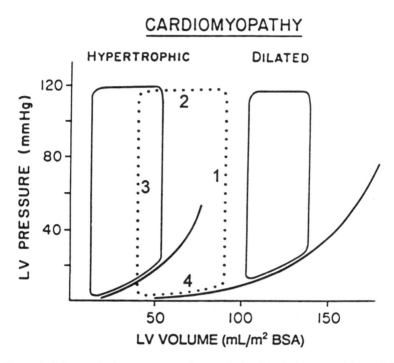

Figure 4. Left ventricular pressure volume relationship in hypertrophic and dilated cardiomyopathy, compared with normal (**dotted outline**). In hypertrophic cardiomyopathy, the diastolic pressure volume curve (**thick line**) is displaced upward. (Reproduced with permission from Reference 7.)

diomyopathy), the phase 4 filling curve is displaced upward so that a higher filling pressure is required for a normal end diastolic volume and stroke volume to be achieved. This is quite distinct from the increase in left ventricular volumes along a normal diastolic filling curve seen in dilated cardiomyopathy. It should be noted that the classic upward displacement of the diastolic pressure volume curve is seen when delivery of blood to the left ventricle is not compromised. It does not apply to the extrinsic filling abnormalities described earlier, nor to intrinsic abnormalities under conditions of limited left ventricular filling. Such conditions apply when patients are hypovolemic due to overdiuresis, are taking vasodilators, or assume the upright position. Under these conditions, cardiac filling is reduced so that the pressure-volume curve moves to the left along an abnormal diastolic border. The result is that the diastolic pressures move toward normal, but cardiac volumes—end diastolic volume, end systolic volume and stroke volume—are low. When patients with left ventricular filling abnormalities are on diuretics and vasodilators, in the upright position cardiac pressures can be entirely normal; the marked pressure-volume shift produces severe abnormalities in stroke volume and cardiac output.

Hypertrophic Cardiomyopathy

The above changes give rise to characteristic responses seen during upright exercise in patients with abnormal left ventricular filling. One of our first observations of this phenomenon was in a group of seven patients who presented with severe heart failure (usually pulmonary edema) despite normal ejection fractions and valve function.[11] Not surprisingly, most patients were hypertensive and elderly. After stabilization of their condition with diuretics and vasodilators, the patients were studied with invasive cardiopulmonary exercise testing performed during upright exercise.

Compared with age-matched normal controls, maximal oxygen uptake ($\dot{V}O_2$max) was reduced by 48%—11.6 versus 22.7 mL/kg/min (Figure 5). Although peak arteriovenous oxygen difference was a little lower (13%) in patients than in normals, most of the 48% decrease in $\dot{V}O_2$max was accounted for by an abnormal cardiac reserve—41% re-

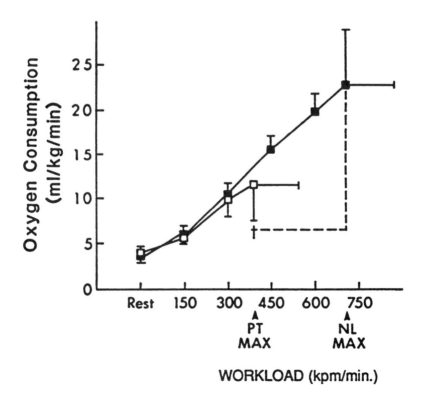

Figure 5. Oxygen consumption at rest and during progressive upright exercise in normal subjects (**closed symbols**) and patients with diastolic heart failure (**open symbols**). † indicates significantly lower maximal $\dot{V}O_2$ consumption for the patient group. (Reproduced with permission from Reference 11.)

duced in patients compared with normals (Figure 6). In the patient group, peak $\dot{V}O_2$ correlated strongly with peak cardiac output ($R = .81$) but not with arteriovenous oxygen difference. In turn, the abnormal cardiac output reserve was accounted for by a failure to increase the stroke volume in response to exercise.

While the left ventricular ejection fraction and end systolic volume were normal in the patient group, they failed to use the Starling mechanism even in the face of an abnormal increase in left ventricular filling pressure as measured by the pulmonary capillary wedge pressure (Figure 7). The abnormal diastolic pressure-volume relationships in these patients are represented in Figure 8. At peak exercise, abnormalities were seen as both an increase in pulmonary capillary wedge pressure and a decrease in cardiac volumes.

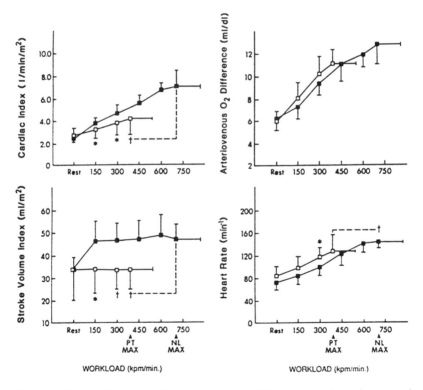

Figure 6. Cardiac index, arteriovenous oxygen difference, stroke volume, and heart rate at rest and during progressive upright exercise in normal subjects and patients with diastolic heart failure. * indicates a significant difference during submaximal workloads. Other symbols are as in Figure 5. (Reproduced with permission from Reference 11.)

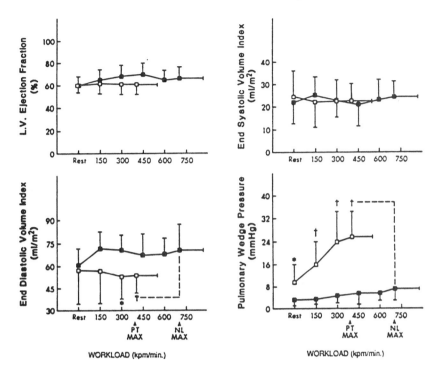

Figure 7. Ejection fraction, end systolic volume index, end diastolic volume index, and pulmonary wedge pressure at rest and during progressive upright exercise in normal subjects and patients with diastolic heart failure. Symbols are as in Figures 5 and 6. (Reproduced with permission from Reference 11.)

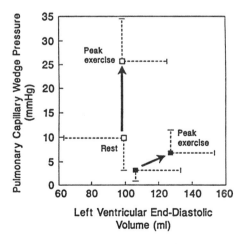

Figure 8. Relationship between left ventricular end diastolic volume and pulmonary capillary wedge pressure at rest and during peak exercise for normal subjects (**closed symbols**) and patients with diastolic heart failure (**open symbols**). Patients achieved no measurable increase in end diastolic volume despite dramatic increases in pulmonary capillary wedge pressure, indicating failure to use the Starling mechanism. (Reproduced with permission from Reference 11.)

Cardiac Transplantation

A similar, though less dramatic, abnormality is seen in another group of cardiac patients with abnormal exercise tolerance despite a normal ejection fraction—cardiac transplant recipients. In a recent study, we examined the response of cardiac pressure and volume in a group of 30 heart transplant recipients, compared with an age-matched control group.[12] In the transplant patients, peak $\dot{V}O_2$ was reduced 46% compared with the age-matched normals—12.3 versus 22.9 mL/kg/min (Figure 9).

The ejection fraction was normal in the transplant recipients, both at rest and during exercise (Figure 10). However, the 46% decrease in peak $\dot{V}O_2$ was related primarily to a 42% reduction in cardiac index (Figure 11). Unlike the previous example, peak arteriovenous oxygen difference was reduced (by 24%), consistent with a contribution from peripheral abnormalities present prior to the transplant, which may now be limiting because of improved cardiac output reserve. The abnormal cardiac output was related, in turn, to a decrease in both heart rate and stroke volume reserves during exercise, with a 79% decrease in heart rate and a 17% decrease in stroke volume index.

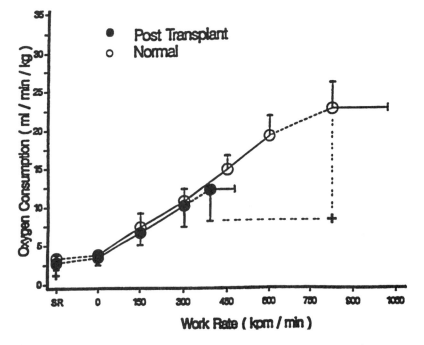

Figure 9. Oxygen consumption during supine rest (SR), upright rest (O), and progressive upright exercise in normal subjects (**open symbols**) and heart transplant recipients (**closed symbols**). + indicates a significantly lower oxygen consumption in transplant recipients. (Reproduced with permission from Reference 12.)

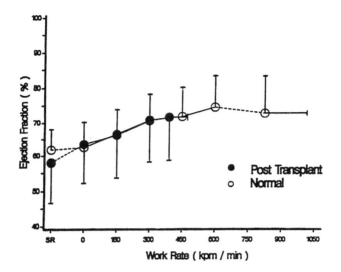

Figure 10. Ejection fraction during supine rest, upright rest, and progressive exercise in normal subjects and heart transplant recipients. Symbols are as in Figure 9. No between group differences are seen. (Reproduced with permission from Reference 12.)

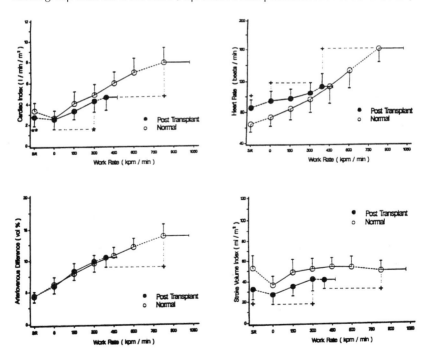

Figure 11. Cardiac index, heart rate, arteriovenous O_2 difference and stroke volume index during supine rest, upright rest, and progressive exercise in normal subjects and heart transplant recipients. Symbols are as in Figures 9 and 10; + indicates significant differences at maximal or submaximal exercise. Peak values for all variables are abnormally low in transplant recipients. (Reproduced with permission from Reference 12.)

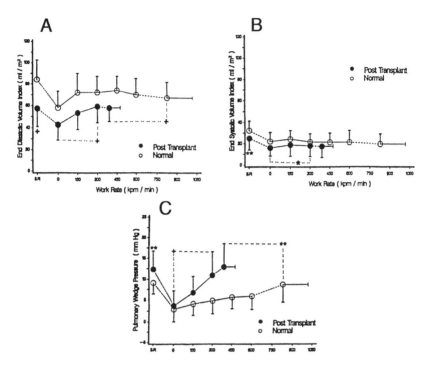

Figure 12. End diastolic volume index, end systolic volume index, and pulmonary wedge pressure during supine rest, upright rest, and progressive exercise in normal subjects and heart transplant recipients. Symbols are as in Figures 9 to 11. Lower diastolic volumes and high pulmonary wedge pressures indicate the abnormal left ventricular filling characteristics of transplant recipients. (Reproduced with permission from Reference 12.)

Why was stroke volume abnormally low, even though it would be expected to be augmented with increased filling time afforded by chronotropic incompetence? As can be seen in Figure 12, an increase in end systolic volume was not the problem. The end diastolic volume was abnormally low, during exercise and even at rest. The Starling mechanism could not be used even though pulmonary capillary wedge pressure was abnormally high. Thus, although peripheral abnormalities and chronotropic incompetence may have added to the decrease in $\dot{V}O_2$max in transplant recipients, the abnormal exercise tolerance reflected an important limitation of left ventricular filling.

Cardiovascular Aging

As mentioned earlier, the aging process itself produces functionally important alterations in left ventricular filling. Abnormalities in left ventricular filling pattern are readily detected in older hearts. Abnormal patterns in the contribution of late atrial to early passive filling (A/E ratios) have been virtually uniformly observed in echocardiographic studies, and are still present when left ventricular pressures are accounted for (Figure 13).[13]

The extent to which changes in left ventricular filling contribute to the decline in exercise tolerance seen in the elderly (as opposed to a decrease in heart rate reserve, peripheral function, or noncardiovascular factors) has been elucidated in our laboratory through age-related comparisons of the left ventricular pressure and volume responses to exercise. We studied 104 normal sedentary subjects aged 20 to 76 years, screened for cardiac disease with rest and exercise radionuclide angiography and echocardiography.[14] During maximal exercise, $\dot{V}O_2$ declined by 48% over the six decades studied; arteriovenous oxygen difference was unchanged across the age range, whereas cardiac index declined by 45% and heart rate declined by 26% (Figure 14). Despite the lower heart rate (which one would have expected to have been accompanied by a compensatory increase in stroke volume), stroke volume decreased by 24% (Figure 15). The inadequate stroke volume reserve resulted from apparent abnormalities in left ventricular con-

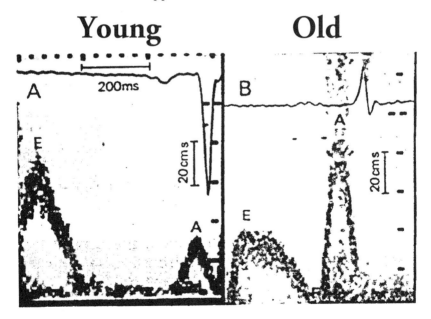

Figure 13. Doppler echocardiographic patterns for young and old subjects, demonstrating the augmented contribution of atrial filling (**A**) in relation to early filling (**E**) in the elderly. (Reproduced with permission. Adapted from Lewis JF, et al. In: Lowenthal DT, ed. *Geriatric Cardiology*. Philadelphia: F.A. Davis Co., 1992.)

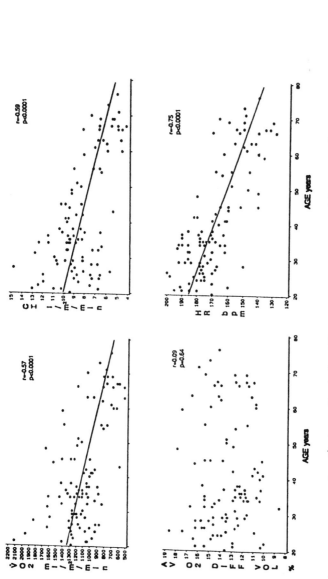

Figure 14. Maximal oxygen consumption ($\dot{V}O_2$), cardiac index (CI), arteriovenous oxygen difference ($A\dot{V}O_2$ Diff), and heart rate (HR) related to age in 104 normal subjects aged 21 to 76 years. The age-related decline in $\dot{V}O_2$max was related to decreases in maximal cardiac output and heart rate, but not to arteriovenous O_2 difference.

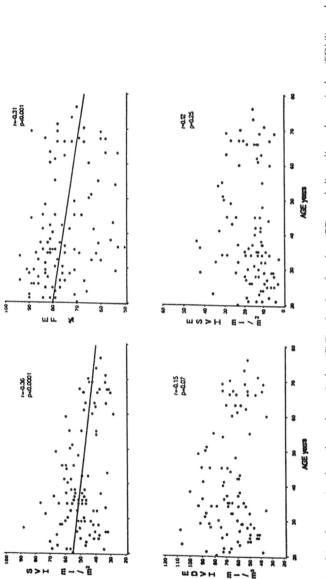

Figure 15. Age relationships for maximal stroke volume index (SVI), ejection fraction (EF), end diastolic volume index (EDVI), and end systolic volume index (ESVI) for 104 normal subjects aged 21 to 76 years. The age-related decline in stroke volume index is accounted for by a decrease in maximal ejection fraction, without a compensatory increase in left ventricular volume.

traction and relaxation: on the one hand, exercise ejection fraction decreased, and on the other end diastolic volume failed to be enhanced, and in fact decreased slightly. As was seen for the previous example of heart transplant recipients, there was a decrease in $\dot{V}O_2$ with age-reflecting failure to use the Starling mechanism to compensate (increased left ventricular shortening) for a decreased exercise heart rate reserve.

Conclusion

By measuring $\dot{V}O_2$max, then, what does cardiopulmonary exercise testing tell us about patients with left ventricular relaxation abnormalities? It can be concluded from the examples presented (and summarized in Figure 16) that $\dot{V}O_2$max is primarily a descriptor of cardiac output reserve rather than of peripheral vascular and metabolic ab-

SIGNIFICANCE OF VO$_2$ MAX

	CO	SV	HR	AVO$_2$D
DCM	+++	++	+	-
HCM	+++	++	-	-
TX	+++	++	+	+
AGE	+++	++	+	-

Figure 16. Summary of the relationship between maximal oxygen consumption ($\dot{V}O_2$max) and hemodynamic variables in various conditions—dilated cardiomyopathy (DCM), hypertrophic cardiomyopathy (HCM), transplant recipients (TX) and advanced age (AGE). In each condition, $\dot{V}O_2$max is strongly related to cardiac output (CO) and stroke volume (SV). Heart rate (HR) is a contributing factor for dilated cardiomyopathy, transplant recipients and advanced age; arteriovenous oxygen difference (A$\dot{V}O_2$D) is related to $\dot{V}O_2$max in transplant recipients only.

normalities. In patients with preserved ejection fractions (as in patients with a low ejection fraction), $\dot{V}O_2$max reflects cardiac output reserve, and as such describes the interaction between stroke volume and heart rate. In such patients, $\dot{V}O_2$max measures the functional impact of left ventricular filling abnormalities on cardiac output reserve, and is therefore a very important measure of diastolic function.

Summary

Abnormalities in left ventricular filling are seen in a wide variety of cardiac disorders, and may account for the observation of heart failure despite a normal ejection fraction.

Altered left ventricular filling has been clearly identified in patients with hypertrophic cardiomyopathy, in heart transplant recipients, and even in elderly subjects who are apparently free of cardiac disease. In each of these conditions, a close relationship has been observed between $\dot{V}O_2$max and maximal cardiac output.

Thus, in patients with left ventricular filling abnormalities peak $\dot{V}O_2$ describes the interaction between stroke volume and heart rate, and is therefore a reliable noninvasive measure of the impact of abnormal left ventricular filling on functional capacity.

References

1. Higginbotham MB, Morris KG, Conn EH, Coleman RE, Cobb FR: Determinants of variable exercise performance among patients with severe left ventricular dysfunction. *Am J Cardiol* 51:52–60, 1983.
2. Froelicher VF: Interpretation of specific exercise test responses. In: Froelicher VF, ed. *Exercise and the Heart,* 2nd edition. Chicago, IL: Year Book Medical Publishers Inc., 83–145, 1987.
3. Massie BM, Conway M, Rajagopalan B, Yonge R, Frostick S, Ledingham J, Sleight P, Radda G: Skeletal muscle metabolism during exercise under ischemic conditions in congestive heart failure: evidence for abnormalities unrelated to blood flow. *Circulation* 78(2):320–326, 1988.
4. Sullivan MJ, Green HJ, Cobb FR: Altered skeletal muscle metabolic response to exercise in chronic heart failure: relation to skeletal muscle aerobic enzyme activity. *Circulation* 84(4):1597–1607, 1991.
5. Kessler KM: Heart failure with normal systolic function: update of prevalence, differential diagnosis, prognosis and therapy. *Arch Intern Med* 148:2109–2111, 1988.
6. Topol EJ, Traill TA, Fortuin NJ: Hypertensive hypertrophic cardiomyopathy of the elderly. *N Engl J Med* 312(5):277–283, 1985.
7. Gaasch WH: Diastolic mechanisms in heart failure. *Heart Failure* 1:195–202, 1985.
8. Brutsaert DL, Sys SU, Gillebert TC: Diastolic failure: pathophysiology and therapeutic implications. *J Am Coll Cardiol* 22(1):318–325, 1993.
9. Gilbert JC, Glantz SA: Determinants of left ventricular filling and of the diastolic pressure-volume relation. *Circ Res* 64(5):827–852, 1989.

10. Mirsky I, Pasipoularides A: Clinical assessment of diastolic function. *Prog Cardiovasc Dis* 32(4):291–318, 1990.
11. Kitzman DW, Higginbotham MB, Cobb FR, Sheikh KH, Sullivan MJ: Exercise intolerance in patients with heart failure and preserved left ventricular systolic function: failure of the Frank-Starling mechanism. *J Am Coll Cardiol* 17(5):1065–1072, 1991.
12. Kao AC, Van Trigt III P, Shaeffer-McCall GS, Shaw JP, Kuzil BB, Page RD, Higginbotham MB: Central and peripheral limitations to upright exercise in untrained cardiac transplant recipients. *Circulation* 89(6):2605–2615, 1994.
13. Kitzman DW, Sheikh KH, Beere PA, Philips JL, Higginbotham MB: Age-related alterations of Doppler left ventricular filling indexes in normal subjects are independent of left ventricular mass, heart rate, contractility and loading conditions. *J Am Coll Cardiol* 18(5):1243–1250, 1991.
14. Kitzman DW, Sullivan MJ, Cobb FR, Higginbotham MB: Exercise cardiac output declines with advancing age in normal subjects. *J Am Coll Cardiol* 13(2):241A, 1989.

4

Cardiopulmonary Exercise Testing and the Evaluation of Systolic Dysfunction

Karl T. Weber, MD

Introduction

Heart failure is a worldwide health problem of increasing proportions related, in part, to the advancing age of our society. The evaluation and management of such patients challenges both the practicing physician and the clinician scientist. One such challenge is having a reliable means to evaluate the severity of heart failure. Another, and given the prevalence of heart disease and chronic airway disease that frequently coexist in the same patient, is based on providing a means whereby exertional breathlessness secondary to either cardiac or ventilatory disease can be distinguished.

In this brief review, the relative merits of cardiopulmonary exercise testing (i.e., the monitoring of breath-by-breath respiratory gas exchange) in addressing these needs are considered. Particular emphasis is placed on addressing systolic dysfunction irrespective of its etiologic basis, and the primary limitation responsible for exertional dyspnea.

Definition of Heart Failure

Heart failure may be defined according to clinical or physiological criteria. In clinical terms, heart failure is defined based on its

From Wasserman, K (ed): *Exercise Gas Exchange in Heart Disease.* Armonk, NY: Futura Publishing Company, Inc., © 1996.

chronicity (i.e., acute versus chronic) or the relative preponderance of signs and symptoms that are in keeping with inadequate right versus left heart pumping function. In physiological terms, heart failure is described as the inability of the heart to deliver oxygen to metabolizing tissues in accordance with prevailing oxygen requirements. This emphasizes the ability of this muscular pump to deliver oxygen (a function of its cardiac output) and is in keeping with its systolic function.

Systolic pump function depends on several factors. These include: the coordinate contraction of atria and ventricles and the right and left heart; chronotropic responsiveness; the ability of blood to enter and leave cardiac chambers while moving in a forward direction; the distensibility of the myocardium, which determines its ability to accommodate blood during filling; and the ability of each ventricle to displace blood. *Circulatory failure* exists when factors extrinsic to the myocardium interfere with its pumping and filling functions. For example, valvular stenosis or incompetence and restrictive pericardial disease each can undermine cardiac output at rest and/or during physical activity. *Cardiac failure,* on the other hand, is due to impaired myocardial contractility (primary systolic dysfunction) or abnormal myocardial stiffness during filling (primary diastolic dysfunction). The focus of this review is on systolic dysfunction in patients with chronic cardiac or circulatory failure. The ability of noninvasive respiratory gas exchange to detect the presence and severity of chronic cardiac or circulatory failure, irrespective of its etiologic basis, is considered.

Maximal Oxygen Uptake, Anaerobic Threshold, and the Severity of Cardiac and/or Circulatory Failure

Symptoms of breathlessness and fatigue appear in patients with chronic cardiac or circulatory failure. These most often occur during physical activity when the need to raise cardiac output is mandated by working skeletal muscle. Such information, which categorizes a patient's functional capacity, can be quite subjective from both the patient's and physician's standpoint. More appealing is the objective evaluation of such symptoms during monitored physical activity. In so doing, an objective means to grade the severity of cardiac or circulatory failure is obtained.

Walking is a nonspecialized skill. A treadmill protocol utilizing gradual increments in muscular work should be selected for patients with chronic cardiac or circulatory failure. For example, if a patient can walk into the doctor's office, he/she can likely walk on the treadmill at 1 mph and 0% grade. This is an extremely slow pace (it takes 1 hour to walk 1 mile) and can be used for stage 1 of the monitored exercise response. Subsequent stages of exercise should invoke additional, gradual increments in work. In this laboratory, a modified Naughton protocol has been found useful for addressing a wide spectrum of patients with cardiac or circulatory failure.[1]

During exercise, oxygen uptake ($\dot{V}O_2$), carbon dioxide production, tidal volume and respiratory rate (whose product equals minute ventilation), and arterial oxygen saturation are monitored noninvasively together with the patient's electrocardiogram and blood pressure. This provides a comprehensive assessment of the patient's cardiac and ventilatory responses and from which the severity of cardiac or circulatory failure can be determined. It does not identify the etiologic basis of failure. This requires careful clinical evaluation together with appropriate laboratory studies.

The severity of cardiac and circulatory failure is gauged according to exercise cardiac output response (or cardiac reserve), as predicted noninvasively using either of two criteria.[2] These include: a) exercise anaerobic threshold, identified when carbon dioxide production exceeds $\dot{V}O_2$ (which is reviewed more extensively in Chapter 1), and b) exercise maximum oxygen uptake($\dot{V}O_2$max), defined as a plateau in oxygen utilization and where $\dot{V}O_2$ remains invariant (<1 mL/kg/min) despite an additional increment in treadmill work.[1]

Invasive hemodynamic and metabolic measurements were used to validate this approach. Seventy-six patients with chronic cardiac failure of diverse etiology and severity were investigated.[3] During upright, incremental treadmill exercise, the following measurements were obtained: right atrial and pulmonary artery pressures; occlusive wedge pressure; cardiac output; pulmonary artery (or mixed venous) oxygen saturation and lactate concentration. Patients were exercised to their $\dot{V}O_2$max. Differences in aerobic capacity, or $\dot{V}O_2$max, were graded according to the following classification[4]: a) little or no impairment in aerobic capacity (Class A) was defined as a $\dot{V}O_2$max of >20 mL/min/kg; b) mild to moderate impairment (Class B) as 16–20 mL/min/kg; c) moderate to severe impairment (Class C) as 10–15 mL/min/kg; and d) severe limitation (Class D) as <10 mL/min/kg. This approach did not take into account differences in age, gender, or physical conditioning. However, even octogenarians have a predicted $\dot{V}O_2$max of >20 mL/min/kg, and patients with cardiac or circulatory failure are not usually exercise trained at the time of clinical presentation. This scheme was therefore felt to offer a starting point. Refinements to this approach will undoubtedly follow.

During incremental exercise the following observations were made. In each patient, irrespective of functional class, arteriovenous oxygen difference increased to >12 vols% at maximal exercise with mixed venous oxygen saturation falling to <30%. In keeping with the theorem of Adolph Fick, it therefore followed that the major determinant of $\dot{V}O_2$max was based on exercise cardiac output response. Exercise cardiac output response for each functional class is shown in Figure 1. The abnormal exercise cardiac output response in Class B, C, and D patients occurred despite marked increments in left ventricular filling pressure as gauged from the rise in wedge pressure (Figure 2). The marked rise in wedge pressure seen in class C and D patients may

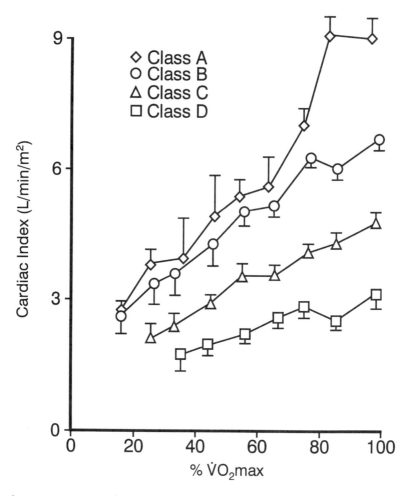

Figure 1. Exercise cardiac index response to upright treadmill exercise in patients with chronic cardiac failure of diverse etiology. Patients were exercised to their maximal oxygen uptake ($\dot{V}O_2$max), which, in turn, was set equal to 100%. This permitted a comparison of each functional class (see text). Exercise cardiac reserve is normal or nearly normal in functional **Class A** while severely impaired in **Class D**. (Reproduced with permission from Reference 3.)

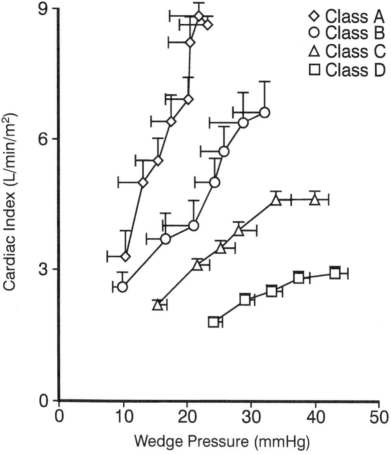

Figure 2. Exercise response in cardiac index and wedge pressure in patients with chronic cardiac failure. Despite marked increments in left ventricular filling pressure, exercise cardiac output response was impaired in **Class B, C,** and **D** patients. (Reproduced with permission from Reference 3.)

suggest the presence of diastolic dysfunction due to intrinsic abnormality in myocardial distensibility or to extrinsic factors, such as ventricular interdependence with increased right ventricular loading or pericardial restraint. The impairment in exercise cardiac output was related to abnormal stroke volume response (Figure 3). The rise in heart rate was considered normal for the level of $\dot{V}O_2$ attained. Noninvasive determination of $\dot{V}O_2$max therefore permits a stratification of differences in exercise cardiac output response and thereby grades the severity of cardiac and circulatory failure (Table).

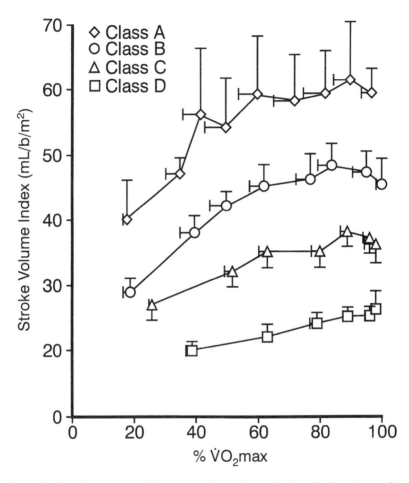

Figure 3. Exercise response in stroke volume for patients with chronic cardiac failure. An inability to raise stroke volume accounted for the abnormal exercise cardiac output response while exercise heart rate (not shown) was normal for the level of work achieved. (Reproduced with permission from Reference 3.)

Anaerobic threshold was defined as that point during exercise where mixed venous lactate concentration rose above 12 mg% representing greater than two standard deviations for normal resting values in the laboratory.[5] This occurred at different levels of work for each functional class as seen in Figure 4 and the Table. The rise in mixed venous lactate also corresponded to the aforementioned response in carbon dioxide production relative to $\dot{V}O_2$. Hence, the noninvasive determination of anaerobic threshold provides another means whereby the severity of cardiac or circulatory failure can be gauged (Table).

Table 1

Exercise Functional Classification Based on
Maximal O_2 Uptake and Anaerobic Threshold

Class	$\dot{V}O_2max$ (mL/min/kg)	AT (mL/min/kg)	CImax (L/min/m²)
A	>20	>14	>8
B	16–20	11–14	6–8
C	10–15	8–11	4–6
D	<10	<8	<4

$\dot{V}O_2max$ = maximal O_2 uptake
AT = anaerobic threshold
CImax = maximal exercise cardiac index

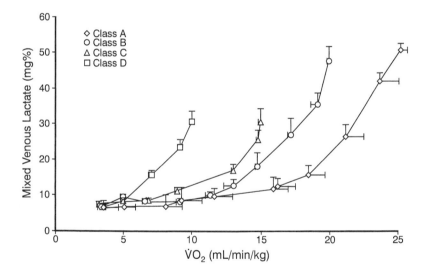

Figure 4. Exercise response in mixed venous (pulmonary artery) lactate concentration to upright treadmill exercise in patients with chronic cardiac failure. For each functional class, mixed venous lactate exceeded 12 mg% at different levels of muscular work, expressed as oxygen uptake ($\dot{V}O_2$). Invasive anaerobic threshold corresponded to noninvasive determination by respiratory gas exchange. (Reproduced with permission from Reference 3.)

Exertional Dyspnea: Cardiac versus Ventilatory Causes

Patients with primary cardiac or circulatory failure are able to cross their anaerobic threshold during incremental exercise, and if motivated by the physician in attendance will attain their $\dot{V}O_2max$. Exertional dyspnea does not prohibit them from achieving these end points. These responses occur without a fall in arterial oxygen saturation. These patients likewise do not use more than 50% of their ventilatory reserve,[2] expressed as their maximum voluntary ventilation obtained during pulmonary function testing or estimated by multiplying their forced expiratory volume at 1 second by 35.

This contrasts to patients with a primary ventilatory limitation to exercise. Such patients become dyspneic and unable to exercise further when they utilize more than 70% of their ventilatory reserve or when arterial oxygen desaturation appears. These patients become symptomatic long before their cardiac reserve is exhausted, and therefore they do not cross their anaerobic threshold and do not attain their $\dot{V}O_2$max.

Summary

Monitoring of respiratory gas exchange during monitored exercise provides a noninvasive, objective means to determine cardiac reserve (exercise cardiac output) in patients with chronic cardiac or circulatory failure of diverse etiology. It also can be used to assess functional capacity over time, response to therapeutic intervention, and as a means to distinguish between primary cardiac or circulatory failure versus ventilatory system failure in patients experiencing exertional dyspnea and in whom there is coexistent heart and lung disease.

References

1. Weber KT, Janicki JS, McElroy PA: Cardiopulmonary exercise (CPX) testing. In: Weber KT, Janicki JS, eds. *Cardiopulmonary Exercise Testing.* Philadelphia: WB Saunders, 151–167, 1986.
2. Weber KT, Kinasewitz GT, Janicki JS, Fishman AP: Oxygen utilization and ventilation during exercise in patients with chronic cardiac failure. *Circulation* 65:1213–1223, 1982.
3. Weber KT, Janicki JS: Cardiopulmonary exercise testing for evaluation of chronic cardiac failure. *Am J Cardiol* 55:22A-31A, 1985.
4. Weber KT, Kinasewitz GT, West JS, Janicki JS, Reichek N, Fishman AP: Long-term vasodilation therapy with trimazosin in chronic cardiac failure. *N Engl J Med* 303:242–250, 1980.
5. Weber KT, Janicki JS: Lactate production during maximal and submaximal exercise in patients with chronic heart failure. *J Am Coll Cardiol* 6:717–724, 1985.

5

Gas Exchange During Recovery from Exercise in Patients with Heart Failure

Mark D. Kraemer, MD

Introduction

The last three decades have seen numerous advances in our understanding of exertional dyspnea and fatigue in heart failure. Nevertheless, despite its fundamental role in the clinical syndrome of heart failure, exercise intolerance has proven difficult to precisely quantify in these patients. There is general agreement that conventional measures of exercise performance, such as maximal oxygen uptake ($\dot{V}O_2$max), provide a means of assessing prognosis, are reproducible, and correlate roughly with functional class. In contrast, these measurements are not particularly sensitive to changes in patients' symptoms over time in response to therapy.[1,2] Perhaps the most dramatic example is the profound improvement in exertional symptoms seen in some patients after cardiac transplantation, which may have no or minimal effect on peak exercise oxygen uptake ($\dot{V}O_2$).

One potential reason for the shortcoming of maximal exercise testing is the lack of similarity to daily activities. Daily life in patients is typically characterized by brief periods of submaximal exercise interspersed between longer periods of inactivity. Studies in normal subjects have shown that metabolic recovery from brief moderate-to-high intensity exercise often takes much longer than the exercise period itself.[3] Furthermore, it has long been observed that some patients with heart failure experience fatigue which persists long after they stop ex-

From Wasserman, K (ed): *Exercise Gas Exchange in Heart Disease*. Armonk, NY: Futura Publishing Company, Inc., © 1996.

ercising. It is thus not difficult to conceive that some patients may actually spend more of their life recovering from exercise than actually performing exercise. Thus, the ability to quantify symptoms related to physical activity may be enhanced by adding an assessment of recovery to currently employed exercise tests.

Though post-exercise respiratory gas exchange has been extensively studied in healthy subjects, data in patients with heart failure are limited. This chapter first briefly reviews the normal physiology of post-exercise gas exchange, with special reference to mechanisms which could theoretically mediate abnormal responses in heart failure. Next, previous studies which have directly examined recovery from exercise in heart failure are reviewed.

Post-Exercise Gas Exchange—Healthy Subjects

Oxygen Uptake

During exercise, $\dot{V}O_2$ reflects the ability of the cardiovascular system to deliver blood to working muscle as well as the capacity and need for oxygen extraction in tissue. During constant workload moderate intensity exercise, $\dot{V}O_2$ rises in a pseudoexponential fashion to approximate a steady state, then falls with similar dynamics back to resting levels during recovery (Figure 1). Classically, the elevation in $\dot{V}O_2$ during recovery has been termed the *oxygen debt,* which implies a strict dependence on the *oxygen deficit* incurred by anaerobic metabolism during exercise. More recently, as the mechanisms which mediate post-exercise $\dot{V}O_2$ have proven more complex, the term *excess post-exercise oxygen consumption* (EPOC) has been used to absolve this entity from a strict dependence on anaerobic metabolism.[4]

During the early period of recovery, oxygen is primarily required for the rephosphorylation of creatine in skeletal muscle, and the early rapid decline in $\dot{V}O_2$ depends upon the rate at which this process occurs. Another determinant of early post-exercise $\dot{V}O_2$ dynamics is the rate of increase in mixed venous oxygen saturation to its resting value,[5] which is in part dependent on hemodynamic factors. Later during recovery, depending on the intensity and duration of exercise, oxygen is required for conversion of lactate to pyruvate.[5] Furthermore, body temperature and tissue catecholamines remain elevated above rest, which may increase systemic oxygen needs (Figure 2). In a recent, well-controlled study, Borsheim et al[6] administered intravenous propranolol to healthy subjects immediately after 60 minutes of heavy exercise (80% maximal $\dot{V}O_2$). With beta-adrenergic blockade, there was a marked reduction in the late component of EPOC compared to control, and total EPOC was reduced by about one-third. In contrast,

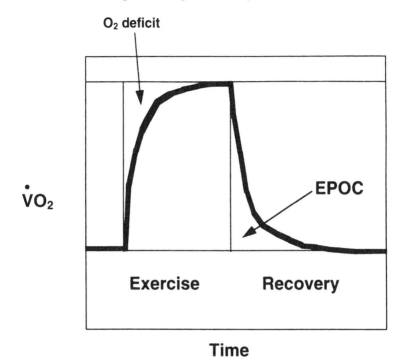

Figure 1. Time course of oxygen uptake ($\dot{V}O_2$) during exercise and recovery for brief constant-load submaximal exercise. The **bold line** represents actual smoothed $\dot{V}O_2$ data from an 8-minute exercise test at 25W in a patient with mild heart failure. The "oxygen deficit" is the difference between steady state $\dot{V}O_2$ and actual $\dot{V}O_2$ integrated over the exercise period. The excess post-exercise oxygen consumption (EPOC, or alternatively "oxygen debt") is the difference between actual $\dot{V}O_2$ and resting $\dot{V}O_2$ integrated over the recovery period.

propranolol had minimal effect on early post-exercise $\dot{V}O_2$ dynamics. Thus, beta-adrenergic stimulation may be an important mechanism for the prolonged component of post-exercise $\dot{V}O_2$. Other putative influences on EPOC include the effects of thyroxine, glucocorticoids, fatty acids, and calcium ions.[4]

In light of the above mechanisms, how might the kinetics of $\dot{V}O_2$ during recovery from exercise be altered in the presence of heart failure? Previous studies using nuclear magnetic resonance spectroscopy have shown a prolonged recovery time for the muscle phosphate-to-phosphocreatine ratio in patients with heart failure after forearm exercise.[7] As early post-exercise $\dot{V}O_2$ is influenced by the need for creatine phosphate repletion, one might predict that the early $\dot{V}O_2$ kinetics during recovery would be slower in heart failure. Though little is known about post-exercise sympathetic activation in heart failure, it has been

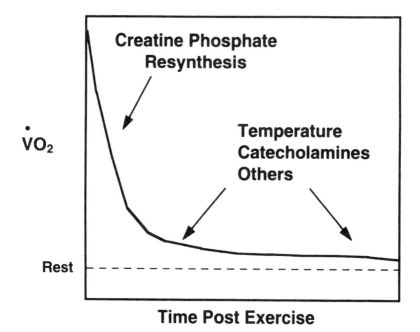

Figure 2. Time course of $\dot{V}O_2$ during recovery from prolonged high-intensity exercise (e.g., 20 minutes at 80% peak $\dot{V}O_2$). $\dot{V}O_2$ kinetics are characterized by an early rapid component and a late slower component. The excess $\dot{V}O_2$ is mediated by the resynthesis of high-energy phosphate stores, sustained elevations in body temperature and catecholamines, and other mechanisms (see text and Reference 4).

well established that plasma catecholamines are elevated in heart failure patients compared to control subjects, both at rest and during exercise at the same absolute workload. If this elevated sympathetic activation persists into the recovery period, one might speculate that the late component of post-exercise $\dot{V}O_2$ kinetics would be slower in heart failure. Finally, regardless of mechanism, the profound deconditioning often seen in patients with heart failure may predispose them to slow $\dot{V}O_2$ kinetics, as it is well established that $\dot{V}O_2$ kinetics are slower in the untrained compared to the trained state.[8]

Carbon Dioxide Output

In normal subjects, carbon dioxide output ($\dot{V}CO_2$) falls much less rapidly than $\dot{V}O_2$ during recovery, accounting for the marked rise in the respiratory exchange ratio ($\dot{V}CO_2 / \dot{V}O_2$) typically seen immediately after moderate or high-intensity exercise. The kinetics of $\dot{V}CO_2$ are also complex, depending both on the rate of carbon dioxide production and elimination. Carbon dioxide is produced mainly as a by-product of tissue acidosis, as lactate, which accumulates during exercise, is buffered by bicarbonate. Carbon dioxide elimination depends not only on intact circulatory and ventilatory systems for removal in the lungs, but also on the metabolism of lactate by various tissues including inactive skeletal muscle.[9,10]

These competing influences complicate any speculation regarding post-exercise $\dot{V}CO_2$ kinetics measured by expired gas analysis in heart failure, and data in these patients are scarce. Nevertheless, lactate generation is higher during exercise at the same absolute workload in heart failure, compared to controls, which could theoretically increase post-exercise carbon dioxide production. The circulatory and ventilatory abnormalities which accompany heart failure might also influence $\dot{V}CO_2$ during recovery.

Minute Ventilation

Minute ventilation ($\dot{V}E$) remains elevated during recovery from exercise in healthy subjects, and is an important means of carbon dioxide removal. Though post-exercise hyperpnea may be mediated in part by carbon dioxide-sensitive chemoreceptors, hemodynamic factors and baroreception are also important.[11] The acute reduction of peripheral blood flow has been shown to depress post-exercise $\dot{V}E$ in humans.[12] In related animal studies, baroreceptor blockade[11] appears to blunt this effect. Thus, the well-known abnormalities of peripheral blood flow and baroreceptor function in heart failure would likely influence post-exercise $\dot{V}E$ in these patients.

Post-Exercise Gas Exchange—Heart Failure

As mentioned earlier, there are few published studies regarding gas exchange during recovery from exercise in patients with heart failure. Nevertheless, post-exercise $\dot{V}O_2$ kinetics have been examined for several different types of exercise, and in several different ways. One approach is to compare the instantaneous $\dot{V}O_2$ at a given time point after exercise. Reddy et al[13] measured systemic $\dot{V}O_2$ using expired gas analysis in patients with heart failure and controls during light forearm exercise and 1 minute post-exercise. There was no significant difference in $\dot{V}O_2$ between groups during exercise, but absolute $\dot{V}O_2$ was significantly elevated in heart failure during the recovery period. Sietsema et al[14] compared post-exercise $\dot{V}O_2$ in normal subjects and patients with mild-to-moderate heart failure (peak $\dot{V}O_2$ 65±20% predicted). Whether after exercise at the same absolute workload or after a "matched" high intensity workload, the normalized $\dot{V}O_2$ (percent change in $\dot{V}O_2$ from rest to the end-exercise value) was higher in heart failure during the first 2 minutes of recovery.

Another approach is to calculate a time constant for $\dot{V}O_2$ using a monexponential curve fit for the first several minutes of recovery. Hayashida et al[15] demonstrated that the $\dot{V}O_2$ time constant is prolonged in heart failure compared to control subjects after maximal upright bicycle exercise. This time constant also appeared to be positively related to the severity of heart failure. The time constant for $\dot{V}E$ during recovery showed a similar relationship. A more recent study has also shown a prolongation in the $\dot{V}O_2$ time constant after constant-load submaximal exercise in patients with cardiac disease.[16] There was a modest correlation (r=0.53) between the time constant for recovery and that for $\dot{V}O_2$ during exercise. This study, however, included only a small number of patients with heart failure, and excluded those in NYHA functional class III and IV.

There is a paucity of data regarding post-exercise $\dot{V}CO_2$ and $\dot{V}E$ in heart failure. As mentioned above and as suggested in another preliminary report,[17] the time-constant for $\dot{V}CO_2$ and $\dot{V}E$ may be prolonged in heart failure after maximal exercise.[15] In a separate uncontrolled study in patients with left ventricular dysfunction due to recent myocardial infarction, $\dot{V}CO_2$ and $\dot{V}E$ measured 5 minutes after supine maximal bicycle ergometry remained elevated at twice the resting value.[18] The significance of this finding is unclear given the lack of an appropriate control group. Furthermore, its applicability to patients with overt chronic heart failure is questionable.

Post-Exercise Symptoms—Heart Failure

In an effort to determine the relationship of altered post-exercise $\dot{V}O_2$ kinetics to exertional symptoms, we compared patients with more advanced heart failure (peak $\dot{V}O_2$ 48±10% predicted) to age and weight matched sedentary control subjects after exercise at three different workloads: (1) maximal bicycle exercise; (2) 8 minutes of constant-load exercise at 25W; and (3) 8 minutes at 85% peak $\dot{V}O_2$. Regardless of exercise level, the post-exercise $\dot{V}O_2$ monoexponential time constant was longer in heart failure. Furthermore, after exercise of similar intensity relative to peak $\dot{V}O_2$ (maximal test and 85% peak $\dot{V}O_2$ test), symptom scores for dyspnea and fatigue, self-assessed using a visual scale, were higher in heart failure patients compared to control subjects.[19] These symptom scores were not significantly different *during* exercise at these levels. In the patient group, the mean fatigue score remained significantly elevated above rest at 20 minutes after exercise, with some patients noting excess fatigue even 45 minutes into recovery. Mean $\dot{V}O_2$, on the other hand, declined back to the resting value even at 10 minutes of recovery. Despite this temporal dissociation between $\dot{V}O_2$ and patient symptoms, there was a significant correlation ($r=0.55$) between individual fatigue scores (averaged over the first 10 minutes of recovery) and the post-exercise $\dot{V}O_2$ time constant. Thus, prolonged $\dot{V}O_2$ kinetics, determined using breath-by-breath gas analysis in the first few minutes of recovery, may be a marker for excess post-exercise fatigue which often persists beyond the period of elevation in $\dot{V}O_2$.

Summary

Gas exchange during recovery from exercise in patients with heart failure is characterized by prolongation of $\dot{V}O_2$ kinetics. There is a slower return toward resting $\dot{V}O_2$ during the first several minutes following brief exercise. This may reflect a slower rate of creatine phosphate repletion, and may relate to deconditioning. The late component of excess post-exercise $\dot{V}O_2$ has not been well-studied in heart failure. This component may be significant following long periods of exercise.

Differences in exertional symptoms between patients with heart failure and healthy subjects appear to be greater during recovery from exercise than during exercise itself. This strengthens the rationale for further study of post-exercise metabolism in heart failure.

Further insights into the pathophysiology of post-exercise fatigue and dyspnea in heart failure might be gained from investigations of acid-base regulation and ventilation following exercise. Ultimately, by incorporating an assessment of recovery from exercise, gas exchange analysis may provide a more accurate gauge of patient symptoms and a more sensitive measure of the response to therapy.

References

1. Francis GS, Rector TS: Maximal exercise tolerance as a therapeutic end point in heart failure—Are we relying on the right measure? *Am J Card* 73:304–306, 1994.
2. Rector TS, Cohn JN: Assessment of patient outcome with the Minnesota Living with Heart Failure Questionnaire: reliability and validity during a randomized, double-blind, placebo-controlled trial of pimobendan. *Am Heart J* 124:1017, 1992.
3. Bahr R, Ingnes I, Vaage O, Sejersted OM, Newsholme EA: Effect of duration of exercise on excess postexercise O_2 consumption. *J Appl Physiol* 62(2): 485–490, 1987.
4. Gaesser GA, Brooks GA: Metabolic basis of excess post-exercise oxygen consumption: a review. *Med Sci Sports Exerc* 16:29–43, 1984.

5. Wasserman K, Van Kessel AL, Burton GG: Interaction of physiological mechanisms during exercise. *J Appl Physiol* 22(1):71–85, 1967.
6. Borsheim E, Bahr R, Hansson P, Gullestad L, Hallen J, Sejersted OM: Effect of β-adrenoceptor blockade on post-exercise oxygen consumption. *Metabolism* 43:565–571, 1994.
7. Mancini DM, Ferro N, Tuchler M, Chance B, Wilson JR: Detection of abnormal calf muscle metabolism in patients with heart failure using phosphorus-31 nuclear magnetic resonance. *Am J Cardiol* 62:1234–1240, 1988.
8. Hagberg JM, Hickson RC, Ehsani A, Holloszy JO: Faster adjustment to and recovery from submaximal exercise in the trained state. *J Appl Physiol* 48(2):218–224, 1980.
9. Kowalchuk JM, Heigenhauser JF, Lindinger MI, Obminski G, Sutton JR, Jones NL: Role of lungs and inactive muscle in acid-base control after maximal exercise. *J Appl Physiol* 65(5):2090–2096, 1988.
10. Stringer W, Casaburi R, Wasserman K. Acid-base regulation during exercise and recovery in humans. *J Appl Physiol* 72(3):954–961, 1992.
11. Huszczuk A, Yeh E, Innes JA, Solarte I, Wasserman K, Whipp BJ: Role of muscle perfusion and baroreception in the hyperpnea following muscle contraction in dog. *Respir Physiol* 91:207–226, 1993.
12. Innes JA, Solarte I, Huszczuk A, Yeh E, Whipp BJ, Wasserman K: Respiration during recovery from exercise: effects of trapping and release of femoral blood flow. *J Appl Physiol* 67:2608–2613, 1989.
13. Reddy HK, Weber KT, Janicki JS, McElroy PA: Hemodynamic, ventilatory and metabolic effects of light isometric exercise in patients with chronic heart failure. *J Am Coll Cardiol* 12:353–358, 1988.
14. Sietsema KE, Ben-Dov I, Zhang YY, Sullivan C, Wasserman K: Dynamics of oxygen uptake for submaximal exercise and recovery in patients with chronic heart failure. *Chest* 105:1693–1700, 1994.
15. Hayashida W, Kumada T, Kohno F, Noda M, Ishikawa N, Kambayashi M, Kawai C: Post-exercise oxygen uptake kinetics in patients with left ventricular dysfunction. *Int J Cardiol* 38:63–72, 1993.
16. Koike A, Yajima T, Adachi H, Shimizu N, Kano H, Sugimoto K, Niwa A, Marumo F, Hiroe M: Evaluation of exercise capacity using submaximal exercise at a constant work rate in patients with cardiovascular disease. *Circulation* 91:1719–1724, 1995.
17. Cohen-Solal A, Geneves M, Laperche T, Dahan M, Ferron B, Aubry N: Kinetics of recovery of ventilation and oxygen uptake after maximal exercise in heart failure: a new index of functional impairment? *Circulation* 88 (suppl):I-591, 1993.
18. Sumimoto T, Sugiura T, Takeuchi M, Yuasa F, Hasegawa T, Nakamura S, Iwasaka T, Inada M: Oxygen utilization, carbon dioxide elimination and ventilation during recovery from supine bicycle exercise 6 to 8 weeks after acute myocardial infarction. *Am J Cardiol* 67:1170–1174, 1991.
19. Kraemer M, Kubo S, Tschumperlin L, Rector T, Bank A: Patients with heart failure demonstrate increased oxygen consumption and symptoms following maximal and submaximal exercise (abstr). *J Am Coll Cardiol* 23:471A, 1994.

6

Analysis of Gas Exchange Dynamics in Patients with Cardiovascular Disease

Kathy E. Sietsema, MD

Analyses of the recovery of oxygen uptake ($\dot{V}O_2$) following exercise in patients with heart failure are based on a classical concept in exercise physiology credited to Hill and Lupton[1] in 1923. These investigators reported that there was a sustained elevation in $\dot{V}O_2$ above baseline levels in the early minutes of recovery from exercise; they called it the *oxygen debt* reasoning that it represented repayment of a *deficit* of $\dot{V}O_2$ relative to metabolic requirements in the early minutes following exercise onset (Figure 1). The observation that cardiovascular disease can alter the magnitude of the oxygen deficit and debt associated with exercise dates back almost as far, having been reported as early as 1927 by Meakens and Long (Figure 2).[2] The role of analysis of exercise $\dot{V}O_2$ dynamics in clinical exercise testing remains to be defined. However, the physiologic responses underlying gas exchange dynamics are of fundamental interest to clinicians treating patients with cardiovascular diseases, and there is therefore good basis to expect that quantifying the dynamic responses to exercise will prove useful in clinical medicine.

Determinants of the Oxygen Deficit

Viewed from the perspective of the oxygen transport process, the oxygen deficit reflects the processes of increasing cardiac output and

From Wasserman, K (ed): *Exercise Gas Exchange in Heart Disease.* Armonk, NY: Futura Publishing Company, Inc., © 1996.

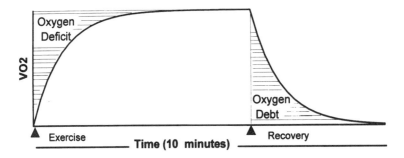

Figure 1. Increase and decrease of oxygen uptake ($\dot{V}O_2$) above baseline during moderate intensity exercise and recovery. **Shaded areas** indicate the oxgyen deficit and debt at exercise onset and recovery onset, respectively.

oxygen extraction to the levels necessary to meet the metabolic requirements of the exercise. This is summarized in the familiar Fick relationship, $\dot{V}O_2 = Q \times c(a–v)O_2$. When a new steady state is attained, the increase in $\dot{V}O_2$ reflects the oxygen consumption cost of the exercise. Because $\dot{V}O_2$ is calculated from respired gases, nonsteady state measures of $\dot{V}O_2$, and therefore the appearance of the oxygen deficit, may be affected by temporal dissociation of oxygen consumption in muscle relative to its replacement by oxygen as venous blood arrives in the pulmonary capillaries. In addition to this transport delay, there must also be a bioenergetic accounting for the muscular work accomplished in the nonsteady state period. Bioenergetic components of the oxygen deficit include work accomplished by use of preformed sources of high energy bonds in the form of phosphocreatine, the use of oxygen stores in capillary blood and myoglobin, and, to the extent that the preceding are insufficient for the energy requirements of the work, the use of non-oxygen consuming metabolic pathways of adenosine triphosphate (ATP) regeneration.[3] Both oxygen transport and oxygen utilization processes come into consideration in the analysis of the oxygen deficit and its repayment.

Characterizing $\dot{V}O_2$ Dynamics

While the concepts of oxygen deficit and debt are not new, the ability to characterize gas exchange dynamics was facilitated by the availability in the 1960s, and thereafter, of rapidly responding gas analyzers and desktop computers. These made breath-by-breath calculations possible and so allowed tracking of rapid changes in $\dot{V}O_2$ during nonsteady state conditions. Modeling of $\dot{V}O_2$ dynamics under various conditions and in response to different exercise stimuli has since given

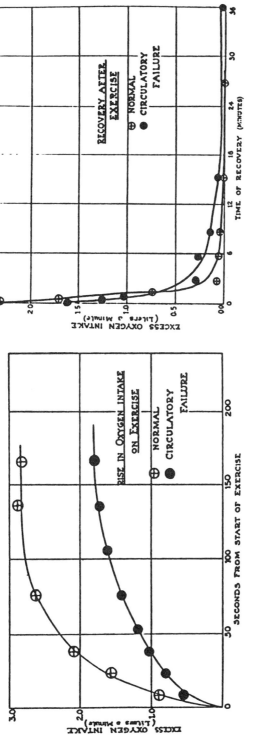
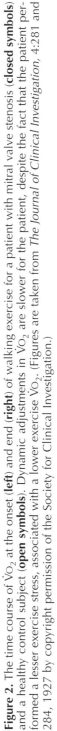

Figure 2. The time course of $\dot{V}O_2$ at the onset (**left**) and end (**right**) of walking exercise for a patient with mitral valve stenosis (**closed symbols**) and a healthy control subject (**open symbols**). Dynamic adjustments in $\dot{V}O_2$ are slower for the patient, despite the fact that the patient performed a lesser exercise stress, associated with a lower exercise $\dot{V}O_2$. (Figures are taken from *The Journal of Clinical Investigation*, 4:281 and 284, 1927 by copyright permission of the Society for Clinical Investigation.)

rise to observations that have relevance to the utilization and interpretation of $\dot{V}O_2$ dynamics in clinical populations.

For moderate intensity exercise, $\dot{V}O_2$ dynamics at exercise onset can be described most simply as an exponential increase.[4] Under certain circumstances, a more precise description of $\dot{V}O_2$ dynamics can be made in which an initial, brief (10 to 20 seconds) component of this response is distinguished from the remaining exponential increase.[5,6] This *cardiodynamic* increase in $\dot{V}O_2$ at the start of exercise appears to reflect primarily a shift of blood volume centrally and is dependent on conditions such as posture and the use of an exercise baseline.[7-9] Meaningful measurement and standardization of this component requires a higher degree of resolution of data than is practical in most clinical exercise laboratories. It is common, therefore, to characterize $\dot{V}O_2$ dynamics for moderate intensity exercise by the time constant of the exponential which best fits the rise in $\dot{V}O_2$ from pre-exercise baseline to exercise steady state. As discussed below, high intensity exercise is characterized by more complex dynamic responses.

Factors Affecting Gas Exchange Dynamics

Gas exchange dynamics are dependent on the intensity of the exercise. Although a monoexponential function describes $\dot{V}O_2$ behavior at the onset of moderate intensity exercise (below the lactate threshold), for higher intensity exercise the dynamics are more complicated, requiring a bi-exponential or higher function to account for the pattern of increasing $\dot{V}O_2$.[5,10-12] Consequently, while $\dot{V}O_2$ reaches a steady state within 3 minutes for moderate exercise, the steady state is delayed or not attained at all when the exercise is above the individual's lactate threshold. The basis for the continued increase in $\dot{V}O_2$ is not well understood, but its magnitude is best correlated with the associated increase in blood lactate.[12-14] The effect of intensity on the characteristics of $\dot{V}O_2$ dynamics has important implications for the use and interpretation of nonsteady state measurements in patients.

First, comparison of dynamic responses from different subjects or groups of subjects requires consideration of whether or not the intensity domains of the studies were comparable. Responses to high intensity exercise by one group of subjects will predictably be different than responses to moderate intensity exercise performed by a comparison group.

Another consequence of the different dynamic responses to differing intensities of exercise relates to the relationship between work rate and $\dot{V}O_2$. If a series of constant work rate tests are undertaken for a range of exercise work rates, the resulting exercise $\dot{V}O_2$ is linearly related to the imposed exercise load only in the domain below the lactate threshold. For work rates above that level, $\dot{V}O_2$ increases asymptotically towards a value higher than what would be predicted for the work rate on the basis of the lower work rate studies.[11] The $\dot{V}O_2$ cost of a work rate, therefore, cannot be predicted for a patient in the domain above his or her lactate threshold by extrapolation from measurements at lower work rates.[15] This has not been widely appreciated, and is not intuitively obvious, for two reasons. First, the relationship between work rate and $\dot{V}O_2$ usually *appears* to be quite linear over the entire range of exercise when graded maximal exercise testing is performed. This apparent linearity results from the nonsteady state nature of the measurements during relatively rapid incrementation of work rate. Secondly, the relationship between $\dot{V}O_2$ and work rate can be evaluated only if a reliable measure of work rate can be made. While work rate is readily determined for exercise on a calibrated cycle ergometer, valid calculation of work rate for treadmill exercise is complicated by factors related to gait and the efficiency of walking on the treadmill. As these factors change during an incremental test, accurate calculation of the external work performed is difficult to accomplish in commonly employed treadmill testing protocols.

In addition to exercise intensity, $\dot{V}O_2$ dynamics are also affected by cardiovascular fitness or conditioning. This is true even within the domain of moderate intensity exercise, and is not simply the consequence of comparing high intensity to moderate intensity exercise. Exercise training of normal subjects results in statistically significant reductions in the $\dot{V}O_2$ time constant.[16–18] Conversely, bedrest-induced deconditioning is associated with slowing of the $\dot{V}O_2$ dynamics.[19]

These observations raise the question of what process is rate-limiting for the increase in $\dot{V}O_2$ at exercise onset. In experiments in which oxygen delivery is reduced in normal subjects, such as by carboxyhemoglobinemia,[20] $\dot{V}O_2$ dynamics for a given exercise task are slowed. Dynamics are also attenuated when heart rate, and therefore presumably cardiac output, responses to exercise are constrained either by β-adrenergic blockade in normal subjects,[21] or by fixing heart rate at the resting level in pacemaker-dependent patients.[22] On the other hand, it has been argued that the normal rate of increase of cardiac output in response to exercise appears to follow a faster time course than that of $\dot{V}O_2$,[23,24] making it unlikely that oxygen delivery is rate-limiting to $\dot{V}O_2$ dynamics under normal circumstances.[25] Therefore, whether it is the oxygen delivery system or the oxygen utilization system which normally limits $\dot{V}O_2$ dynamics remains a subject of debate. The debate underscores that, like other parameters of exercise function, dynamic characteristics of gas exchange involve both central circulatory and peripheral tissue factors. The relative importance of these two factors may depend on the fitness status and cardiovascular health of the individual subject relative to the exercise task.

$\dot{V}O_2$ Dynamics in Cardiovascular Disease

The patients reported by Meakins and Long in 1927[2] to have a slow rise in $\dot{V}O_2$ following exercise onset had diagnoses of rheumatic mitral valve disease. In the 1970's, Auchincloss and colleagues correlated breath-by-breath increases of $\dot{V}O_2$ with concomitant nonsteady state cardiac output during the exercise transition in normal subjects.[26] They later reported slower than normal $\dot{V}O_2$ dynamics (reflected in a lower $\dot{V}O_2$ value at 1 minute following onset of exercise) in patients with rheumatic heart disease[27] and in 21 of 40 patients studied with coronary artery disease.[28] Slowed $\dot{V}O_2$ kinetics have more recently been described for patients with chronic heart failure,[29,30] cyanotic congenital heart diseases,[31] and pulmonary vascular diseases.[32,33] There is ample evidence, therefore, that chronic cardiovascular diseases can reduce the rate at which $\dot{V}O_2$ increases with exercise, in addition to reducing the maximal level which can be attained.

Interpretation of dynamic responses in clinical populations is complicated by the issue of exercise intensity discussed above. Delayed attainment of steady state $\dot{V}O_2$ in patients compared to controls could be due to the same exercise stimulus being above the lactate threshold for patients and below the threshold of the controls. If the purpose of the investigation is to demonstrate physiologic responses to a particular task (e.g., walking at a given speed), then the differences in responses between groups are of interest regardless of whether or not they can be attributed to differences in the relative work intensity represented by the task. However, if the comparison is made to draw conclusions regarding fundamental differences in underlying metabolic responses to a moderate exercise stress, then careful matching of the exercise intensity is important.

To address the question of whether $\dot{V}O_2$ dynamics were slowed in chronic heart failure at the same relative intensity of exercise as well as the same absolute work rate, we measured dynamic responses to exercise in 18 patients with heart failure and 10 age-matched controls.[29] The patients' $\dot{V}O_2$ dynamics were significantly slower than control subjects' when exercising to the same absolute work rates, but the difference was not statistically significant when both groups exercised at the same relative intensity above the lactate threshold. Recovery rates following exercise were nevertheless slower for the patients at both matched work rates and matched work intensities (Figure 3). Exercise intensity could therefore account for some, but not all, of the slow dynamics of $\dot{V}O_2$ in these patients with heart failure.

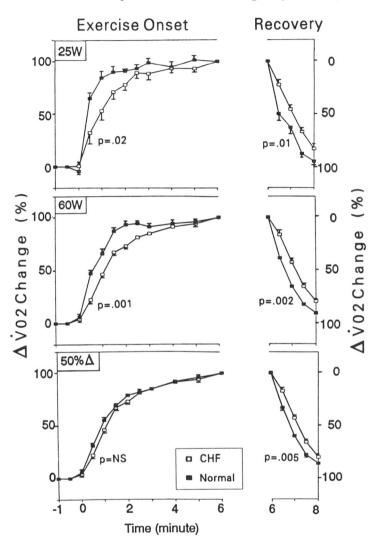

Figure 3. Oxygen uptake ($\dot{V}O_2$) for constant work rate exercise performed by patients with chronic compensated heart failure (**open symbols,** n=18) and age matched control subjects (**closed symbols,** n=10). $\dot{V}O_2$ was normalized to the rest-to-exercise increase ($\Delta \dot{V}O_2$ change) and averaged over 30-second intervals; values are shown as group means ± 1 SE. For matched work rates of 25 and 60 watts, the increase in $\dot{V}O_2$ is slower for the patients than the normals. For a matched work intensity midway between the subjects' lactate thresholds and maximal exercise capacity, onset dynamics for $\dot{V}O_2$ for the two groups are not different. During recovery, however, $\dot{V}O_2$ decreases more slowly for the patients both at matched work rates and at the matched work intensity. (Reproduced with permission from Reference 26.)

In summary, both cardiovascular disease and cardiovascular deconditioning are associated with a reduction in the rate of adjustment to and recovery from the gas exchange requirements of submaximal exercise. Dynamic responses to exercise therefore appear to be another index of cardiovascular health or fitness.

Potential Clinical Significance and Application of Measurements of $\dot{V}O_2$ Dynamics

There are technical difficulties in quantifying gas exchange dynamics in clinical populations. Low work rates may need to be employed because of limited exercise capacity, and very low work rates may be needed if the exercise is intended to be of moderate intensity. With a low absolute work rate, regardless of the corresponding intensity, $\dot{V}O_2$ is also low and the poor signal-to-noise ratio for the measurements results in wide confidence limits for derived parameters.[34] Improvement in signal-to-noise characteristics may be accomplished by the averaging of multiple replicates of a test,[35] but this is not always practical. There are as of yet limited data reported concerning the test-retest reproducibility of parameters of dynamic responses from studies in clinical populations.

Although maximal $\dot{V}O_2$ is the single most physiologically meaningful and reproducible parameter of cardiovascular function, its measurement may sometimes entail risk for patients with cardiovascular diseases. Furthermore, maximal capacity as measured in the laboratory may not be the most important aspect of exercise performance with respect to a patient's functional status. With the exceptions of severely impaired patients and athletes training at high intensities, most people don't regularly utilize their maximal exercise capacity. Rather, activities of daily living are comprised of brief, intermittent, submaximal bouts of exercise. Exercise testing protocols which utilize submaximal exercise and recovery, therefore, reflect the type of exercise stress that makes up spontaneous activity patterns. Delayed attainment of steady state conditions and prolonged recovery times may have direct correlates to the symptomatic expression of exercise intolerance, and may therefore be important aspects of exercise function for understanding how cardiovascular disease affects the quality of life. If these responses can be readily and reproducibly quantified, they may provide a useful index for expression of exercise intolerance that does not rely on maximal exercise performance.

Summary

$\dot{V}O_2$ does not increase to the exercise requirement instantaneously. Rather, its rate of increase reflects the rates of increase in cardiac output and of oxygen extraction and utilization by exercising muscle. There is thus a deficit of $\dot{V}O_2$ relative to work early in exercise. Similarly, at the end of exercise, the rate of decrease of $\dot{V}O_2$ is dictated by the need to replenish stores of oxygen and high energy compounds utilized in the nonsteady state. Results of modeling of respiratory gas exchange dynamics in normal subjects provide a framework for qualitative and quantitative characterization of these responses and their relationship to exercise intensity. Given the importance of cardiovascular processes in mediating respiratory gas exchange, it is not surprising that gas exchange dynamics have been found to be slowed in patients with a variety of cardiovascular diseases. Because normal activity patterns are comprised of repeated transitions between submaximal levels of exercise, these responses are directly relevant to daily life function. Understanding dynamic responses may therefore prove to be as important as maximal exercise capacity to the understanding of exercise intolerance in heart disease. The utility of these measurements in evaluation of clinical populations is as yet incompletely explored.

References

1. Hill AV, Lupton H: Muscular exercise, lactic acid, and the supply utilization of oxygen. Q J Med 16:135–171, 1923.
2. Meakins J, Long CNH: Oxygen consumption, oxygen debt and lactic acid in circulatory failure. J Clin Invest 4:273–293, 1927.
3. Piiper J, DiPrampero PE, Cerretelli P: Oxygen debt and high-energy phosphates in gastrocnemius muscle of the dog. J Appl Physiol 215:523–531, 1968.
4. Whipp BJ, Mahler M: Dynamics of pulmonary gas exchange during exercise. In: West JB, ed. Pulmonary Gas Exchange. Organism and Environment. New York: Academic Press, Inc., vol. 2; 33–96, 1980.
5. Linnarson D: Dynamics of pulmonary gas exchange and heart rate changes at start and end of exercise. Acta Physiol Scand (suppl) 415:1–68, 1974.
6. Sietsema KE, Daly JA, Wasserman K: Early dynamics of $\dot{V}O_2$ uptake and heart rate as affected by exercise work rate. J Appl Physiol 67:2535–2541, 1989.
7. Whipp BJ, Davis JA, Torres F, Wasserman K: A test to determine parameters of aerobic function during exercise. J Appl Physiol 50:217–221, 1981.
8. Weissman ML, Jones PW, Oren A, Lamarra N, Whipp BJ, Wasserman K: Cardiac output increase and gas exchange at the start of exercise. J Appl Physiol 52:236–244, 1982.
9. Weiler-Ravell D, Whipp BJ, Cooper DM, Wasserman K: The control of breathing at the start of exercise as influenced by posture. J Appl Physiol 55:1460–1466, 1983.
10. Whipp BJ, Ward SA, Lamarra N, Davis JA, Wasserman K: Parameters of ventilatory and gas exchange dynamics during exercise. J Appl Physiol 52:1506–1513, 1982.
11. Barstow TJ, Mole PA: Linear and nonlinear characteristics of oxygen uptake kinetics during heavy exercise. J Appl Physiol 71:2099–2106, 1991.

12. Casaburi R, Barstow TJ, Robinson T, Wasserman K: Influence of work rate on ventilatory and gas exchange kinetics. *J Appl Physiol* 67:547–555, 1989.

13. Roston WL, Whipp BJ, Davis JA, Cunningham DA, Effros RM, Wasserman K: Oxygen uptake kinetics and lactate concentration during exercise in humans. *Am Rev Respir Dis* 135:1080–1084, 1987.

14. Casaburi R, Storer TW, Ben-Dov I, Wasserman K: Effect of endurance training on possible determinants of $\dot{V}O_2$ during heavy exercise. *J Appl Physiol* 62:199–207, 1987.

15. Solal AC, Chabernaud JM, Gourgon R: Comparison of oxygen uptake during bicycle exercise in patients with chronic heart failure and normal subjects. *J Am Coll Cardiol* 16:80–85, 1990.

16. Hickson RC, Bomze HA, Holloszy JO: Faster adjustment of O_2 uptake to the energy requirement of exercise in the trained state. *J Appl Physiol* 44:877–881, 1978.

17. Hagberg JM, Hickson RC, Ehsani AA, Holloszy JO: Faster adjustment to and recovery from submaximal exercise in the trained state. *J Appl Physiol* 48:218–224, 1980.

18. Yoshida T, Udo M, Ohmori T, Matsumoto Y, Uramoto T, Yamamoto K: Day-to-day changes in oxygen uptake kinetics at the onset of exercise during strenuous endurance training. *Eur J Appl Physiol* 64:78–83, 1992.

19. Convertino VA, Goldwater DJ, Sandler H: $\dot{V}O_2$ kinetics of constant-load exercise following bed-rest-induced deconditioning. *J Appl Physiol* 57:1545–1550, 1984.

20. Koike A, Wasserman K, McKenzie DK, Zanconato S, Weiler-Ravell D: Evidence that diffusion limitation determines oxygen uptake kinetics during exercise in humans. *J Clin Invest* 86:1698–1706, 1990.

21. Hughson RL, Smyth GA: Slower adaptation of $\dot{V}O_2$ to steady state of submaximal exercise with β-blockade. *Eur J Appl Physiol* 52:107–110, 1983.

22. Casaburi R, Spitzer S, Haskell R, Wasserman K: Effect of altering heart rate on oxygen uptake at exercise onset. *Chest* 95:6–12, 1989.

23. Inman MD, Hughson RL, Weisiger KH, Swanson GD: Estimate of mean tissue $\dot{V}O_2$ consumption at onset of exercise in males. *J Appl Physiol* 63:1578–1585, 1987.

24. Miyamoto Y, Hiura T, Tamura T, Nakamura T, Higuchi J, Mikami T: Dynamics of cardiac, respiratory and metabolic function in men in response to step work load. *J Appl Physiol* 52:1198–1208, 1982.

25. Barstow TJ, Lamarra N, and Whipp BJ: Modulation of muscle and pulmonary oxygen uptake by circulatory dynamics during exercise. *J Appl Physiol* 68:979–989, 1990.

26. Gilbert R, Auchincloss JH Jr: Comparison of cardiovascular response to steady and unsteady state exercise. *J Appl Physiol* 30:388–393, 1971.

27. Auchincloss JH Jr, Gilbert R, Baule GH: Unsteady state measurement of oxygen transfer in patients with rheumatic heart disease. *Clin Sci* 39:21–37, 1970.

28. Auchincloss Jr JH, Gilbert R, Bowman BA: Response of oxygen uptake to exercise in coronary artery disease. *Chest* 65:500–506, 1974.

29. Sietsema KE, Ben-Dov I, Zhang YY, Sullivan C, Wasserman K: Dynamics of oxygen uptake for submaximal exercise and recovery in patients with chronic heart failure. *Chest* 105:1693–1700, 1994.

30. Riley M, Porszasz J, Stanford CF, Nicholls DP: Gas exchange responses to constant work rate exercise in chronic heart failure. *Br Heart J* 72:150–155, 1994.

31. Sietsema KE, Cooper DM, Perloff JK, et al: Dynamics of oxygen uptake during exercise in adults with cyanotic congenital heart disease. *Circulation* 73:1137–1144, 1986.
32. Sietsema KE: Oxygen uptake kinetics in response to exercise in patients with pulmonary vascular disease. *Am Rev Respir Dis* 145:1052–1057, 1992.
33. Nery L, Wasserman K, Andrews JD, Huntsman DJ, Hansen JE, Whipp BJ: Ventilatory and gas exchange kinetics during exercise in chronic airways obstruction. *J Appl Physiol* 56:1594–1602, 1982.
34. Lamarra N, Whipp BJ, Ward SA, Wasserman K: Effect of inter-breath fluctuations on characterizing exercise gas exchange kinetics. *J Appl Physiol* 62:2003–2012, 1987.
35. Beaver WL, Wasserman K: Transients in ventilation at start and end of exercise. *J Appl Physiol* 25:390–399, 1968.

Section 3

The Ventilatory Response to Exercise in Patients with Heart Disease

---

7

The Relation Between Muscle Function and Increased Ventilation in Heart Failure

Philip A. Poole-Wilson, MD

Introduction

Heart failure is a clinical syndrome rather than a diagnosis. Many definitions have been proffered during the current century.[1] Definitions based on physiological or biochemical parameters have in general not been universally accepted because they do not envelop the broad spectrum of disease which is encompassed by the generic term heart failure. Heart failure is a clinical syndrome caused by an abnormality of the heart and recognized by a characteristic pattern of hemodynamic, renal, neural, and hormonal responses.[1,2] A simpler definition is ventricular dysfunction with symptoms. Such definitions do allow the possibility of epidemiologic studies on heart failure. For heart failure to be present in a patient, symptoms should be elicited, the ventricle should be shown to be abnormal in its function, and preferably the patient should be on treatment for heart failure or have responded to treatment. The diagnosis of heart failure based solely on symptoms and clinical examination by a primary physician in the community is often in error, notably in females.[3] The problem is that many noncardiac causes exist for breathlessness and swollen ankles.

Recent trials have demonstrated that certain interventions in heart failure improve prognosis.[4–6] This fundamental finding has distracted physicians from an unresolved and key problem, namely the alleviation of symptoms. Any approach to the treatment of symptoms should

From Wasserman, K (ed): *Exercise Gas Exchange in Heart Disease.* Armonk, NY: Futura Publishing Company, Inc., © 1996.

be based on an understanding of the cause of those symptoms. Whereas traditionally symptoms in heart failure have been attributed to a low cardiac output or raised left ventricular end-diastolic pressure, recent evidence suggests that symptoms have their origins in the periphery[7-10] and are the consequences of the long-term body response to heart failure. This idea has important clinical consequences, the most significant being that many treatments would not be expected immediately to benefit patients; the benefit would only be manifest after several weeks or months of treatment. Such a delayed response to treatment is observed after heart transplantation[11] and after cardioversion.[12]

Causes of Symptoms

Putative mechanisms for the origin of symptoms in heart failure are shown in Table 1. The retention of salt and water in the body is a cardinal feature of untreated advanced heart failure.[13] The increased fluid volumes are the consequence of failure of the kidney to excrete salt and water which is attributable to a low perfusion pressure (the old concept of forward failure),[14] to the effect of an increased venous pressure (the old concept of backward failure),[15] or to intrarenal changes brought about by activation of neurohumoral and cytokine systems within the body.

The symptoms, or possibly more accurately the signs, of swollen ankles and ascites are easily explained by fluid retention. Far more difficult to account for are the common limiting symptoms of exercise,

---

Table 1

Origin of Symptoms on Exercise in Chronic Heart Failure

1.	**Lungs**	increased stiffness due to raised venous pressure and lymphatic distension
		increased left atrial pressure
		increased physiological dead space
		increased respiratory rate
		weakness of diaphragm
		increased bronchial reactivity
2.	**Circulation**	reduced blood flow to skeletal muscle
		increased production of metabolites
		altered response to metabolites
3.	**Skeletal muscle**	rest atrophy
		ischemic atrophy
		specific abnormality

namely shortness of breath and fatigue. Even the clinical elucidation of these symptoms in patients is difficult. Sensations in the chest are described differently by various patients. Confusion can commonly exist among both patients and physicians between the sensations brought about by myocardial ischemia, conventionally referred to as angina, and those symptoms brought about by a limitation of exercise in the absence of angina and usually referred to as breathlessness. Furthermore, breathlessness and fatigue can be elicited as the limiting symptom in an individual patient by undertaking different forms of exercise (Table 2).[16] Fast exercise tests are usually limited by breathlessness, whereas long exercise programs are commonly terminated by fatigue.[16] Any explanation for symptoms in heart failure must explain that simple observation. Altered hemodynamic responses are not a sufficient explanation.[8]

The simplest idea would be that breathlessness is due to abnormality in the lung (Table 1). The most popular hypothesis in the past was that breathlessness was a consequence of a raised left atrial pressure which activated receptors in the lung[17] or increased lung stiffness and lung work. More recently, other abnormalities[7] have been emphasized such as an increased respiratory rate, muscle weakness in the chest wall and diaphragm, bronchial reactivity, and an increased physiological dead space. An alternative hypothesis has related breathlessness to changes in the peripheral circulation and in particular to changes in the skeletal muscle.[9] Signals might arise from the skeletal muscle which are interpreted by the brain as fatigue or breathlessness.

Table 2

Symptoms and Physiology During Different Forms of Exercise

10 patients, NYHA II or III Undergoing Both Tests			
	Fast Test	Slow Test	p
Limiting symptom	Breathlessness	Fatigue	
Exercise time (min)	<4	31	
$M\dot{V}O_2 (mL/kg^{-1}/min^{-1})$	17	15	0.001
$AT(mL/kg^{-1}/min^{-1})$	12	11	0.002
$V_E(L/min^{-1})$	51	47	0.003
$CI(L/min^{-1})$	4.7	4.0	0.03
Mean BP (mm Hg)	87	87	ns
PWP (mm Hg)	25	26	ns
Change arterial pH	0.06	0.02	0.005
Change Part CO_2	−1	−1	ns
Lactate (mmol/L^{-1})	3.7	2.2	0.001

(Reproduced with permission from Reference 16.)

Ventilation in Heart Failure

The pattern and nature of breathing in heart failure has been the subject of extensive investigation in the last two decades. Certain key points have emerged which must be accounted for by any explanation of the changes which take place. The first is that the blood gases in patients with heart failure change little, if at all, either at rest or at exercise.[18–22] In particular, the partial pressure of carbon dioxide (P_{CO_2})is not increased at peak exercise (Table 3).[23] Indeed in some studies, the P_{CO_2} at peak exercise is reduced. Desaturation does not occur. In a recent paper, evidence of desaturation in three patients was attributable to either pulmonary emboli, lung disease, or a right-to-left shunt.[23] These entities should always be sought when desaturation is a major feature in a patient with heart failure. Some patients have small reductions in saturation occurring transiently at night.[24]

The second major observation is that for any given level of carbon dioxide production during exercise in patients with heart failure, ventilation is increased in comparison to normal persons.[19,25–31] The increase in ventilation relates to the severity of heart failure, and can be used as a method to estimate the severity of heart failure without having to reach peak exercise.[25] The increased ventilation cannot be accounted for by an increase in anatomic dead space associated with an altered respiratory pattern. The abnormality has been attributed to an increase in the physiological dead space. The idea was put forward that a proportion of alveoli were ventilated, but not perfused. Such a change could have been brought about either as a response within the pulmonary circulation to the raised left atrial pressure, or more probably to the altered neurohumoral and cytokine response to heart failure.

A major and key difficulty with the hypothesis that the increased ventilation was attributable to an abnormality in the lung is that such a change would need a stimulus. The stimulus could not be carbon dioxide itself because the arterial P_{CO_2} at peak exercise was normal or reduced rather than increased. A metabolic acidosis could be a contributory stimulant to the increased ventilation (Table 3).[23] An alternative, and very different, hypothesis is that the increased ventilation is due to neural signals arising from exercising skeletal muscle.[9,27] According to this hypothesis, the failure to observe a large fall in arterial P_{CO_2} would be attributable to alterations in the microcirculation within the lung and to the complex interaction between the different storage compartments for carbon dioxide in the body during non-steady state exercise. This hypothesis would suggest that the symptoms of heart failure emanate largely from signals from the periphery, and that the changes in the ventilation are a response to those signals rather than local factors in the lung being the lead cause.

Table 3

Arterial Blood Gases on Exercise in Heart Failure

34 Patients, 59 Years, 22 IHD & 12 DCM, EF = 24.5%, Mean (SEM)			
	Rest	Peak Exercise	Recovery
PaO_2(kPa)	12.9 (0.3)	13.3 (0.3)	14.8 (0.3)**
$PaCO_2$(kPa)	4.9 (0.1)	4.6 (0.1)*	4.6 (0.1)
Arterial pH	7.43 (0.006)	7.40 (0.007)**	7.38 (0.009)*

*p < 0.005; **p < 0.001 compared with the column to the left.
(Reproduced with permission from Reference 23.)

Skeletal Muscle in Heart Failure

The nature of changes in skeletal muscle in patients with heart failure has been extensively investigated in the last 10 years (Table 4). Histologic studies have been extensive.[32–37] What has become evident is that skeletal muscle is grossly abnormal; the nature of the abnormality is less clear. A switch in fiber type has been claimed, but a major difficulty exists because of fiber type variability in the control group with which the heart failure patients were compared. The variation in the proportion of type 1 and type 2 fibers is normally so great that it is unlikely that changes could be detected in a small group of patients with heart failure. Longitudinal studies are necessary.

Nevertheless, both type 1 and type 2 fibers are grossly atrophic. Increased variation in fiber size, the presence of lipid droplets, reversion to neonatal isoforms of myosin, altered morphology of mitochondria, and

Table 4

Skeletal Muscle in Heart Failure

Morphology	Quantity	Loss of muscle mass (or bulk)
	Site	Localized to legs or general abnormality
		Orientation and fiber position
	Quality	Atrophy, damage and/or necrosis
		Change of fiber type
Blood flow		mL/min reduced, mL/min/100mL variable
Metabolism		An inevitable consequence of atrophy and damage, or a specific change
Function		Weakness and/or increased fatigue

abnormalities of enzyme function have all been reported. These abnormalities occur not only in the large muscles of the leg, but also in the strap muscles of the chest wall and in the diaphragm.[38,39] The changes are more common in patients with idiopathic cardiomyopathy suggesting that some of these patients have a generalized myopathy. Changes have been reported in patients whose heart failure is attributable to ischemic heart disease and this cannot be explained by generalized myopathy.

The cause of the histologic changes is neither rest atrophy nor multiple episodes of ischemia. The changes are specific to heart failure and are probably the result of the cytokine activation which occurs in heart failure. Increased plasma levels of Tumor Necrosis Factor, other cytokines, and the development of insulin resistance may be key factors. A major consequence of these histologic abnormalities is that virtually all other functions of the major muscles of the leg would be expected to be abnormal. This includes gross measurements of function, fatigue, or metabolism.

The function of limb muscles in patients with heart failure has been assessed.[40-42] The small muscles of the hand appear not to be greatly affected in heart failure, but fatigue occurs more easily than in control patients. On the other hand, the strength of the major muscles such as the quadriceps is reduced. This is partly attributable to atrophy and a reduction in muscle mass. Muscle mass is a key determinant of oxygen consumption and thus of peak oxygen consumption during exercise. The use of peak oxygen consumption to measure the severity of heart failure has an important limitation since it is not entirely attributable to the function of the cardiovascular system, and is influenced by motivation and muscle mass (atrophy).

The metabolism of skeletal muscle in heart failure is abnormal.[43] These abnormalities have been demonstrated by magnetic resonance both in the presence of blood flow and after occlusion of blood flow. The latter is important because, otherwise, changes could have been explained by small alterations of blood flow. A major problem remains as to whether these metabolic abnormalities are merely a consequence of the histologic abnormalities, including atrophy, or whether they represent a specific metabolic change. Most of the described abnormalities are probably the consequence of the body's response to heart failure and may have much in common with the changes which occur in other chronic diseases.

The peripheral resistance is increased in heart failure.[44-47] Some of that increase in resistance is merely the consequence of atrophy of muscle. A mouse inevitably has a higher resistance than a human. Part of the increased resistance is explained by activation of neurohumoral systems, and in particular the sympathetic system and the renin-angiotensin system. There is little evidence for anatomic abnormalities of the vessel wall. The only anatomic change which has been demonstrated is a thickening of the basement membrane of capillaries.[48,49] A major problem with the interpretation of blood flow measurements is how they have been measured. Measurements of whole blood flow and resistance to a limb will be substantially altered by the presence of atrophy. Measurements made by plethysmography are recorded as blood flow per 100 mL of water. The evidence that this is reduced in heart failure is controversial. It is probable that a reduction of blood flow per unit mass of muscle is a feature of terminal heart failure accompanied by cardiac cachexia.

Muscle Hypothesis

A proposal on how these various measurements might be brought together is outlined in the Figure. This is called the muscle hypothesis.[9] According to this proposal, the initial abnormality in heart failure is a reduction in the function of the heart as a pump. As a consequence, there are complex body responses. These include activation of the neuroendocrine system and of numerous cytokine systems. Initially, a reduction in muscle strength may result and eventually, over time, there is a progressive deterioration not only in muscle strength, but also in

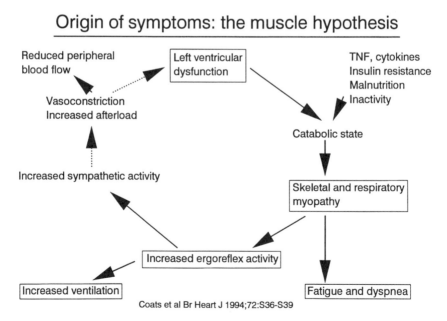

Coats et al Br Heart J 1994;72:S36-S39

Figure. The muscle hypothesis for the origin of symptoms in heart failure. TNF = Tumor Necrosis Factor

the anatomy of the muscle, namely muscle atrophy. This atrophy may be the consequence of cytokine accumulation and could involve the process of apoptosis. The initial determinant for the activation of the body's response to heart failure is the attempt by the body to maintain the blood pressure at rest and during exercise.[14,50,51] The changes in the body are a long-term adverse effect of this reflex body response. The changes in the peripheral muscles lead to activation of ergore-flexes,[52,53] and these contribute to further activation of the sympathetic system and may eventually even worsen left ventricular dysfunction. A major advantage of this hypothesis is that it brings together the symptoms of breathlessness and fatigue. Fatigue and breathlessness are to a large extent a consequence of abnormal muscle function both in skeletal muscle and in the muscles of the chest wall and diaphragm. The sensation of breathlessness is a result of the increased ventilation and this emanates from the signals initiated in skeletal muscle. Thus, there is a direct relationship between muscle function and increased ventilation in patients with heart failure.

Summary

Heart failure is initiated by an abnormality of cardiac function, but many of the symptoms are a consequence of the complex response affecting many organs in the body. Atrophy and functional abnormalities of skeletal muscle may lead to neurological signals during exercise which are interpreted by the brain as fatigue or shortness of breath. These ideas have led to the *muscle hypothesis* of the origin of symptoms in heart failure.

References

1. Poole-Wilson PA: Chronic heart failure: cause, pathophysiology, prognosis, clinical manifestations, investigations. In: Julian DG, Camm AJ, Fox KF, Hall RJC, Poole-Wilson PA, eds. *Diseases of the Heart*. London: Balliere-Tindall, 24–36, 1989.
2. Poole-Wilson PA: Heart failure. *Med Int* 2:866–871, 1985.
3. Remes I, Miettinen H, Reunanen A, Pyorala K: Validity of clinical diagnosis of heart failure in primary health care. *Eur Heart J* 12:315–321, 1991.
4. The CONSENSUS Trial Study Group: Effects of enalapril on mortality in severe congestive heart failure: results of the Cooperative North Scandinavian Enalapril Survival Study (CONSENSUS). *N Engl J Med* 316:1429–1435, 1987.
5. Cohn JN, Archibald DG, Ziesche S, et al: Effect of vasodilator therapy on mortality in chronic congestive heart failure: results of a Veterans Administration Cooperative Study. *N Engl J Med* 314:1547–1552, 1986.
6. The SOLVD Investigators: Effect of enalapril on survival in patients with reduced left ventricular ejection fractions and congestive heart failure. *N Engl J Med* 325:293–302, 1991.

7. Poole-Wilson PA, Buller NP: Causes of symptoms in chronic congestive heart failure and implications for treatment. *Am J Cardiol* 62:31A–34A, 1988.
8. Lipkin DP, Poole-Wilson PA: Symptoms limiting exercise in chronic heart failure [editorial]. *Br Med J* 292:1030–1031, 1986.
9. Coats AJS, Clark AL, Piepoli M, Volterrani M, Poole-Wilson PA: Symptoms and quality of life in heart failure: the muscle hypothesis. *Br Heart J* 72:36–39, 1994.
10. Poole-Wilson PA, Buller NP, Lipkin DP: Regional blood flow, muscle strength and skeletal muscle histology in severe congestive heart failure. *Am J Cardiol* 62:49E–52E, 1988.
11. Sinoway LI, Minotti JR, Davis D, et al: Delayed reversal of impaired vasodilation in congestive heart failure after heart transplantation. *Am J Cardiol* 61:1076–1079, 1988.
12. Lipkin DP, Frenneaux M, Stewart R, Joshi J, Lowe T, McKenna WJ: Delayed improvement in exercise capacity after cardioversion of atrial fibrillation to sinus rhythm. *Br Heart J* 59:572–577, 1988.
13. Anand IS, Ferrari R, Kalra GS, Wahi PL, Poole-Wilson PA, Harris PC: Edema of cardiac origin: studies of body water and sodium, renal function, hemodynamic indexes, and plasma hormones in untreated congestive cardiac failure. *Circulation* 80:299–305, 1989.
14. Harris P: Evolution and the cardiac patient. *Cardiovasc Res* 17:437–445, 1983.
15. Firth JD, Raine AE, Ledingham JG: Raised venous pressure: a direct cause of renal sodium retention in oedema? *Lancet* 1:1033–1035, 1988.
16. Lipkin DP, Canepa-Anson R, Stephens MR, Poole-Wilson PA: Factors determining symptoms in heart failure: comparison of fast and slow exercise tests. *Br Heart J* 55:439–445, 1986.
17. Paintal AS: Mechanism of stimulation of type J pulmonary receptors. *J Physiol* 203:511–532, 1969.
18. Sullivan MJ, Higginbotham MB, Cobb FR: Increased exercise ventilation in patients with chronic heart failure: intact ventilatory control despite hemodynamic and pulmonary abnormalities. *Circulation* 77:552–559, 1988.
19. Roubin GS, Anderson SD, Shen WF, et al: Hemodynamic and metabolic basis of impaired exercise tolerance in patients with severe left ventricular dysfunction [see comments]. *J Am Coll Cardiol* 15:986–994, 1990.
20. Barlow CW, Qayyum MS, Davey PP, Conway J, Paterson DJ, Robbins PA: Effect of physical training on exercise-induced hyperkalemia in chronic heart failure: relation with ventilation and catecholamines. *Circulation* 89:1144–1152, 1994.
21. Anand IS, Kalra GS, Harris P, et al: Diuretics as initial and sole treatment in chronic heart failure. *Cardioscience* 2:273–278, 1991.
22. Moore DP, Weston AR, Hughes JMB, Oakley CM, Cleland JGF: Effects of increased inspired oxygen concentrations on exercise performance in chronic heart failure. *Lancet* 339:850–853, 1992.
23. Clark AL, Coats AJS: Usefulness of arterial blood gas estimations during exercise in patients with chronic heart failure. *Br Heart J* 71:528–530, 1994.
24. Davies SW, John LM, Wedzicha JA, Lipkin D: Overnight studies in severe chronic left heart failure: arrhythmias and oxygen desaturation. *Br Heart J* 65:77–83, 1991.
25. Buller NP, Poole-Wilson PA: Mechanism of the increased ventilatory response to exercise in patients with chronic heart failure. *Br Heart J* 63:281–283, 1990.
26. Clark AL, Poole-Wilson PA, Coats AJS : The relationship between ventilation and carbon dioxide production in patients with chronic heart failure. *J Am Coll Cardiol* 20:1326–1332, 1992.

27. Clark A, Coats A: The mechanisms underlying the increased ventilatory response to exercise in chronic stable heart failure. *Eur Heart J* 13:1698–1708, 1992.
28. Fink LI, Wilson JR, Ferraro N: Exercise ventilation and pulmonary artery wedge pressure in chronic stable congestive heart failure. *Am J Cardiol* 57:249–253, 1986.
29. Franciosa JA: Exercise testing in chronic congestive heart failure. *Am J Cardiol* 53:1447–1450, 1984.
30. Higginbotham MB, Morris KG, Conn EH, Coleman RE, Cobb FR: Determinants of variable exercise performance among patients with severe left ventricular dysfunction. *Am J Cardiol* 51:52–60, 1983.
31. Rubin SA, Brown HV, Swan HJ: Arterial oxygenation and arterial oxygen transport in chronic myocardial failure at rest, during exercise and after hydralazine treatment. *Circulation* 66:143–148, 1982.
32. Lipkin DP, Jones DA, Round JM, Poole-Wilson PA: Abnormalities of skeletal muscle in patients with chronic heart failure [published errata in *Int J Cardiol* Jun;19(3):396, 1988 and *Int J Cardiol* Jul;20(1):161, 1988]. *Int J Cardiol* 18:187–195, 1988.
33. Sullivan MJ, Green HJ, Cobb FR: Skeletal muscle biochemistry and histology in ambulatory patients with long-term heart failure. *Circulation* 81:518–527, 1990.
34. Drexler H, Hiroi M, Riede U, Banhardt U, Meinertz T, Just H: Skeletal muscle blood flow, metabolism, and morphology in chronic congestive heart failure and effects of short- and long-term angiotensin-converting enzyme inhibition. *Am J Cardiol* 62:82E–85E, 1988.
35. Mancini DM, Walter G, Reichek N, et al: Contribution of skeletal muscle atrophy to exercise intolerance and altered muscle metabolism in heart failure. *Circulation* 85:1364–1373, 1992.
36. Drexler H, Riede U, Munzel T, Konig H, Funke E, Just H: Alteration of skeletal muscle in chronic heart failure. *Circulation* 85:1751–1759, 1992.
37. Dunnigan A, Staley NA, Smith SA, et al: Cardiac and skeletal muscle abnormalities in cardiomyopathy: comparison of patients with ventricular tachycardia or congestive heart failure. *J Am Coll Cardiol* 10:608–618, 1987.
38. Lindsay DC, Lovegrove CA, Dunn MJ, et al: Histological abnormalities of diaphragmatic muscle may contribute to dyspnea in heart failure. *Circulation* (suppl I)86:515, 1992.
39. Mancini DM, Henson D, LaManca J, Levine S: Respiratory muscle function and dyspnea in patients with chronic congestive heart failure. *Circulation* 86:909–918, 1992.
40. Buller NP, Jones D, Poole-Wilson PA: Direct measurement of skeletal muscle fatigue in patients with chronic heart failure. *Br Heart J* 65:20–24, 1991.
41. Wilson JR, Mancini DM, Dunkman WB: Exertional fatigue due to skeletal muscle dysfunction in patients with heart failure. *Circulation* 87:470–475, 1993.
42. Minotti JR, Pillay P, Chang L, Wells L, Massie BM: Neurophysiological assessment of skeletal muscle fatigue in patients with congestive heart failure. *Circulation* 86:903–908, 1992.
43. Massie BM, Conway M, Rajagopalan B, et al: Skeletal muscle metabolism during exercise under ischemic conditions in congestive heart failure: evidence for abnormalities unrelated to blood flow. *Circulation* 78:320–326, 1988.
44. Wade OL, Bishop JM: *Cardiac Output and Regional Blood Flow.* Oxford: Blackwell, 1962.

45. LeJemtel TH, Maskin CS, Lucido D, Chadwick BJ: Failure to augment maximal limb blood flow in response to one leg versus two leg exercise in patients with severe heart failure. *Circulation* 74:245–251, 1986.
46. Zelis R, Flaim SF: Alterations in vasomotor tone in congestive heart failure. *Prog Cardiovasc Dis* 24:437–459, 1982.
47. Wilson JR, Wiener DH, Fink LI, Ferraro N: Vasodilatory behavior skeletal muscle arterioles in patients with nonedematous chronic heart failure. *Circulation* 74:775–779, 1986.
48. Longhurst J, Capone RJ, Zelis R: Evaluation of skeletal muscle capillary basement membrane thickness in congestive heart failure. *Chest* 67:195–198, 1975.
49. Lindsay DC, Anand IS, Bennett JG, et al: Ultrastructural analysis of skeletal muscle: microvascular dimensions and basement membrane thickness in chronic heart failure. *Eur Heart J* 15:1470–1476, 1994.
50. Harris P: Congestive cardiac failure: central role of the arterial blood pressure. *Br Heart J* 58:190–203, 1987.
51. Harris P: Role of arterial pressure in the oedema of heart disease. *Lancet* 1:1036–1038, 1988.
52. Piepoli M, Clark AL, Volterrani M, et al: Muscle ergoreflex role in exertional dyspnea in chronic heart failure patients. *J Am Coll Cardiol* (suppl A)21:480A, 1993.
53. Asmussen E, Nielsen M: Experiments on nervous factors controlling respiration and circulation during exercise employing blocking of the blood flow. *Acta Physiol Scand* 60:103–111, 1964.

8

Dyspnea in Heart Failure

Franz X. Kleber, MD; Irmingard Reindl, MD
Klaus D. Wernecke, MD; Gert Baumann, MD

Introduction

Pulmonary abnormalities in heart failure have been observed for many decades. Reduced vital capacity, increased dead space, arterial hypoxemia,[1,2] abnormal distribution of alveolar ventilation, and hypoxic vasoconstriction[3] may contribute to the increased ventilation. The isocapnic exercise hyperpnea[4,5,6] in heart failure has so far not been broadly investigated. Since it is one of the key features in patients with dyspnea, it deserves major scientific effort to further clarify the hitherto incompletely understood pathophysiology of dyspnea in heart failure.[7] This chapter reviews our current knowledge about dyspnea in heart failure.

Awareness and Measurement of Dyspnea

Dyspnea, like fatigue, is a complex symptom. Both are not represented by measurement of one physiological variable. Both are leading symptoms of patients with heart failure and probably are interreleated. Like fatigue, dyspnea is incompletely understood. In order to measure it semiquantitatively, several scaling systems have been implemented. The New York Heart Association (NYHA) classification and the Borg scale are being broadly used by general practitioners and cardiologists. The variability of unpleasant feelings that are summarized in the term dyspnea suggests different pathophysiologies caus-

From Wasserman, K (ed): *Exercise Gas Exchange in Heart Disease.* Armonk, NY: Futura Publishing Company, Inc., © 1996.

ing the discomfort. Simon et al[8] tried to differentiate the various forms of dyspnea, and described the interrelationship between various complaints and the underlying cause. The major discomforts described as dyspnea according to their investigation are: shortness of breath, problems with expiration, difficulty taking a deep breath (shallow breathing pattern), increased breathing effort, feeling of suffocation, air hunger or breathlessness, tightness of chest, or a very deep and heavy breathing sensation. In various disease entities, there is a wide variety of symptoms. Dyspnea in heart failure was associated with a rapid breathing pattern, a suffocating discomfort, and air hunger.

Probably the most important scaling system for dyspnea was introduced by Borg[9] in 1982. Among several physiological variables, the effort of breathing, the oxygen consumption of the respiratory muscles, and the work of breathing correlated especially well with the Borg scale.[10] Respiratory muscle strength as measured by maximal inspiratory or expiratory pressure and maximal expiratory flow rates correlated negatively with the Borg scale value.[10]

Thus, in further analyses, it is important to clarify which pathophysiological changes increase the work of breathing.

Cardiac Asthma

The term cardiac asthma was introduced by Hope in 1935.[11] Overt airway obstruction limiting exercise capacity is rarely seen in mild and moderate heart failure, but it might complicate severe pulmonary congestion.[12] However, some degree of bronchial hyperresponsiveness has been described in a large proporation of patients with heart failure (Cabanes 1989). Its pathogenesis is not entirely clear. Congestion can lead to airway constriction. Unmyelinated C fibers of the vagus nerve with endings in lung parenchyma (J-receptors) and bronchi and similar fibers in the pulmonary vasculature are stimulated by edema and distention of the vascular tree (overview Reference 12). Reflexes are transmitted via the vagus. In addition, local axon reflexes, leading to liberation of substance P, have also been suggested.[12] Since the small airways' bronchial circulation drains via pulmonary veins into the left atrium,[13] an increase in pulmonary venous pressure, as seen in left heart failure, can cause congestion and swelling of the bronchial mucosa.[14] This congestion probably is seldom severe enough to cause a decrease in airflow, but by initiating reflex bronchial contraction, might lead to bronchial hyperresponsiveness or even manifest obstructive physiology. Cabanes et al[15] were able to suppress the bronchial hyperresponsiveness to inhaled metacholine by administration of the alpha-adrenergic vasoconstrictor, methoxamine. These investigators were able to improve exercise endurance and reduce dyspnea by inhalation of this drug. The effect of methoxamine on submaximal or maximal oxygen consumption, however, was almost negligible. The role of bronchial hyperresponsiveness in exercise limitation in most patients with heart failure is, therefore, probably rather small.

Exercise Hyperpnea

Of all the variables associated with dyspnea, exercise hyperpnea and reduction in ventilatory efficiency are the most striking. Exercise hyperpnea is the increase in ventilation in relation to work performed. Ventilatory efficiency is the increase in ventilation in relation to gas exchange. Since carbon dioxide production is increased in heart failure by early lactic acidosis with additional carbon dioxide production through buffering of lactic acid by bicarbonate,[16] and ventilation is driven by it, ventilatory efficiency relative to oxygen uptake ($\dot{V}O_2$) is reduced. This, however, is a normal reaction to the abnormality in metabolism and does not reflect pulmonary pathophysiology. Therefore, the relationship between ventilation and $\dot{V}O_2$ cannot correctly reflect ventilatory efficiency of the lungs. We therefore used the relationship between minute ventilation and carbon dioxide production during exercise to measure ventilatory efficiency during the period of exercise when arterial PCO_2 ($PaCO_2$) does not change. Only a change in the PCO_2 setpoint can change the slope of this relationship in the absence of changing the ventilatory dead space/tidal volume ratio. $PaCO_2$ decrease occurs in response to lactate acidosis. This factor as a cause of a change in slope can be avoided in patients who exercise until exhaustion by excluding the last part of ventilatory measurements, when endtidal PCO_2 may decrease, from the slope analysis. Several questions arise from the observation of exercise hyperpnea: What is the contribution of reduced ventilatory efficiency? To what extent are the metabolic changes with early lactic acidosis contributing to it? Does it limit exercise performance? Does an abnormality in the diffusive characteristics of the alveolo-capillary membrane contribute to it? What is the contribution of ventilation-perfusion mismatch? Is the ventilation-perfusion mismatch reversible, or is it caused by irreversible structural pulmonary abnormalities?

The Contribution of Reduced Ventilatory Efficiency to Exercise Hyperpnea

Exercise hyperpnea driven by early lactic acidosis causes a terminal slope increase in the linear relationship between minute ventilation ($\dot{V}E$)

and $\dot{V}O_2$. The increase in the slope of the relationship $\dot{V}E$ versus $\dot{V}O_2$ is, therefore, seen before the decrease in arterial pH. Up to that level of the individual exercise capacity, the observed exercise hyperpnea is caused solely by reduction of ventilatory efficiency. Above the anaerobic threshold (AT), the contribution of anaerobic metabolism to ventilatory drive is represented by the increase in $\dot{V}E/\dot{V}O_2$ after the anaerobic threshold ($\dot{V}O_2AT$) is reached. Patients with chronic heart failure (CHF) often stop exercise early after $\dot{V}O_2AT$ and thus, in most patients, the contribution of early anaerobic metabolism to exercise ventilation is less important than the contribution of ventilation-perfusion mismatch.

Is the Reduction in Ventilatory Efficiency Limiting Exercise Performance?

Only recently, normal values for ventilatory efficiency for various ages and both sexes have been presented.[17] There has been considerable debate about the importance of ventilation increase in determining exercise capacity.[18,19] The main reason is the high ventilatory reserve at maximal exercise in heart failure patients.[6] In patients with pulmonary limitations, the breathing reserve is minimal, the ratio of maximal exercise ventilation to maximal voluntary ventilation (as measured from forced vital capacity multiplied by an experimentally determined factor of 41[20]) often approaching 100%. Patients with heart failure usually do not reach this level and thus have considerable ventilatory reserve left. In addition, Yokoyama reported that the addition of artificial dead space does not further acutely limit exercise performance.[21] However, a ventilation in excess of 30% to 50% of maximal voluntary ventilation (MVV) may cause symptoms of breathlessness,[22] and therefore will be avoided by patients whenever possible. Due to the inefficiency of ventilation, patients with heart failure might easily reach this level of the MVV during daily activities.

A group of 71 patients with heart failure of various causes (dilated cardiomyopathy n=56; coronary heart disease n=11; valvular heart disease n=4), with left ventricular ejection fraction of 28 ± 11%, median NYHA functional class III, was prospectively divided into two groups: patients with normal ventilatory efficiency ($\dot{V}E$ versus $\dot{V}CO_2$ slope 35 or less), and those with reduced ventilatory efficiency ($\dot{V}E$ versus $\dot{V}CO_2$ slope above 35). We exercised these patients on a modified Naughton protocol. Patients with reduced ventilatory efficiency had significantly lower ejection fractions (25.5 ± 8.7 versus 31.5 ± 11.9%, p<0.05), significantly lower $\dot{V}O_2$ at the AT (8.7 ± 2.2 versus 13.5 ± 3.3 mL/kg/min, p<0.05), at peak exercise (12.2 ± 3.1 versus 20.8 ± 5.6 mL/kg/min, p<0.05), and a higher median NYHA class (III versus II). This study[23] showed that ventilatory efficiency is at least tightly related to impairment in exercise capacity. The mathematically close correlation between $\dot{V}E$ versus $\dot{V}CO_2$ slope and oxygen consumption (own unpublished results) further strengthens the idea of a pathophysiological role of impairment of ventilatory efficiency in heart failure in limiting exercise capacity. One explanation for this could be that patients, in order to avoid breathlessness, reduce their activity and thereby their oxidative capacity. A direct influence of training on ventilatory efficiency has been described,[24] but is very limited in its extent. Another idea is that the endurance capacity of the respiratory muscles is unable to maintain the high level of exercise ventilation, and that respiratory muscle fatigue causes the sensation of dyspnea. This hypothesis is in agreement with the temporal dissociation between ventilatory response to exercise and the sensation of dyspnea as well as the marked dyspnea which occurs after the end of exercise despite a reduction in ventilatory minute volumes.[25] Furthermore, respiratory work approaches levels that have been shown to generate respiratory muscle fatigue.[26] Selective training of respiratory muscles can not only improve maximal ventilation during exercise,[27] but also improves oxygen consumption, further supporting the evidence for respiratory muscle fatigue as one limiting factor in heart failure.[28] This concept would be in good agreement with the findings of respiratory muscle abnormalities found by Piepoli[29] and the respiratory muscle deoxygenation found by Mancini.[30] The contribution of the respiratory muscles to total oxygen consumption and to lactic acidosis can also be more than trivial. For these reasons, a decrease in the level of ventilation by improvement of ventilatory efficiency may improve exercise capacity (see below). The ability to reduce global ventilation-perfusion mismatch, as demonstrated with gamma camera imaging (81m-Krypton gas and iv 99m-Technetium macro aggregated albumin),[31] is in accordance with our own results and those of others[32] which closely relate ventilatory efficiency to exercise capacity. Ultimate proof of the influence of ventilatory efficiency on exercise capacity, however, is impossible without demonstrating improvement of exercise capacity when ventilatory efficiency improves.

Is the Reduction in Ventilatory Efficiency Reversible in Chronic Heart Failure?

To test the reversibility of reduction of ventilatory efficiency, we investigated 17 patients, ages 35 to 73, median 59 years with median NYHA class III due to impaired left ventricular performance (mean left ventricular ejection fraction 27 [range 13–40]%). $\dot{V}O_2AT$ was 8.6 ± 3.3 mL/kg/min and peak $\dot{V}O_2$ was 12.9 ± 4.9 mL/kg/min.[33] All patients were regarded as being suboptimally treated. The new therapeutic intervention consisted of Angiotensin Converting Enzyme (ACE) inhibitors or an increase in the dose of ACE inhibitors. In three patients, in addition, we either started or increased diuretics. Follow-up was performed with cardiopulmonary exercise testing after 4 weeks. Patients who improved ventilatory efficiency, measured as the $\dot{V}E$ versus $\dot{V}CO_2$ slope of at least 5, had a large increase in oxygen consumption ($\dot{V}O_2$max from 11.2 ± 2.8 to 17.4 ± 5.3 mL/kg/min, p<0.005) (Figure 1). In contrast, patients with no or small improvement in ventilatory efficiency had no improvement in $\dot{V}O_2$max. The improvement in ventilatory efficiency was only in a small part due to an improvement of anatomic dead space (by improving the rapid and shallow breathing pattern of heart failure). Subtracting anatomic dead space ventilation (as derived by body weight $\times$ 2.2 + age (years) $\times$ respiratory rate) revealed that the improvement of ventilatory efficiency was to a large extent due to a decrease of physiological dead space from 38% to 28% of total exercise ventilation. Both factors resulted in a considerable increase in effective alveolar ventilation (Figure 2). Thus, exercise hyperpnea can be reduced in a considerable proportion of patients with heart failure. The improvement seen by administration of vasodilators results from a decrease in physiological dead space. The improvement in ventilatory efficiency accompanies the improvement in exercise capacity.

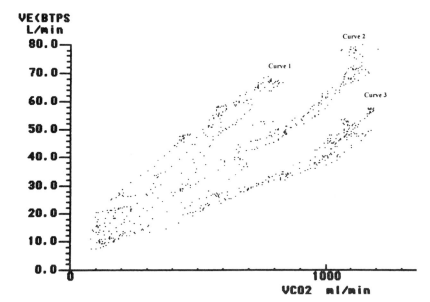

Figure 1. Decrease in the minute ventilation ($\dot{V}E$) versus carbon dioxide output ($\dot{V}CO_2$) slope in a patient during improvement of heart failure symptoms by drug therapy. **Curve 1:** before treatment; **Curve 2:** after 4 weeks of afterload reduction; **Curve 3:** after 8 weeks of afterload reduction.

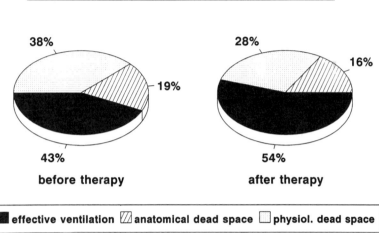

REDUCTION OF DEAD SPACE VENTILATION
in responders

38%	28%
19%	16%
43%	54%
before therapy	after therapy

■ effective ventilation ▨ anatomical dead space ☐ physiol. dead space

Figure 2. Change in contribution of alveolar (effective) ventilation, anatomic and physiological dead space ventilation as a result of treatment in patients who improve their minute ventilation ($\dot{V}E$) versus carbon dioxide output ($\dot{V}CO_2$) slope after pharmacotherapy (=responders). Results are the average of 9 subjects. (See text for details.)

Is an Abnormality of the Diffusive Membrane Seen?

By applying the Roughton and Forster formula,[34] Puri et al described an impairment of the diffusive membrane in heart failure.[35] This formula is used to partition the diffusion abnormalities into two specific resistances to gas exchange: the diffusive membrane and the capillary blood volume. By measuring the carbon monoxide transfer at different inspiratory oxygen concentrations, the equation yields the relative contribution of both constituents to the diffusion abnormality. The equation assumes that the pulmonary capillary blood volume is unchanged by a short exposure to a high inspiratory oxygen concentration. Structural changes in the pulmonary alveolo-capillary membrane are thought to cause the calculated change in membrane resistance. The failure of the diffusive membrane characteristics to return to normal readily after heart transplantation[36] supports this concept.

The contribution of the diffusion abnormalities of carbon monoxide to exercise hyperpnea is unknown. After heart transplantation, patients normalize their ventilatory efficiency (own unpublished results) despite the residual diffusion abnormalities.[36] To further clarify these interrelationships between hyperpnea and the diffusion capacity measurement, we investigated pulmonary function in the above described group of 71 patients.

The transfer factor for carbon monoxide was significantly different in patients with normal (n=46) as compared to abnormal (n=25)
ventilatory efficiency. This difference was due to a combination of a reduced capillary blood volume and altered membrane characteristics.
This suggested a pathophysiological relationship between diffusion
abnormalities and reduction of ventilatory efficiency. However, further analyses showed a lack of correlation between the diffusion abnormality and the $\dot{V}E$ versus $\dot{V}CO_2$ slope in patients with slope values
above 35 (Figure 3). Thus, the correlation was absent in the pathophysiological state suggesting an association of these two phenomena
instead of a causative connection. So hemodynamic explanations for
the reduction in ventilatory efficiency with alveolar hypoperfusion or
alveolar shutdown became even more likely.

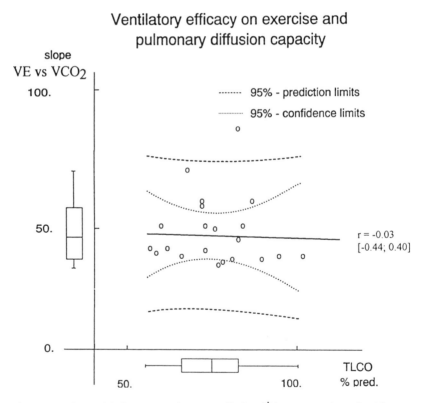

Figure 3. Relationship between minute ventilation ($\dot{V}E$) versus carbon dioxide output ($\dot{V}CO_2$) slope and diffusion capacity for carbon monoxide (TLCO) in percent of
predicted values in patients with compromised ventilatory efficiency ($\dot{V}E$ versus
$\dot{V}CO_2$ slope >35). **Box plot:** line through rectangle is median value, boundary of
rectangles are the 25% and 75% percentiles, and the lines extending from the rectangle represent minimal and maximal values excluding outlayers. Correlation
coefficient r: values in brackets are the 95% confidence limits of r.

Does Exercise Hyperpnea Reflect Alveolar Hypoperfusion in Heart Failure?

If alveolar hypoperfusion is linked to hyperpnea or increased $\dot{V}E$ versus $\dot{V}CO_2$ slope, then pulmonary artery pressure and pulmonary vascular resistance should be closely correlated. However, Sullivan[37] was unable to find such a correlation. His group of patients, however, had only slightly elevated $\dot{V}E/\dot{V}CO_2$ values. In a group of 25 patients with heart failure (LVEF 32.6 ± 15.0%) with a $\dot{V}E$ versus $\dot{V}CO_2$ slope range between 24 and 85 (median 36), we measured hemodynamics by right heart catheterization and obtained blood specimens from the pulmonary artery, the aorta, and the femoral vein for determination of plasma concentrations of catecholamines and endothelin. In close time correlation, we performed cardiopulmonary exercise testing. Pulmonary artery pressure (Figure 4) and pulmonary capillary wedge

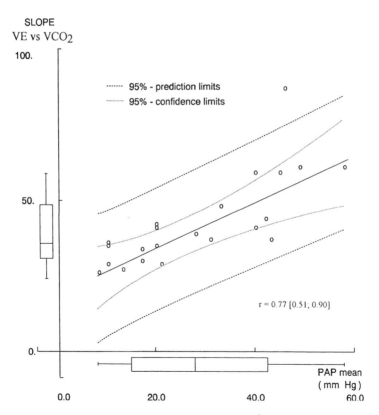

Figrue 4. Relationship between minute ventilation ($\dot{V}E$) versus carbon dioxide output ($\dot{V}CO_2$) slope and pulmonary artery mean pressure (PAP mean), mmHg. Box plot and correlation coefficient: see Figure 3.

pressure as well as cardiac output correlated with ventilatory efficiency. Also, the slope of the $\dot{V}E$ versus $\dot{V}CO_2$ relationship correlated significantly with norepinephrine in the pulmonary artery and aorta and endothelin in the aorta, whereas epinephrine and dopamine plasma concentrations did not. The correlations of endothelin as well as of norepinephrine with the $\dot{V}E$ versus $\dot{V}CO_2$ slope were quite weak and 95% confidence intervals of the correlation crossed zero. Despite the close relationship with central hemodynamics, vasoconstrictors do not appear to play a major role in mediating the alveolar hypoperfusion. However, mediators other than those tested or defective endothelial vasodilatory mechanisms[38,39] might play a significant role in mediating alveolar hypoperfusion.

Summary

Dyspnea and fatigue are the two predominant symptoms of patients with CHF. Both are not completely represented by measurement of one specific physiological variable. Both seem also to share common pathways in their pathophysiology. The most prominent measurable physiological signs of dyspnea are bronchial hyperresponsiveness and cardiac asthma, reduced respiratory strength, and increased respiratory work as well as hyperpnea. By far the greatest spontaneous differences from normal have been shown in ventilatory minute volumes on exercise. Exercise hyperpnea in CHF is mainly caused by increased and earlier excessive production of carbon dioxide and uneven distribution between ventilation and perfusion within the lung (ventilation-perfusion mismatch). This uneven distribution leads to a reduction of ventilatory efficiency with wasted ventilation in areas of underperfusion. It represents the only reason for excessive ventilation at rest and at work rates below the *AT,* and contributes a major and often the largest part to exercise hyperpnea after onset of anaerobic metabolism. A decrease in diffusion capacity, as measured by the transfer of carbon monoxide from the airways to the blood, is probably not a causative factor for the disturbance of ventilatory efficiency. A close correlation of exercise hyperpnea and pulmonary artery pressures at rest is observed. However, pulmonary artery and aortic plasma levels of major vasoconstrictors do not closely correlate with ventilatory efficiency. Disturbance of ventilatory efficiency is not caused solely by structural abnormalities. The $\dot{V}E$ versus $\dot{V}CO_2$ slope can be improved by vasodilator therapy in a considerable number of heart failure patients. The contribution of exercise-induced increase of airway resistance to hyperpnea and dyspnea remains to be evaluated, although preliminary therapeutic results with vasoconstrictors (methoxamine) are encouraging. We conclude that disturbance of ventilatory efficiency plays a key role in the pathophysiology and management of dyspnea.

Acknowledgments

The authors thank Dr. Karlman Wasserman for his invaluable advice and for reviewing this manuscript. We are indebted to Mrs. Linda Bunk for expert secretarial assistance in preparing this manuscript. The work presented was in part supported by a grant of the German Federal Government, Bundesministerium fur Forschung und Technologie (BMFT Grant Nr. 9814337).

References

1. Frank NR, Lyons HA, Siebens AA, Nealon TF: Pulmonary compliance in patients with cardiac disease. *Am J Med* 22:516, 1957.
2. Friedmann BL, Macias DJ, Yu PN: Pulmonary function studies in patients with mitral stenosis. *Am Rev Tuberc* 79:265, 1959.
3. Raine J, Bishop JM: The distribution of alveolar ventilation in mitral stenosis at rest and after exercise. *Clin Sci* 24:63, 1963.
4. Sullivan MJ, Higginbotham MB, Cobb FR: Increased exercise ventilation in patients with chronic heart failure: intact ventilatory control despite hemodynamic and pulmonary abnormalities. *Circulation* 77:552–559, 1988.
5. Franciosa JA, Leddy CL, Wilen M, Schwartz DE: Relation between hemodynamic and ventilatory responses in determining exercise capacity in severe congestive heart failure. *Am J Cardiol* 53:127–134, 1984.
6. Rajfer SI, Nemanich JW, Schurman AJ, Rossen JD: Metabolic responses to exercise in patients with heart failure. *Circulation* (suppl VI)76:46–53, 1987.
7. Szidon JP: Pathophysiology of the congested lung. *Cardiology Clin* 7:39–48, 1989.
8. Simon P, Schwartzstein RM, Weiss JW, Fencl V, Teghtsoonian M, Weinberger SE: Distinguishable types of dyspnea in patients with shortness of breath. *Am Rev Respir Dis* 142:1009–1014, 1990.
9. Borg GV: Psychophysical bases of perceived exertion. *Med Sci Sports Exerc* 14:377–381, 1982.
10. Mancini DM, Henson D, LaManca J, Levine S: Respiratory muscle function and dyspnea in patients with chronic congestive heart failure. *Circulation* 86:909–918, 1992.
11. Hope J: *A Treatise on the Diseases of the Heart and Great Vessels*. 2nd ed. London: W. Kidd, 1935.
12. Snashall PD, Fan Chung K: Airway obstruction and bronchial hyperresponsiveness in left ventricular failure and mitral stenosis. *Am Rev Respir Dis* 144:945–956, 1991.
13. Deffebach ME, Charan NB, Lakshminarayan S, Butler J: The bronchial circulation: small, but a vital attribute of the lung. *Am Rev Respir Dis* 135:463–481, 1987.
14. Cabanes LR, Weber SN, Matran R, et al: Bronchial hyperresponsiveness to methacholine in patients with impaired left ventricular function. *N Engl J Med* 320:1317–1322, 1989.

15. Cabanes L, Costes F, Weber S: Improvement in exercise performance by inhalation of methoxamine in patients with impaired left ventricular function. *N Engl J Med* 326:1661–1665, 1992.
16. Wasserman K, Zhang Y, Riley ML: Ventilation during exercise in chronic heart failure. *Basic Res Cardiol* 1995. (In press.)
17. Habedank D, Reindl I, Sonntag CF, Kleber FX: Ventilatory efficacy in healthy volunteers during cardiopulmonary exercise testing. *Eur J Appl Physiol* (suppl 3)69:14, 1994.
18. Wilson JR, Mancini DM, Farrell L: Excessive ventilatory levels do not limit the exercise capacity of patients with heart failure. *Circulation* (suppl I)86:I–399, 1992.
19. Metra M, Dei Cas L, Panina G, Visioli O: Exercise hyperventilation in chronic congestive heart failure, and its relation to functional capacity and hemodynamics. *Am J Cardiol* 70:1007–1008, 1992.
20. Miller WF, Scacci R, Gast LR: *Laboratory Evaluation of Pulmonary Function.* Philadelphia: JB Lippincott Co., 300, 1987.
21. Yokoyama H, Sato H, Ozaki H, et al: Role of reduced ventilatory efficiency in exercise intolerance in patients with chronic heart failure(abstr). *Heart Failure* 1:713, 1993.
22. Cournand A, Richard DW: Pulmonary insufficiency: discussion of a physiological classification and presentation of clinical tests. *Am Rev Tuberc* 44:26–41, 1941.
23. Reindl I, Kleber FX, Felix SB, et al: Exertional hyperpnoea in patients with chronic heart failure is associated with impairment of pulmonary gas transfer (abstr). *Eur Heart J* (suppl)15:240, 1994.
24. Coats AJS, Adamopoulos S, Radaelli A, et al: Controlled trial of physical training in chronic heart failure: exercise performance, hemodynamics, ventilation, and autonomic function. *Circulation* 85:2119–2131, 1992.
25. Davies SW, Jordan SL, Lipkin DP: Does increased dead space ventilation during exercise explain dyspnoea in chronic left heart failure? *J of Heart Failure* 1:890, 1993.
26. Mancini DM, Henson D, LaManca J, Levine S: Respiratory muscle function and dyspnea in patients with chronic congestive heart failure. *Circulation* 86:909–918, 1992.
27. Mancini DM, Donchez LJ, LaManca J, Henson D, Mandak JS, Levine S: Respiratory muscle training improves exercise performance in patients with heart failure(abstr). *Circulation* 88:I–415, 1993.
28. McParland C, Krishnan B, Wang Y, Gallagher C: Inspiratory muscle weakness and dyspnea in chronic heart failure. *Am Rev Respir Dis* 146:467–472, 1992.
29. Piepoli M, Clark A, Volterrani M, et al: Muscle ergoreflex role in exertional dyspnea in chronic heart failure patients(abstr). *J Am Coll Cardiol* 21:480A, 1993.
30. Mancini D, Ferraro N, Nazzaro D, Chance B, Wilson JR: Respiratory muscle deoxygenation during exercise in patients with heart failure demonstrated with near-infrared spectroscopy. *J Am Coll Cardiol* 18:492–498, 1991.
31. Uren NG, Davies SW, Agnew JE, et al: The ability to reduce global ventilation-perfusion mismatch on exercise is related to exercise capacity in chronic heart failure(abstr). *Eur Heart J* 13:100, 1992.
32. Davey P, Meyer T, Coats A, et al: Ventilation in chronic heart failure: effects of physical training. *Br Heart J* 68:473–477, 1992.
33. Reindl I, Kleber FX: Exertional hyperpnea in patients with chronic heart failure is a reversible cause of exercise intolerance. *Basic Res Cardiol* 1995. (In press.)

34. Roughton FJW, Forster FR: Relative importance of diffusion and chemical reaction rates in determining rate of exchange of gases in human lung, with special reference to true diffusing capacity of pulmonary membrane and volume of blood in the lung capillaries. *J Appl Physiol* 11:290–302, 1957.
35. Puri S, Cleland JF: Abnormal alveolar-capillary membrane gas transfer in chronic heart failure. Submitted to *Basic Research Cardiology*, 1994.
36. Ohar J, Osterloh J, Ahmed N, Miller L: Diffusing capacity decreases after heart transplantation. *Chest* 103:857–861, 1993.
37. Sullivan MJ, Higginbotham MB, Cobb FR: Increased exercise ventilation in patients with chronic heart failure: intact ventilatory control despite hemodynamic and pulmonary abnormalities. *Circulation* 77:552–559, 1988.
38. Kleber FX, Wensel R, Felix SB, Reindl I, Baumann G: Acetylcholine causes dose-dependent increase in pulmonary flow in patients with chronic heart failure and elevated pulmonary vascular resistances. *Basic Res Cardiol* 1996. (In press.)
39. Cleland JF: Increased alveolar-capillary membrane resistance can predict maximal exercise capacity in chronic heart failure. *Circulation* (suppl)88: I–213, 1993.

9

Increased Ventilatory Response to Exercise as Related to Functional Capacity

Akira Koike, MD; Michiaki Hiroe, MD
Fumiaki Marumo, MD

Exertional dyspnea, which results from increased ventilation during exercise, is the main symptom of patients with heart failure. However, pathophysiologic mechanisms for this increased ventilation have not been fully clarified.[1-3] Neurogenic, humoral, or cardiodynamic reflex has been considered to be a possible stimulus of exercise hyperpnea.[1] It has also been reported that potassium released during muscle contraction causes an increase in ventilation during exercise by stimulating carotid bodies.[3-5] Although ventilation during exercise may be controlled mainly by a combination of neural and humoral drives, considerable controversy exists as to relative contributions of these factors.[3] This chapter focuses on our recent studies[6,7] which have addressed the issue of humoral reflex, especially on the relation between the lactic acidosis and exercise hyperpnea in patients with cardiovascular disease.

Effects of Acute Reduction in Oxygen Transport on Ventilatory Control

The binding of hemoglobin by carbon monoxide reversibly decreases the blood oxygen carrying capacity, without changing the ar-

From Wasserman, K (ed): *Exercise Gas Exchange in Heart Disease.* Armonk, NY: Futura Publishing Company, Inc., © 1996.

terial partial pressure of oxygen (PO_2), producing a useful reversible model to study impaired oxygen transport.[8-14] Carbon monoxide has been shown not to have a direct effect on the carotid bodies and the ventilatory control mechanisms.[15-17] Using the carbon monoxide model, effects of acute reduction in oxygen transport on exercise ventilation were evaluated in 10 normal subjects.[6]

Each subject was studied on three different days, one without added carbon monoxide (control), one with approximately 11% carboxyhemoglobin, and one with approximately 20% carboxyhemoglobin. The order was randomized. On each day, an incremental exercise test to the symptom limited maximum and two (moderate and heavy) constant work-rate exercises for 6 minutes were performed by each subject on a cycle ergometer. To keep the carboxyhemoglobin levels, the subjects breathed 0.02% carbon monoxide in air during exercise.

The lactic acidosis threshold (*LAT*) and maximal work rate were previously determined for each subject from an incremental cycle ergometer exercise test while breathing room air without added carbon monoxide. The *LAT* was determined noninvasively as the break point in the carbon dioxide output ($\dot{V}CO_2$) versus oxygen uptake ($\dot{V}O_2$) plot, i.e., the V-slope method.[14,18,19] The $\dot{V}O_2$ at this break point has been shown to correlate well with the $\dot{V}O_2$ at which blood bicarbonate level starts to decrease.[18,19] The moderate-intensity constant work rate was determined to correspond to $\dot{V}O_2$ at 80% of the *LAT*. For heavy-intensity exercise, the difference between the work rate at the *LAT* and that at peak exercise was first calculated; the work rate of heavy-intensity exercise was then determined by adding 40% of this difference to the work rate at the *LAT*. The subjects performed the same work rate tests for all three levels of carboxyhemoglobin.

The mean response of ventilation with respect to $\dot{V}O_2$ at rest, the *LAT*, respiratory compensation point, and maximum work rate is shown in Figure 1 for the 10 subjects studied. Both maximum work rate and exercise duration were significantly decreased with increased carboxyhemoglobin. Peak $\dot{V}O_2$ and the *LAT* were also significantly decreased with increased carboxyhemoglobin (Figure 1). There was no difference in $\dot{V}O_2$ or ventilation at rest for the three levels of carboxyhemoglobin. The slope of the increase in ventilation relative to $\dot{V}O_2$ below each *LAT* was the same for all three carboxyhemoglobin levels. However, ventilation increased more steeply above the *LAT*, the higher the carboxyhemoglobin.

Figure 2 shows the response of ventilation during 6 minutes of constant work-rate exercise and venous lactate concentration 2 minutes after exercise in one representative subject. The venous lactate concentration measured 2 minutes after heavy-intensity exercise was 2.3 mM/L for the control, and was increased to 5.1 mM/L and 8.0 mM/L for the 11% and 20% carboxyhemoglobin, respectively. Venti-

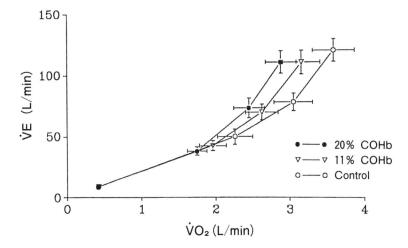

Figure 1. Ventilation ($\dot{V}_E$) at rest, lactic acidosis threshold, respiratory compensation point (oxygen uptake at which $\dot{V}_E$ increases disproportionately to carbon dioxide output) and peak exercise going from lowest to highest oxygen uptake ($\dot{V}_{O_2}$), respectively, in 10 subjects at the three levels of carboxyhemoglobin (COHb) indicated. **Points** and **bars** represent mean ± SE. (Modified from Reference 6.)

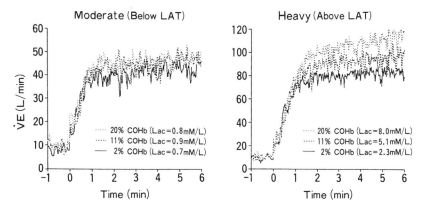

Figure 2. Effects of increased carboxyhemoglobin (COHb) on ventilation ($\dot{V}_E$) response during moderate (145 W) and heavy (260 W) work intensities in one normal subject (32-year-old male). Venous lactate concentration (Lac) was obtained 2 minutes after each exercise test. (Modified from Reference 6.)

lation during heavy exercise was also higher with increased carboxyhemoglobin. For the moderate exercise, however, there was no appreciable change in ventilation or lactate concentration in spite of the increased carboxyhemoglobin. These results indicate a tight relationship between the increase in lactate and increase in ventilation. The relationship between the increase in ventilation at the end of exercise with 11% and 20% carboxyhemoglobin from that of the control test, and the corresponding increase in venous lactate concentration 2 minutes after exercise is shown in Figure 3 for each subject. The increase in ventilation and lactate concentration showed a good positive correlation (r=0.83, P<0.0001).

For the incremental exercise test of this study, a significant increase in ventilation was noted by increasing carboxyhemoglobin up to 20% only during exercise above the *LAT* (Figure 1). The amount of the increase in ventilation was correlated with the increase in carboxyhemoglobin, i.e., the reduction in arterial oxygen content. However, there was no additional stimulus to ventilation at work rates below the *LAT*. These findings are consistent with the hypothesis that the additional lactic acidosis caused by decreased oxygen transport due to the

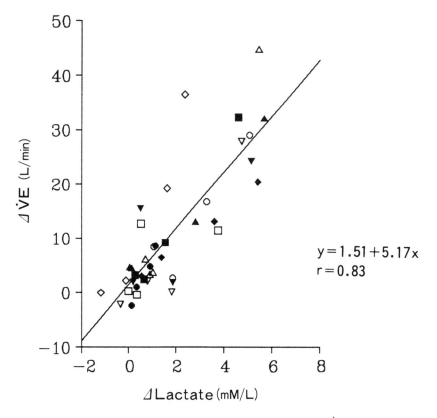

Figure 3. Relationship between the increase in ventilation (ΔV̇E) at the end of constant work rate tests with 11% and 20% carboxyhemoglobin from that of the control test, and the corresponding increase in venous lactate concentration (ΔLactate) 2 minutes after exercise for each subject. (Reproduced with permission from Reference 6).

increased carboxyhemoglobin level accounts for the increased ventilation at work rates above the *LAT,* and not the carboxyhemoglobin
level, itself. This hypothesis is strongly supported by the positive correlation of ventilation increase and the lactate increase during constant
work-rate exercise (Figure 3).

Changes in Lactate and Bicarbonate Levels during Exercise in Cardiac Patients

Figure 4 shows the pattern of the increase in arterial lactate and
the decrease in bicarbonate in trained subjects, sedentary healthy subjects and in cardiac patients.[20] The lactate level started to increase at
the lower $\dot{V}O_2$ in cardiac patients, as compared to normal subjects. The
slope of the increase in lactate concentration to the increase in $\dot{V}O_2$ was

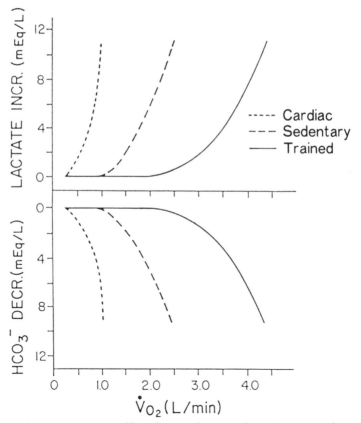

Figure 4. Lactate increase and bicarbonate decrease during incremental exercise
in trained and sedentary normal subjects and cardiac patients. (Reproduced with
permission from Reference 20.)

also steeper in cardiac patients. Plasma bicarbonate decreased in a close reciprocal relationship with lactate increase (lower panel of Figure 4). Thus, the metabolic acidosis due to the production of lactic acid during exercise must occur earlier and be more severe in cardiac patients compared to normal subjects. This metabolic acidosis would cause exercise hyperpnea by stimulating peripheral or central chemoreceptors in these patients, as shown in the normal subjects whose oxygen transport was acutely reduced by breathing carbon monoxide (Figure 1). $\dot{V}CO_2$ must also increase more rapidly above the *LAT* with the increasing severity of heart failure, because an additional 22 mL of carbon dioxide over that produced by aerobic metabolism must be generated from each milliequivalent of lactic acid buffered by bicarbonate.[21]

Carbon Dioxide Production During Exercise in Cardiac Patients

The pattern of increase in $\dot{V}CO_2$ was compared between 42 healthy subjects without evidence of heart disease [age: 40 ± 17 (SD) yr], and 106 patients with cardiovascular disease[22]; 47 patients (55 ± 10 yr) were in New York Heart Association functional class I, 47 patients (57 ± 9 yr) in class II, and 12 patients (65 ± 12 yr) in class III. Their diagnoses were coronary artery disease (n=30), valvular heart disease (n=26), hypertensive heart disease (n=25), dilated cardiomyopathy (n=7), and other heart disease (n=18).

Each subject performed a symptom limited incremental exercise test on a cycle ergometer. The exercise test was begun with a 4-minute warm up at 20 watts, 60 rpm, followed by a progressive increase in work rate (10, 15 or 20 W/min) in a ramp pattern. *LAT* was determined using the V-slope method.[14,18,19]

In the lower panel of Figure 5, $\dot{V}CO_2$ is plotted as a function of $\dot{V}O_2$ during the incremental exercise in a typical patient with cardiovascular disease. The slope of the linear increase in $\dot{V}CO_2$ with respect to $\dot{V}O_2$ is approximately 1 below the *LAT*.[21] Above the threshold, the slope abruptly increases,[14,18,19,21,23] because additional $\dot{V}CO_2$ is generated as bicarbonate buffers lactic acid.[21] The *LAT*, therefore, can be determined as the intersection of the lower and upper slopes with the latter having a value greater than 1 (V-slope method[14,18,19]). The slope of the increase in $\dot{V}CO_2$ to the increase in $\dot{V}O_2$ below and above the *LAT* was calculated for each subject.[22] In this study, we hypothesized that $\dot{V}CO_2$ in cardiac patients would be higher only during exercise above the *LAT* as compared to normal subjects, according to the severity of heart failure.

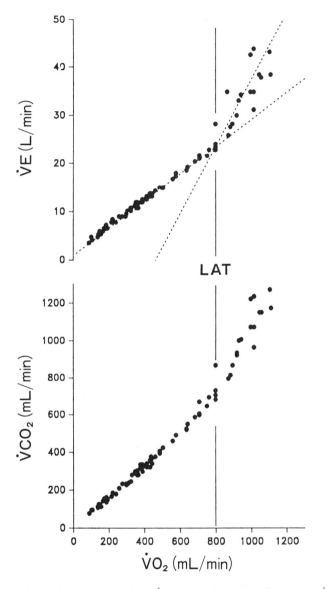

Figure 5. Relationship of ventilation ($\dot{V}E$) and carbon dioxide output ($\dot{V}CO_2$) to oxygen uptake ($\dot{V}O_2$) at rest and during exercise in a 65-year-old female cardiac patient. The **vertical line** indicates the lactic acidosis threshold (*LAT*) determined as the break point in the $\dot{V}CO_2$-$\dot{V}O_2$ plot (**lower panel**). **Dotted lines** indicate the slope of the increase in $\dot{V}E$ to the increase in $\dot{V}O_2$ below and above the *LAT*. Although $\dot{V}E$ increased linearly with the increase in $\dot{V}O_2$ below the *LAT*, the slope of the increase in $\dot{V}E$ to the increase in $\dot{V}O_2$ became steeper at work rates above the *LAT*. (Reproduced with permission from Reference 22.)

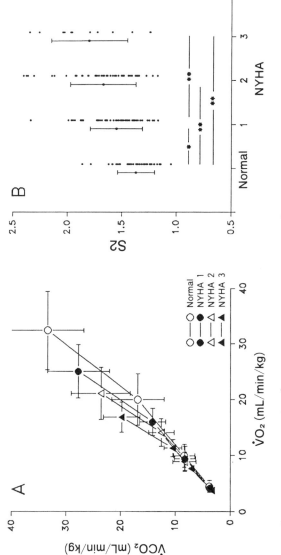

Figure 6. Oxygen uptake ($\dot{V}O_2$) and carbon dioxide output ($\dot{V}CO_2$) at rest, during warm up (20 W), at the lactic acidosis threshold and during peak exercise, progressing from the lowest to highest $\dot{V}O_2$ (**panel A**), and the slope of the increase in $\dot{V}CO_2$ with respect to $\dot{V}O_2$ above the lactic acidosis threshold (S2) in all subjects (**panel B**). *p<0.05, **p<0.01 by the Newman-Keuls multiple range test. NYHA = New York Heart Association functional class. **Points** and **bars** represent mean ± SD. (Reproduced with permission from Reference 7.)

Figure 6A shows the values for $\dot{V}O_2$ and $\dot{V}CO_2$ at rest and at 20 watts, the *LAT* and peak exercise in normal subjects and patients with cardiovascular disease. The peak $\dot{V}O_2$ normalized to each subject's body weight was 32.4 ± 7.1 mL/min/kg in the normal subjects. The value was significantly decreased below normal to 25.1 ± 4.8, 21.1 ± 4.7 and 16.9 ± 2.7 mL/min/kg in patients in class I, class II and class III, respectively. Similarly, *LAT*, which was 20.0 ± 4.6 mL/min/kg in normal subjects, was significantly decreased with increasing severity of heart disease: 16.0 ± 2.4, 14.1 ± 2.5 and 11.3 ± 1.5 mL/min/kg, respectively, in patients in functional class I, class II and class III.

The slope of the increase in $\dot{V}CO_2$ to the increase in $\dot{V}O_2$ above the *LAT* (S2) was 1.37 ± 0.17 in normal subjects (Figure 6B). The slope was significantly increased with the increasing severity of heart disease; 1.55 ± 0.24 in class I patients, 1.67 ± 0.30 in class II patients, and 1.80 ± 0.35 in class III patients. However, the lower slope of the increase in $\dot{V}CO_2$ to the increase in $\dot{V}O_2$ was approximately 0.9 and did not differ between normal subjects and patients with either functional class I, II or III heart failure.

Although the slope of the increase in work rate was selected as 10 W/min, 15 W/min, or 20 W/min randomly in this study, this slope was found to have no influence on the slope of the increase in $\dot{V}CO_2$ to the increase in $\dot{V}O_2$ above or below the *LAT*.[22] There was no relationship between age and this slope above the *LAT*,[22] although it is well known that the *LAT* and peak $\dot{V}O_2$ decline with age.[24]

The steeper slope of the increase in $\dot{V}CO_2$ to the increase in $\dot{V}O_2$ above the *LAT* in patients with heart failure must indicate that additional carbon dioxide over that produced by aerobic metabolism was generated from buffering of lactic acid by bicarbonate. Thus, the slope of the increase in $\dot{V}CO_2$ with respect to $\dot{V}O_2$ reflects the degree of lactic acidosis in heart failure patients. Lactic acidosis during exercise must also influence ventilation in these patients, according to the severity of heart failure.

Ventilatory Response to Exercise as Related to Functional Capacity in Patients with Cardiovascular Disease

The upper panel of Figure 5 shows the relationship between ventilation and $\dot{V}O_2$. At work rates below the *LAT*, ventilation increases linearly as the $\dot{V}O_2$ increases. However, the slope of the increase in ventilation relative to the increase in $\dot{V}O_2$ becomes steeper at work rates above the *LAT*. Therefore, we compared the slopes of the increase in ventilation as a function of the increase in $\dot{V}O_2$ above the *LAT*, for normal subjects and patients in New York Heart Association functional class I, II and III. In this comparison, a subset of our original population was evaluated. This subset consisted of 48 patients with cardiovascular disease (19 patients in class I, 22 patients in class II, and 7 patients in class III) and 16 normal subjects of similar age, who all had performed a 10 W/min ramp test to the symptom limited maximum.[7] The slopes of the increase in ventilation to the increase in $\dot{V}O_2$ were calculated below and above the *LAT* for each subject.

Figure 7A shows the relation between ventilation and $\dot{V}O_2$ during the incremental exercise in normal subjects and patients with cardiovascular disease. The peak $\dot{V}O_2$ and $\dot{V}O_2$ at the *LAT* were significantly decreased as the severity of heart failure increased. The slope of the increase in ventilation to the increase in $\dot{V}O_2$ at work rates below the *LAT* did not differ between normal subjects and patients in either class I, II or III: it was 28.4 ± 8.8, 27.2 ± 7.0, 25.0 ± 10.7, and 28.3 ± 7.7 respectively. The slope of the increase in ventilation to the increase in $\dot{V}O_2$ above the *LAT* was 46.6 ± 13.5 in normal subjects, 46.1 ± 10.3 (N.S.) in class I patients, 60.8 ± 17.9 ($P<0.05$) in class II patients, and 66.5 ± 21.2 ($P<0.01$) in class III patients.

There was no statistical difference in the slope of the increase in ventilation to the increase in $\dot{V}CO_2$ either below or above the *LAT* between normal subjects and cardiac patients (Figure 7B), although it tended to be steeper in patients with class III heart failure especially above the *LAT*.

Normal subjects and patients with functional class I heart failure need approximately 400 mL/min/kg of ventilation to perform exercise which corresponds to 15 mL/min/kg of $\dot{V}O_2$ (Figure 7A). However, cardiac patients in class III require approximately 600 mL/min/kg of ventilation to perform this level of exercise because it exceeds their *LAT*. This amount of ventilation is almost one and one-half times as much ventilation as normal subjects. Thus, the excess exercise ventilation in heart failure patients appears to be mainly due to the worsening of exercise lactic acidosis.

Figure 8 shows the ventilatory equivalent for oxygen and carbon dioxide in all the subjects at rest, during 20 watts of warm up, at the *LAT*, and at peak exercise. The ventilatory equivalent for carbon dioxide, which decreased initially, was stable during exercise in spite of the work rate increase. In contrast, while the ventilatory equivalent for oxygen also decreased initially, it reached a minimum value at the *LAT* and then increased in every group. The ventilatory equivalent for oxygen at peak exercise was significantly higher in class III patients than in normal subjects or patients in class I. Although not significant, ventilatory equivalent for carbon dioxide in class III patients tended to be higher during exercise. This may be related to an increase in the ratio of pulmonary dead space to tidal volume or a decrease in the arterial

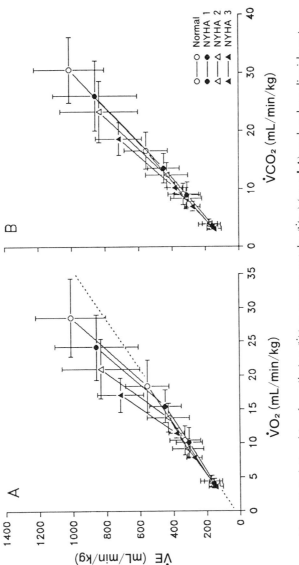

Figure 7. Relationship of ventilation ($\dot{V}E$) to oxygen uptake ($\dot{V}O_2$) (**panel A**) and carbon dioxide output ($\dot{V}CO_2$) (**panel B**). Data were obtained at rest, during warm up (20 W), at the lactic acidosis threshold and during peak exercise, going from lowest to highest $\dot{V}O_2$ (or $\dot{V}CO_2$). **Dotted line** in panel A indicates the mean slope of the increase in $\dot{V}E$ to the increase in $\dot{V}O_2$ below the lactic acidosis threshold in four groups. **Points** and **bars** represent mean ± SD. (Reproduced with permission from Reference 7.)

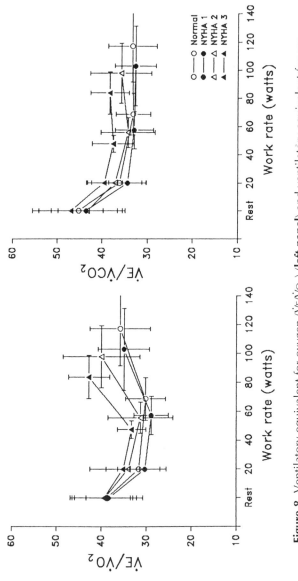

Figure 8. Ventilatory equivalent for oxygen ($\dot{V}_E/\dot{V}_{O_2}$) **(left panel)** and ventilatory equivalent for carbon dioxide ($\dot{V}_E/\dot{V}_{CO_2}$) **(right panel)** at rest, during warm up (20 W), at the lactic acidosis threshold and during peak exercise, progressing from the lowest to the highest work rate. **Points** and **bars** represent mean ± SD. (Reproduced with permission from Reference 7.)

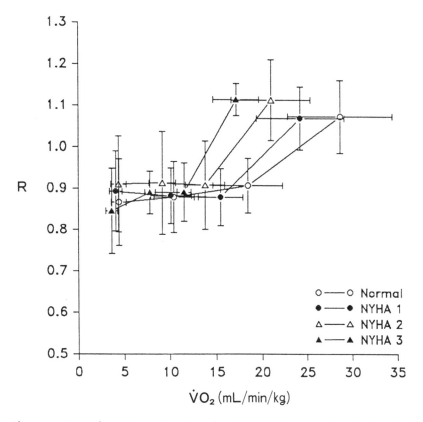

Figure 9. Gas exchange ratio (R) at rest, during warm up (20 W), at the lactic aci-dosis threshold, and during peak exercise, going from the lowest to the highest oxygen uptake ($\dot{V}O_2$). **Points** and **bars** represent mean ± SD. (Reproduced with permission from Reference 7.)

partial pressure of carbon dioxide (PCO_2) regulatory set point in these patients.

Figure 9 shows the change in gas exchange ratio during the incremental exercise test. The gas exchange ratio, which did not differ among the groups below the *LAT*, increased abruptly at work rates above the *LAT*. This reflects the increased rate of carbon dioxide production at work rates above the *LAT*.

Summary

Although many theories have been raised on ventilatory control during exercise for over a century,[1,3] the mechanism of exercise hyperpnea in patients with cardiovascular disease has not been well understood. We hypothesized that if increased ventilation in these patients resulted from exercise lactic acidosis, this increase in ventilation would be manifest only at work rates above the *LAT*—not below the threshold. There was no difference in the slope of the increase in ventilation to the increase in $\dot{V}O_2$ below the *LAT* between normal subjects and cardiac patients or among cardiac patients. This must indicate that the required ventilation is the same among normal subjects and cardiac patients despite the difference in the severity of heart failure, when performing exercise by aerobic metabolism alone. However, the slope of the increase in ventilation to the increase in $\dot{V}O_2$ at work rates above the *LAT* was significantly higher in heart failure patients than in normal subjects. These findings are consistent with the results of normal subjects, in whom oxygen transport was experimentally reduced by increasing carboxyhemoglobin levels. Exercise lactic acidosis in patients with cardiovascular disease must be caused by decreased oxygen transport to the working muscles and/or by decreased ability to use oxygen efficiently due to skeletal muscle deconditioning. The hydrogen ion produced during the lactic acidosis is probably the main respiratory stimulus at work rates above the *LAT* in these patients. These data strongly suggest that the increased ventilation during exercise, which must contribute to the symptom of exertional dyspnea in heart failure patients, is primarily the consequence of stimuli to regulate arterial pH.

References

1. Wasserman K, Whipp BJ, Casaburi R: Respiratory control during exercise. In: Fishman AP, ed. *Handbook of Physiology*. Bethesda, Maryland: American Physiological Society, 595–619, 1986.
2. Sullivan MJ, Higginbotham MB, Cobb FR: Increased exercise ventilation in patients with chronic heart failure: intact ventilatory control despite hemodynamic and pulmonary abnormalities. *Circulation* 77:552–559, 1988.
3. Paterson DJ: Potassium and ventilation in exercise. *J Appl Physiol* 72:811–820, 1992.
4. Linton RAF, Band DM: The effect of potassium on carotid chemoreceptor activity and ventilation in the cat. *Respir Physiol* 59:65–70, 1985.
5. Paterson DJ, Friedland JS, Bascom ID, et al: Changes in arterial K^+ and ventilation during exercise in normal subjects and subjects with McArdle's syndrome. *J Physiol* (London) 429:339–348, 1990.
6. Koike A, Wasserman K, Armon Y, et al: The work-rate-dependent effect of carbon monoxide on ventilatory control during exercise. *Respir Physiol* 85:169–183, 1991.
7. Koike A, Hiroe M, Taniguchi K, et al: Respiratory control during exercise in patients with cardiovascular disease. *Am Rev Respir Dis* 147:425–429, 1993.
8. Pirnay F, Dujardin J, Deroanne R, et al: Muscular exercise during intoxication by carbon monoxide. *J Appl Physiol* 31:573–575, 1971.
9. Ekblom B, Huot R: Response to submaximal and maximal exercise at different levels of carboxyhemoglobin. *Acta Physiol Scand* 86:474–482, 1972.

10. Vogel JA, Gleser MA: Effect of carbon monoxide on oxygen transport during exercise. *J Appl Physiol* 32:234–239, 1972.
11. Raven PB, Drinkwater BL, Ruhling RO, et al: Effect of carbon monoxide and peroxyacetyl nitrate on man's maximal aerobic capacity. *J Appl Physiol* 36:288–293, 1974.
12. Horvath SM, Bedi JF, Wagner JA, et al: Maximal aerobic capacity at several ambient concentrations of CO at several altitudes. *J Appl Physiol* 65: 2696–2708, 1988.
13. Koike A, Wasserman K, McKenzie DK, et al: Evidence that diffusion limitation determines oxygen uptake kinetics during exercise in humans. *J Clin Invest* 86:1698–1706, 1990.
14. Koike A, Weiler-Ravell D, McKenzie DK, et al: Evidence that the metabolic acidosis threshold is the anaerobic threshold. *J Appl Physiol* 68:2521–2526, 1990.
15. Comroe JH Jr, Schmidt CF: The part played by reflexes from the carotid body in the chemical regulation of respiration in the dog. *Am J Physiol* 121: 75–97, 1938.
16. Chiodi H, Dill DB, Consolazio F, et al: Respiratory and circulatory responses to acute carbon monoxide poisoning. *Am J Physiol* 134:683–693, 1941.
17. Duke HN, Green JH, Neil E: Carotid chemoreceptor impulse activity during inhalation of carbon monoxide mixtures. *J Physiol* (London) 118: 520–527, 1952.
18. Beaver WL, Wasserman K, Whipp BJ: A new method for detecting anaerobic threshold by gas exchange. *J Appl Physiol* 60:2020–2027, 1986.
19. Sue DY, Wasserman K, Moricca RB, et al: Metabolic acidosis during exercise in patients with chronic obstructive pulmonary disease. *Chest* 94:931–938, 1988.
20. Wasserman K: Physiologic basis of exercise testing. In: Fishman AP, ed. *Pulmonary Diseases and Disorders*. New York: McGraw-Hill Book Company, 337–347, 1980.
21. Wasserman K: New concepts in assessing cardiovascular function. *Circulation* 78:1060–1071, 1988.
22. Koike A, Hiroe M, Adachi H, et al: Anaerobic metabolism as an indicator of aerobic function during exercise in cardiac patients. *J Am Coll Cardiol* 20:120–126, 1992.
23. Wasserman K, Beaver WL, Whipp BJ: Gas exchange theory and the lactic acidosis (anaerobic) threshold. *Circulation* (suppl II)81:14–30, 1990.
24. Itoh H, Koike A, Taniguchi K, et al: Severity and pathophysiology of heart failure on the basis of anaerobic threshold (*AT*) and related parameters. *Jpn Circulation J* 53:146–154, 1989.

10

Ventilatory and Arterial Blood Gas Changes During Exercise in Heart Failure

Marco Metra, MD; Domenica Raccagni, MD
Gianni Carini, MD; Fulvio Orzan, MD
Antimo Papa, MD; Savina Nodari, MD
Robert J. Cody, MD; Livio Dei Cas, MD

Exertional dyspnea and fatigue are the main symptoms of patients with chronic heart failure (HF). Their pathogenesis is complex as it depends on the interaction of many hemodynamic, pulmonary, vascular, muscular, and humoral factors.[1-3] Among them, the ventilatory response to exercise occupies an important role as shown both by its correlation with exercise capacity, and by its changes after interventions which improve functional capacity.

Patients with HF have, compared with normal subjects, an increased minute ventilation ($\dot{V}E$) at matched workloads. In contrast, at peak exercise, because of the lower workload attained, they reach a lower $\dot{V}E$.[3-15] This exercise hyperpnea is mainly caused by an increased respiratory rate, whereas tidal volume may not be significantly changed in comparison with normal subjects.[5,8,11,14] Patients with HF, therefore, use a pattern of rapid, shallow breathing which is less efficient than normal. As many investigators have shown,[5,9,11,13] this increase in the ventilatory response relative to the workload, oxygen uptake and carbon dioxide output ($\dot{V}O_2$ and $\dot{V}CO_2$) values attained, occurs throughout exercise both below and above the anaerobic thresh-

From Wasserman, K (ed): *Exercise Gas Exchange in Heart Disease*. Armonk, NY: Futura Publishing Company, Inc., © 1996.

old (*AT*). Therefore, it cannot be related to an earlier than normal metabolic acidosis, but rather to other mechanisms operating in HF.

Assessment of the Ventilatory Response to Exercise

The $\dot{V}E$ attained at peak exercise is highly dependent on the peak exercise workload and peak $\dot{V}O_2$. Peak exercise $\dot{V}E$ is reduced in patients with HF, compared with normal subjects, and may increase following interventions which increase peak exercise capacity.[16–18] Peak exercise $\dot{V}E$, however, cannot be considered as an index of the ventilatory response to exercise. The ventilatory response to exercise is determined by a complex interaction of many factors (Table 1) and, thus, $\dot{V}E$ should not be assessed as an absolute value without reference to metabolic or work-rate status. As one of the most important factors is maintenance of the constancy of arterial blood gases, namely arterial carbon dioxide partial pressure ($PaCO_2$),[19,20] the ventilatory response to exercise is often assessed using the relation between $\dot{V}E$ and $\dot{V}CO_2$ during exercise (Table 2).[7–12]

During exercise, $\dot{V}E$ increases linearly with $\dot{V}CO_2$ up to high work rates, above the *AT*, when lactic acidosis becomes prominent enough to cause a further increase of $\dot{V}E$ disproportionate to $\dot{V}CO_2$.[19,20] As $\dot{V}E$ is closely and linearly related with $\dot{V}CO_2$, the ventilatory response to exercise can be estimated using the slope of $\dot{V}E$ versus $\dot{V}CO_2$ (Figure 1).[9–11] This slope is significantly steeper in patients with HF compared with

---

Table 1

Determinants of the Ventilatory Response to Exercise

- Hemodynamics
  Pulmonary pressures
    Lung compliance
    Juxtacapillary receptor stimulation
  Exercise cardiac output
    Ventilation/ perfusion mismatch
- Arterial chemoreceptors control (maintenance of arterial blood gases and pH constancy)
  Pulmonary dead space/ tidal volume ratio
    Pulmonary ventilation/ perfusion mismatch (hemodynamics)
    Alveolar-capillary gas diffusion capacity
    Breathing pattern
  Skeletal muscle lactic acidosis
- Arterial chemoreceptor sensitivity
- Central nervous system control
- Plasma potassium
- Skeletal muscle dependent mechanisms (metaboreceptors? mechanoreceptors?)

Table 2

Variables Used to Assess the Ventilatory Response to Exercise

- Peak exercise minute ventilation ($\dot{V}E$)(L/min) (16–18)
- Peak exercise $\dot{V}E/\dot{V}CO_2$ (8)
- Calculated $\dot{V}E$ at $\dot{V}CO_2 = 1$ L/min (7)
- Slope of the relation between $\dot{V}E$ and $\dot{V}CO_2$ (9–11)
- Final/rest $\dot{V}E/\dot{V}CO_2$ ratio (12)

normal subjects[9–11] and is inversely related to other variables which measure maximal exercise capacity, namely peak $\dot{V}O_2$.[9,11] We found significant inverse correlations between the slope of $\dot{V}E$ versus $\dot{V}CO_2$ and peak exercise workload, peak $\dot{V}O_2$, and the AT in a group of 68 patients with HF.[11] Similar results were obtained in a larger group of 266 consecutive patients with left ventricular dysfunction (ejection fraction $\leq 45\%$) (r value between the slope of $\dot{V}E$ versus $\dot{V}CO_2$ and peak $\dot{V}O_2 = -0.41$; p< 0.001) (Figure 2). It must be noted, however, that this correlation was present mainly in the 185 patients with an impaired functional capacity

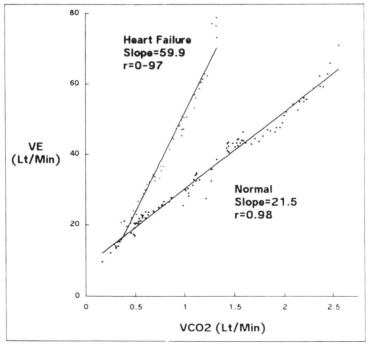

Figure 1. Assessment of the slope of the $\dot{V}E$ versus $\dot{V}CO_2$ relation in a normal subject and a patient with chronic heart failure. (Reproduced with permission from Reference 11.)

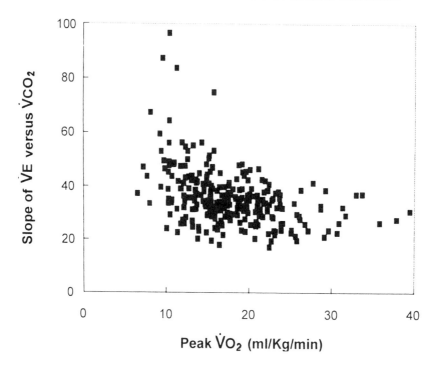

Figure 2. Correlation between the slope of exercise ventilation versus carbon dioxide production and peak $\dot{V}O_2$, normalized to body weight, in 266 patients with chronic heart failure (left ventricular ejection fraction < 45%).

(peak $\dot{V}O_2$ < 20 mL/kg/min) (r value = −0.35; p<0.001) whereas it was not significant in the remaining patients with a peak $\dot{V}O_2$ ⩾ 20 mL/kg/ min. This is in accordance with previous studies which showed the absence of a significant relation between the slope of $\dot{V}E$ versus $\dot{V}CO_2$ and peak $\dot{V}O_2$ in normal subjects,[10,11,21] and suggests that maximal exercise performance becomes dependent on ventilation only when exercise capacity is severely limited, but not in healthy subjects or patients with left ventricular dysfunction and normal functional capacity.

Unlike peak $\dot{V}O_2$, which is significantly related to age,[22,23] the slope of the relation between $\dot{V}E$ and $\dot{V}CO_2$ is not influenced by age. In our study group of 266 patients with left ventricular dysfunction, peak $\dot{V}O_2$ was related to age (r = −0.33; p<0.001), but the slope of $\dot{V}E$ versus $\dot{V}CO_2$ was not (r = 0.07; n.s.).

The slope of $\dot{V}E$ versus $\dot{V}CO_2$ during exercise may be used as an objective measure of the functional capacity of patients with HF. However, its values may differ when maximal or submaximal, below *AT*, efforts are performed. In fact, the $\dot{V}E/\dot{V}CO_2$ ratio does not remain constant during exercise, but rather, by the end of exercise, $\dot{V}E$ tends to rise more steeply than $\dot{V}CO_2$ with a consequent increase of the $\dot{V}E/\dot{V}CO_2$ ratio. This was first described in normal subjects in whom a phase of respiratory compensation for lactic acidosis follows the isocapnic buffering period at high work rates, [19,20] and a similar or even more evident pattern was observed in patients with chronic HF.[12] This increase of the $\dot{V}E/\dot{V}CO_2$ ratio at the end of exercise is also reflected in the slope of $\dot{V}E$ versus $\dot{V}CO_2$. In fact, we[11] and other investigators[24] have shown that the value of this slope is underestimated when data from only the first part of exercise are used compared with all the data from a maximal exercise test. Despite these limits, the slope of $\dot{V}E$ versus $\dot{V}CO_2$ has been widely used to assess the ventilatory response to exercise and has been shown to be sensitive to interventions which improve functional capacity like physical training[25–27] and heart transplantation.[28]

Another measure proposed to overcome the limits of the slope of $\dot{V}E$ versus $\dot{V}CO_2$ is the ratio between the $\dot{V}E/\dot{V}CO_2$ at the end of exercise compared to the resting value.[12] This parameter has been shown to correlate with exercise capacity.[12] However, it is dependent on the resting $\dot{V}E/\dot{V}CO_2$ ratio which is often relatively high, because of hyperventilation, presumably caused by patient anxiety and unrelated to the patient's clinical or hemodynamic condition.

Mechanisms of Exercise Hyperpnea in Heart Failure

The control of the ventilatory response to exercise is complex, as many factors may contribute to it (Table 1). Some of the factors unique to HF are summarized in the next paragraphs.

Pulmonary Pressures

Pulmonary hypertension might stimulate the ventilatory response to exercise both through a reduction of lung compliance and the activation of pulmonary juxtacapillary receptors which may sense the increased intravascular pressures.[1] These mechanisms probably operate in patients with mitral valve disease,[4,29] but do not seem to be active in patients with HF caused by postinfarction or idiopathic dilated cardiomyopathy. In fact, no significant relationship was found between both pulmonary arterial and pulmonary capillary pressures and the ventilatory response to exercise in these patients.[7,8,11] Moreover, the ventilatory response to exercise is not modified by an acute reduction of pulmonary pressures obtained after the administration of either dobutamine or prazosin.[7]

Two other mechanisms might cause the abnormal ventilatory response to exercise of the patients with HF: mechanisms aimed to maintain constancy of arterial blood gases and pH and/or mechanisms which stimulate ventilation independently from any control of arterial blood gases. If the first were active, we should postulate that the patients with HF present a normal respiratory control, and that the increase of the ventilatory response to exercise compensates other abnormalities, such as an increase in the pulmonary dead space to tidal volume ratio, which should tend to alter arterial blood gas composition.[8] In contrast, if non-CO_2, non-pH dependent mechanisms were active, patients should present an increase of $\dot{V}E$ unrelated to arterial blood gas homeostasis.

Increased Pulmonary Dead Space

Many mechanisms may alter the arterial blood gas composition and pH during exercise in the patients with HF. The reduced cardiac output response to exercise of the patients with HF may cause uneven lung perfusion with a secondary increase of the ventilation/perfusion mismatch. This will cause the pulmonary physiological dead space to tidal volume ratio (VD/VT) to increase. In accordance with this hypothesis, peak exercise cardiac output has been shown to correlate inversely with VD/VT.[8] In our experience, peak exercise cardiac output and VD/VT were the only two variables independently related, at multivariate regression analysis, to the slope of $\dot{V}E$ versus $\dot{V}CO_2$.[11] The increase in VD/VT in patients with HF may impair pulmonary gas exchange with secondary arterial hypoxemia and/or hypercapnia which, sensed by the arterial chemoreceptors, might increase the ventilatory drive. Accordingly, the ability to decrease the ventilation/perfusion mismatch during exercise has been shown to be related to a better functional capacity in patients with HF.[15]

Another factor which might impair pulmonary gas exchange is a reduction in the alveolar-capillary gas diffusion capacity. Patients with HF may have a reduction in the resting pulmonary diffusion capacity to carbon monoxide [30–32] and this measurement is directly related to peak $\dot{V}O_2$.[33] It has been shown that the reduction of lung gas diffusion capacity is not caused by a decreased pulmonary capillary blood volume, but rather by reduced permeability of the alveolar-capillary membrane to carbon monoxide, presumably secondary to interstitial edema and/or fibrosis.[34,35]

A third factor which might increase the VD/VT during exercise in patients with HF is an abnormal breathing pattern. Because these patients tend to have an increased respiratory rate with a small increase in tidal volume, compared with normal subjects,[5,8,10,11,14] VD/VT may not decrease normally during exercise.

Thus, if maintenance of arterial blood gas homeostasis were the main mechanism stimulating ventilation in HF, we should speculate that the uneven lung perfusion, reduction in the alveolar diffusion capacity, and abnormal breathing pattern determine an increase of V_D/V_T with secondary arterial hypoxemia and/or hypercapnia which, sensed by the carotid bodies, increases the ventilatory drive. In accordance with this hypothesis, many investigators have found an increase in the V_D/V_T in patients with HF with a significant direct correlation between this variable and the ventilatory response to exercise.[6,10,11,13,16,36] In our study, peak exercise V_D/V_T was the single most important determinant of the $\dot{V}_E$ versus $\dot{V}_{CO_2}$ slope at multivariate stepwise regression analysis (Figure 3).[11] Similar results were obtained in a previous study.[8]

However, the finding of a significant correlation between V_D/V_T and the ventilatory response to exercise does not necessarily mean the existence of a cause and effect relationship. It might be that both variables, V_D/V_T and $\dot{V}_E$, are dependent on some other common factor.[37] For example, an abnormal increase of $\dot{V}_E$ during exercise, caused by a non-CO_2, non-pH dependent mechanism, might alter the respiratory pattern so that the increase of V_D/V_T is secondary to, and not a cause of, increased $\dot{V}_E$.[38] Both the increased V_D/V_T and increased ventilatory drive might be expressions of a more advanced HF state with a greater

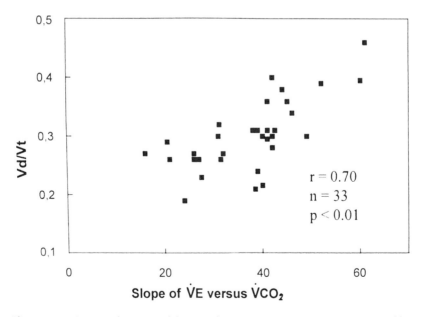

Figure 3. V_D/V_T as a function of the ventilatory response to exercise, assessed by the slope of $\dot{V}_E$ versus $\dot{V}_{CO_2}$ during exercise, in patients with heart failure.

impairment of cardiac output, reflex control mechanisms, and a greater alteration of skeletal muscle function.

Exercise Arterial Blood Gas Changes in Heart Failure

If the increase in VD/VT was the only mechanism which stimulates the ventilatory drive, arterial hypoxemia and hypercapnia may develop during exercise in patients with HF. In contrast, arterial oxygen saturation tends to remain constant whereas PaO_2 tends to increase and $PaCO_2$ to decrease without an increase in pH (no respiratory alkalosis), from rest to exercise, in the majority of the studies performed in patients with HF (Table 3).[8,11,36,39–43] Moreover, in the studies in which exercise blood gases were compared between patients with HF and normal subjects, no significant difference was found except for a tendency to a lower $PaCO_2$ and a higher pH during exercise in patients with HF, compared with normal subjects (Table 4).[8,39,40,42] These changes are opposite to what should happen if uneven ventila-

---

Table 3

Exercise Induced Changes of Arterial Blood Gases in Patients with Chronic Heart Failure: Comparison with Resting Data

Author	SaO_2	PaO_2	$PaCO_2$	pH
Rajfer et al., 1987 (36)		▲	▽	=
Sullivan et al., 1988 (8)		▲	(▽)	=
Roubin et al., 1990 (39)	=	=	=	=
Hachamovitch et al., 1991 (40)	=	=	▽	=
Moore et al., 1992 (41)	(▽)			
Metra et al., 1992 (11)	=		(▽)	=
Barlow et al., 1994 (42)		=	=	=
Clark and Coats, 1994 (43)	=	=	▽	▽

Table 4

Arterial Blood Gases in Patients with Chronic Heart Failure vs. Normal Subjects

Author	SaO_2	PaO_2	$PaCO_2$	pH
Sullivan et al., 1990 (8)	=	▽ (rest)	=	▲ (ex)
Roubin et al., 1990 (39)	=	=	▽ (ex)	▲ (ex)
Hachamovitch et al., 1991 (40)	=	=	=	▲
Barlow et al., 1994 (42)	=	=		▲

tion/perfusion matching was the only factor affecting blood gases and the ventilatory response to exercise in patients with HF.

Metabolic Acidosis

Studies conducted using phosphorus-31 nuclear magnetic resonance have definitively shown that patients with HF present an earlier and greater metabolic acidosis during exercise compared with normal subjects.[3,44,45] These changes are more evident in patients with a more severe functional limitation and are related to inadequate skeletal muscle perfusion, reduced muscle mass, and biochemical abnormalities occurring in the skeletal muscle.[3] As arterial chemoreceptors are highly sensitive to metabolic acidosis, this might be one of the main causes of the heightened ventilatory drive of patients with HF.

In accordance with this last hypothesis, in one study, the $\dot{V}E/\dot{V}O_2$ ratio was found to be increased, in comparison with normal subjects, only at a $\dot{V}O_2$ above the AT, with a steeper increase in the patients with more severe functional limitation.[46] These data suggest that the increase of $\dot{V}E$ in HF is a compensatory mechanism to a greater lactic acidosis. However, in this study, the majority of HF patients had NYHA functional class I–II. In contrast, patients with a more severe functional limitation may present an increased ventilatory drive also at low work rates, below the AT,[5,9,11,13] as shown both by an increase of their $\dot{V}E$ relative to $\dot{V}CO_2$ (Figure 1) and by an increase of the slope of $\dot{V}E$ versus $\dot{V}CO_2$ calculated using data from the entire exercise test (Figure 2). Moreover, despite the earlier and greater lactic acidosis occurring in their skeletal muscle, patients with a more severe functional limitation do not generally develop a greater decrease of systemic arterial pH during exercise (Table 4).[8,39,41,42] Thus, non-pH dependent mechanisms must be considered as possible factors contributing to the heightened ventilatory drive of patients with more severe HF.

Non-CO$_2$, Non-pH Dependent Mechanisms

Many non-CO$_2$, non-pH dependent mechanisms can stimulate ventilation[20]; however, data which can definitively clarify their role are still lacking. An impairment of the control of respiration by the central nervous system does not seem to be present in HF, as arterial blood gases tend to remain normal during exercise (Tables 3 and 4).[8,11,36,39–43] Differences may, however, be present between patients with a normal or slightly decreased functional capacity and those more severely limited. While ventilatory control appears to be normal at low work rates in patients with mild HF,[10,11,46] exercise hyperpnea in patients with more severe HF might be explained by an altered regulation of $\dot{V}E$ by a lower than normal central $PaCO_2$ "set point" and / or by an increased sensitivity of carotid bodies and aortic chemoreceptors accompanying a reduced PaO_2.

Another mechanism stimulating ventilation might be an increased plasma potassium during exercise. Potassium is released from the skeletal muscles during exercise with a consequent hyperkalemia which has been correlated with the ventilatory response.[42,47,48] Moreover, the improvement of functional capacity obtained after physical training is accompanied both by a reduction of the ventilatory response to exercise, and by a decrease of plasma potassium levels in patients with HF.[42]

Skeletal muscles might also influence ventilation. Muscular receptors, sensitive to either stretching (mechanoreceptors), acidosis, or other metabolic abnormalities (metaboreceptors), might stimulate the ventilatory response to exercise.[49,50] These receptors seem to have a limited role, or no role at all, in the control of ventilation in normal subjects.[20] In fact, no change of $\dot{V}E$ was detected when nervous transmission or blood flow from skeletal muscles was interrupted.[51,52] However, as skeletal muscles undergo deep biochemical and functional changes in patients with HF,[3,45,53–5] they might become able to stimulate ventilation. In accordance with this hypothesis, it has been shown that independent from any change in $\dot{V}O_2$, $\dot{V}E$ can be influenced by the muscle group performing the work, in patients with HF.[56] The existence of a link between skeletal muscle function and $\dot{V}E$ is also suggested by the observation that the ventilatory response to exercise can be reduced by whole-body training,[25–27] but not by selective respiratory muscle training,[57] despite the increase in exercise capacity with both methods.

Relationship Between the Ventilatory Response to Exercise and Hemodynamics, Functional Capacity, and Exercise Arterial Blood Gases of Patients with Heart Failure

An important limitation of previous HF studies is that patients were considered as a homogeneous study group despite the existence of high variability in their functional capacity.[1,5,11,33,39,58–60] Differences in the severity of HF might have influenced the ventilatory responses to exercise and might explain differences between studies. We therefore evaluated the hemodynamic, respiratory, and arterial blood gas changes during exercise in a group of patients with chronic stable HF subdivided on the basis of their ventilatory response.

We studied 21 patients with chronic HF caused by postinfarction (9 patients) or idiopathic dilated (12 patients) cardiomyopathy who were clinically stable in the 3 months before the study. All patients had significant left ventricular dysfunction, shown by an ejection fraction ≤35%. They had no major arrhythmias or signs of myocardial ischemia on at least two preliminary cardiopulmonary exercise tests.

All patients underwent right heart catheterization and radial artery cannulation to obtain central hemodynamic variables, systemic arterial and mixed venous blood gases during exercise. Bicycle cardiopulmonary exercise testing was performed with workload increments of 20W/2min up to limiting fatigue and/or dyspnea. Minute ventilation, $\dot{V}O_2$, and $\dot{V}CO_2$ were obtained breath-by-breath (2001 Medical Graphics equipment). Hemodynamic variables, systemic, and pulmonary arterial blood sampling were obtained at each workload.

The ventilatory response to exercise was quantified by the slope of $\dot{V}E$ versus $\dot{V}CO_2$.[11] Pulmonary VD/VT was calculated using the Bohr equation.[61] Effective alveolar ventilation (VA) was calculated as $VA = \dot{V}E \times (1 - VD/VT)$ using the modified alveolar gas equation $\dot{V}E = 863 \times \dot{V}CO_2/(PaCO_2 \times (1 - VD/VT))$[20]; this allowed calculation of the $VA/\dot{V}CO_2$ ratio.[61] Measurements of VD/VT, $\dot{V}E$ and its derived parameters were obtained after subtraction of the volume of the apparatus dead space.

Patients were subdivided into two groups on the basis of the mean value of the slope of the $\dot{V}E$ versus $\dot{V}CO_2$ relation: patients in the first group had a normal or slightly increased ventilatory response to exercise with a slope < 40 (range 21 to 37); patients in the second group had a slope > 40 (range 41 to 64). Baseline characteristics of the patient group are summarized in Table 5. Resting and peak exercise hemodynamic data, and arterial blood gas values in patients considered globally and subdivided on the basis of their $\dot{V}E/\dot{V}CO_2$ slope, are summarized in Tables 6 and 7, respectively.

In our study group, the 11 patients with HF showing an increased ventilatory response to exercise (slope of $\dot{V}E$ versus $\dot{V}CO_2$ > 40) had worse clinical and functional features (Table 5), hemodynamics (Table 6), and gas exchange efficiency (Table 7) in comparison with the others (slope of $\dot{V}E$ versus $\dot{V}CO_2$ < 40). Also, regulation of arterial acid-base balance during exercise was significantly different (Table 7). In patients with an excessive ventilatory response, the $\dot{V}E/\dot{V}CO_2$ ratio remained high throughout exercise with a tendency to a further rise by the end of exercise (Table 7); in contrast, in patients with a slope of $\dot{V}E$ versus $\dot{V}CO_2$ < 40, the $\dot{V}E/\dot{V}E_2$ ratio decreased at the start and remained low during exercise. These different behaviors have been previously described by Clark et al.[12] As expected, because of the close correlation between VD/VT and the ventilatory response to exercise,[8,11,13,38] the

Table 5

Clinical and Functional Features for Total Group (n = 21) and for Those Patients with a Slope of $\dot{V}E$ Versus $\dot{V}CO_2$ < 40 (n = 10) and > 40 (n = 11)

	Total	Slope <40	Slope >40	Significance
Age (years)	54 ± 14	53 ± 17	54 ± 13	n.s.
NYHA Class	2.48 ± 0.60	2.00 ± 0.50	2.83 ± 0.39	0.001
LV Ejection Fraction (%)	17 ± 8	23 ± 9	13 ± 3	0.012
Peak $\dot{V}O_2$ (mL/kg/min)	16 ± 5	20 ± 3	14 ± 4	0.001
Peak $\dot{V}O_2$ (% predicted)	58 ± 20	76 ± 17	44 ± 7	0.0003
AT (mL/kg/min)	11 ± 3	13 ± 2	10 ± 3	0.05
Peak $\dot{V}CO_2/\dot{V}O_2$	1.09 ± 0.07	1.08 ± 0.07	1.09 ± 0.08	n.s.
Slope of $\dot{V}E$ versus $\dot{V}CO_2$	41 ± 12	30 ± 6	49 ± 8	<0.0001

Abbreviations: Slope = slope of the relation between $\dot{V}E$ and $\dot{V}CO_2$ during exercise; AT = anaerobic threshold; significance = significance between data of patients with $\dot{V}E$ versus $\dot{V}CO_2$ slope < and > 40.

Table 6

Hemodynamic Variables at Rest and Peak Exercise for Total group (n = 21) and for Those Patients with a Slope of $\dot{V}E$ Versus $\dot{V}CO_2$ < 40 (n = 10) and > 40 (n = 11)

	Total	Slope <40	Slope >40	Significance
Heart rate (beats/min)				
Rest	84 ± 15	75 ± 11	93 ± 13	0.003
Peak Exercise	145 ± 22	142 ± 25	149 ± 20	n.s.
MAP (mHg)				
Rest	90 ± 11	95 ± 11	85 ± 9	0.04
Peak exercise	105 ± 16	112 ± 19	98 ± 11	0.05
CI (L/min/m²)				
Rest	2.26 ± 0.43	2.45 ± 0.42	2.09 ± 0.38	0.05
Peak exercise	5.06 ± 1.90	6.24 ± 1.88	3.98 ± 1.19	0.005
PWP (mmHg)				
Rest	19 ± 6	16 ± 6	21 ± 6	n.s.
Peak exercise	42 ± 14	40 ± 17	43 ± 11	n.s.
RAP (mmHg)				
Rest	3 ± 3	2 ± 2	5 ± 4	0.05
Peak exercise	9 ± 5	7 ± 3	11 ± 5	0.05

Abbreviations: MAP = mean arterial pressure; CI = cardiac index; PWP = pulmonary wedge pressure; RAP = right atrial pressure; other abbreviations as in Table 5.

Table 7

Respiratory Variables and Arterial Blood Gasses During Exercise for Total Group (n = 21) and for Those Patients with a Slope of $\dot{V}E$ Versus $\dot{V}CO_2 < 40$ (n = 10) and > 40 (n = 11)

	Total	Slope <40	Slope >40	Significance
$\dot{V}E/\dot{V}CO_2$				
Rest	51 ± 12	47 ± 13	54 ± 11	n.s.
40% exercise	43 ± 10	37 ± 7	49 ± 8	0.002
80% exercise	42 ± 9	34 ± 6	48 ± 6	<0.0001
Peak exercise	45 ± 13	34 ± 6	55 ± 7	<0.0001
Vd/Vt				
Rest	0.49 ± 0.10	0.47 ± 0.10	0.50 ± 0.11	n.s.
400% exercise	0.38 ± 0.12	0.33 ± 0.12	0.42 ± 0.10	n.s.
80% exercise	0.33 ± 0.11	0.27 ± 0.11	0.38 ± 0.08	0.02
Peak exercise	0.31 ± 0.16	0.19 ± 0.12	0.42 ± 0.09	<0.0001
$Va/\dot{V}CO_2$				
Rest	25 ± 3	24 ± 4	26 ± 3	n.s.
40% exercise	26 ± 4	24 ± 3	28 ± 4	0.03
80% exercise	27 ± 4	25 ± 3	30 ± 4	0.007
Peak exercise	29 ± 4	27 ± 3	32 ± 5	0.01
PaO_2 (mmHg)				
Rest	94 ± 8	92 ± 7	95 ± 9	n.s.
40% exercise	98 ± 11	98 ± 9	99 ± 12	n.s.
80% exercise	103 ± 11	103 ± 9	103 ± 13	n.s.
Peak exercise	106 ± 12	105 ± 9	107 ± 14	n.s.
$PaCO_2$ (mmHg)				
Rest	35 ± 5	37 ± 6	33 ± 4	n.s.
40% exercise	34 ± 5	36 ± 4	32 ± 5	n.s.
80% exercise	32 ± 5	35 ± 4	30 ± 4	n.s.
Peak exercise	30 ± 4	32 ± 3	28 ± 5	0.03
pH				
Rest	7.43 ± 0.04	7.44 ± 0.06	7.41 ± 0.02	n.s.
40% exercise	7.41 ± 0.03	7.40 ± 0.04	7.42 ± 0.02	n.s.
80% exercise	7.38 ± 0.08	7.33 ± 0.10	7.42 ± 0.01	0.02
Peak exercise	7.37 ± 0.01	7.31 ± 0.12	7.42 ± 0.02	0.02
HCO_{3-} (mEq/L)				
Rest	22 ± 2	23 ± 2	21 ± 2	n.s.
40% exercise	22 ± 2	23 ± 2	21 ± 2	n.s.
80% exercise	20 ± 3	20 ± 3	20 ± 3	n.s.
Peak exercise	18 ± 3	18 ± 2	19 ± 3	n.s.

exercise-induced changes of VD/VT were similar to those of the $\dot{V}E/\dot{V}CO_2$ ratio. Patients with an excessive ventilatory response to exercise presented also an increase of the $VA/\dot{V}CO_2$ ratio (Table 7). Our results differ from those obtained by Sullivan et al[62]; this could be explained by differences in the study groups, with ours including patients with more advanced HF.

Arterial blood gas analysis confirmed that patients with HF and an increase of the slope of $\dot{V}E$ versus $\dot{V}CO_2$ had a high gain ventilatory drive. In fact, while the patients with a normal or slightly increased ventilatory response developed metabolic acidosis by the end of exercise, similar to that described in normal subjects,[19,20] no significant pH change during exercise was observed by arterial blood gas analysis in the patients with increased exercise hyperpnea (Table 7).

These findings are not in contrast to the results of previous studies which show that patients with more advanced HF develop an earlier and greater metabolic acidosis during exercise, measured at the level of the skeletal muscle by nuclear magnetic resonance.[3,44,45] It is possible that patients with more advanced HF have metabolic changes in the skeletal muscles which, during exercise, are accompanied by an excessive stimulation of the ventilatory drive which masks development of arterial metabolic acidosis as measured by arterial blood gas analysis. The cause of this increased ventilatory drive remains to be explained.

Clinical Meaning of the Ventilatory Response to Exercise in Patients with Heart Failure

Despite the controversies regarding its methods of measurement and mechanisms, exercise hyperpnea seems to have an important role in the functional limitation of patients with HF. The ventilatory response to exercise, evaluated both as the peak exercise $\dot{V}E/\dot{V}CO_2$ ratio[8,13] or as the slope of $\dot{V}E$ versus $\dot{V}CO_2$ (Figure 1),[9–11] is inversely related to peak exercise capacity. Interestingly, this relationship is not present in normal subjects.[10,11] Thus, the increased ventilatory response to exercise may be a mechanism limiting exercise capacity in patients with HF.

Lipkin et al[63] first suggested that the excessive ventilatory response to exercise may contribute to the symptom of exertional dyspnea. In their study, the responses to two exercise protocols, based on a rapid or a slow increment of the workload, respectively, were compared. The exercise performed with a rapid workload increment was stopped because of dyspnea in all of the patients and was associated with a significantly increased ventilatory response.[63] A mechanism by which the excessive ventilatory response to exercise can cause the sensation of dyspnea has been suggested by the studies of Mancini et al.[3,14,64] Exercise hyperpnea may cause an increase in the work of the respiratory muscles of patients with HF.[64] An increased oxygen demand by the respiratory muscles concomitant with the reduction of the cardiac output response to exercise may cause hypoperfusion and deoxygenation of the respiratory muscles[14] with the sensation of dyspnea. Accordingly, selective respiratory muscle training has been shown to reduce the sensation of exertional dyspnea in patients with HF.[57] The role of the ventilatory response to exercise is also shown by its improvement after interventions which increase functional capacity, as with angiotensin converting enzyme inhibitor therapy,[65] physical rehabilitation,[25–27] and heart transplantation.[28]

Conclusions

Patients with HF have an increased ventilatory response to exercise shown by the increase in $\dot{V}E$ relative to the workload, $\dot{V}O_2$, and $\dot{V}CO_2$ attained. This ventilatory response can be quantified by the slope of the relation between $\dot{V}E$ aud $\dot{V}CO_2$ during exercise.

The mechanisms of exercise hyperpnea in HF are still unsettled. A first hypothesis was that it is a compensatory response to increased VD/VT in order to maintain arterial blood gas and pH constancy. However, other mechanisms, namely an increased sensitivity of the arterial chemoreceptors and/or the activation of reflexes by the abnormal skeletal muscles, may be important.

The excessive ventilatory response to exercise is probably one of the main factors contributing to the limitation of the functional capacity of patients with HF. This is shown by the inverse relation between it and peak exercise capacity in patients with HF, and by its reduction concomitant with an improvement of functional capacity after physical training or heart transplantation. Exercise hyperpnea may increase the work of the respiratory muscles which, in association with their reduced perfusion, may cause sufficient muscle deoxygenation to contribute to the sensation of dyspnea.

Summary

Patients with heart failure (HF) present an increased ventilatory response to exercise with an increase in minute ventilation ($\dot{V}E$) relative to workload, $\dot{V}O_2$, and $\dot{V}CO_2$. Minute ventilation should not be measured in absolute units, but relative to one of its main determinants, e.g., $\dot{V}CO_2$. As $\dot{V}E$ is closely correlated to $\dot{V}CO_2$ during exercise, the ventilatory response to exercise has been quantified using the slope of the relation of $\dot{V}E$ versus $\dot{V}CO_2$. This slope is significantly steeper in patients with HF compared with normal subjects, and is inversely correlated with peak $\dot{V}O_2$ in patients with HF with a significant impairment of exercise capacity.

The mechanisms of exercise hyperpnea in HF are still unclear. A first hypothesis is that hyperpnea is a compensatory response to the increased physiological dead space to tidal volume ratio (VD/VT) in order to maintain a constant arterial pH. However, as the patients with more marked exercise hyperpnea do not develop arterial acidemia, it is possible that other mechanisms, namely an increased sensitivity of the arterial chemoreceptors and/or the activation of reflexes by the abnormal skeletal muscles, stimulate their ventilatory response, keeping arterial pH relatively constant. The excessive ventilatory response to exercise is probably one of the main factors contributing to the reduction of the functional capacity of patients with HF. This is shown by the inverse relationship between it and peak exercise capacity of patients with HF, and by its reduction concomitant with an improvement in functional capacity after physical training or heart transplantation. In fact, exercise hyperpnea may cause an increase in the work of the respiratory muscles which, in the presence of their reduced perfusion, may sustain their deoxygenation and the sensation of dyspnea.

References

1. Myers J, Froelicher VF: Hemodynamic determinants of exercise capacity in chronic heart failure. *Ann Intern Med* 115:377–386, 1991.
2. Clark A, Coats A: The mechanisms underlying the increased ventilatory response to exercise in chronic stable heart failure. *Eur Heart J* 13:1698–1708, 1992.
3. Wilson JR, Mancini DM: Factors contributing to the exercise limitation of heart failure. *J Am Coll Cardiol* (suppl A)22:93A–98A, 1993.
4. Gazetopolous N, Davies H, Oliver C, Deuchan D: Ventilation and haemodynamics in heart disease. *Br Heart J* 77:552–559, 1966.
5. Weber KT, Kinasewitz GT, Janicki JS, Fishman AP: Oxygen utilization and ventilation during exercise in patients with chronic cardiac failure. *Circulation* 65:1213–1223, 1982.
6. Rubin SA, Brown HV: Ventilation and gas exchange during exercise among patients with severe chronic heart failure. *Am Rev Respir Dis* (suppl)129:563–564, 1984.
7. Fink LI, Wilson JR, Ferraro N: Exercise ventilation and pulmonary artery wedge pressure in chronic stable congestive heart failure. *Am J Cardiol* 57:249–253, 1986.
8. Sullivan MJ, Higginbotham MB, Cobb FR: Increased exercise ventilation in patients with chronic heart failure: intact ventilatory control despite hemodynamic and pulmonary abnormalities. *Circulation* 77:552–559, 1988.
9. Buller NP, Poole-Wilson PA: Mechanism of the increased ventilatory response to exercise in patients with chronic heart failure. *Br Heart J* 63:281–283, 1990.

10. Davies SW, Emery TM, Watling MIL, et al: A critical threshold of exercise capacity in the ventilatory response to exercise in heart failure. *Br Heart J* 65:179–183, 1991.

11. Metra M, Dei Cas L, Panina G, Visioli O: Exercise hyperventilation in chronic congestive heart failure, and its relation to functional capacity and hemodynamics. *Am J Cardiol* 70:622–628, 1992.

12. Clark AL, Poole-Wilson PA, Coats AJS: Relation between ventilation and carbon dioxide production in patients with chronic heart failure. *J Am Coll Cardiol* 20:1326–1332, 1992.

13. Myers J, Salleh A, Buhanan N, et al: Ventilatory mechanisms of exercise intolerance in chronic heart failure. *Am Heart J* 124:709–710, 1992.

14. Mancini DM, Ferraro N, Nazzaro D, et al: Respiratory muscle deoxygenation during exercise in patients with heart failure demonstrated with near-infrared spectroscopy. *J Am Coll Cardiol* 18:492–498, 1991.

15. Uren NG, Davies SW, Agnew JE, et al: Reduction of mismatch of global ventilation and perfusion on exercise is related to exercise capacity of chronic heart failure. *Br Heart J* 70:241–246, 1993.

16. Sullivan M, Atwood E, Myers J, et al: Increased exercise capacity after digoxin administration in patients with heart failure. *J Am Coll Cardiol* 13:1138–1143, 1989.

17. Metra M, Cannella G, La Canna G, et al: Improvement in exercise capacity after correction of anemia in patients with end-stage renal failure. *Am J Cardiol* 68:1060–1066, 1991.

18. Agostoni PG, Marenzi GC, Pepi M, et al: Isolated ultrafiltration in moderate congestive heart failure. *J Am Coll Cardiol* 21:424–431, 1993.

19. Wasserman K, Whipp BJ, Casaburi R: Respiratory control during exercise. In: Cherniak NS, Widdicombe JG, eds. *Handbook of Physiology,* Vol. 2. Bethesda, MD: American Physiological Society, 595–619, 1986.

20. Wasserman K, Hansen JE, Sue DY, Whipp BJ, Casaburi R: Physiology of exercise. In: Wasserman K, Hansen JE, Sue DY, Whipp BJ, Casaburi R, eds. *Principles of Exercise Testing and Interpretation.* Philadelphia: Lea and Febiger, 9–51, 1994.

21. Clark AL, Swan JW, Laney R, et al: The role of right and left ventricular function in the ventilatory response to exercise in chronic heart failure. *Circulation* 89:2062–2069, 1994.

22. Metra M, Raddino R, Nodari S, et al: Influence of age on the parameters used to quantitate functional capacity in the patients with heart failure (abstr). *Eur Heart J* (suppl)11:213, 1990.

23. Mabee SW, Metra M, Reed DE, et al: Age related changes in hemodynamic response to exercise in patients with chronic congestive heart failure (abstr). *J Am Coll Cardiol* (suppl)23:122A, 1994.

24. Clark AL, Poole-Wilson PA, Coats AJS: Effects of motivation of the patient on indices of exercise capacity in chronic heart failure. *Br Heart J* 71:162–165, 1994.

25. Sullivan MJ, Higginbotham MB, Cobb FR: Exercise training in patients with chronic heart failure delays ventilatory anaerobic threshold and improves submaximal exercise performance. *Circulation* 79:324–329, 1989.

26. Coats AJS, Adamopoulos S, Radaelli A, et al: Controlled trial of physical training in chronic heart failure: exercise performance, hemodynamics, ventilation, and autonomic function. *Circulation* 85:2119–2131, 1992.

27. Davey P, Meyer T, Coats A, et al: Ventilation in chronic heart failure: effects of physical training. *Br Heart J* 68:473–477, 1992.

28. Marzo KP, Wilson JR, Mancini DM: Effects of cardiac transplantation on ventilatory response to exercise. *Am J Cardiol* 69:547–553, 1992.

29. Reed JW, Ablett M, Cotes JE: Ventilatory responses to exercise and to carbon dioxide in mitral stenosis before and after valvulotomy: causes of tachypnoea. *Clin Sci Molecular Med* 54:9–16, 1987.
30. Siegel JL, Miller A, Brown LK, et al: Pulmonary diffusing capacity in left ventricular failure. *Chest* 98:550–553, 1990.
31. Wright RS, Levine MS, Bellamy PE, et al: Ventilatory and diffusion abnormalities in potential heart transplant recipients. *Chest* 98:816–820, 1990.
32. Naum CC, Sciurba FC, Rogers RM: Pulmonary function abnormalities in chronic severe cardiomyopathy preceding cardiac transplantation. *Am Rev Respir Dis* 145:1334–1338, 1992.
33. Kraemer MD, Kubo SH, Rector TS, et al: Pulmonary and peripheral vascular factors are important determinants of peak exercise oxygen uptake in patients with heart failure. *J Am Coll Cardiol* 21:641–648, 1993.
34. Davies SW, Bailey J, Keegan J, et al: Reduced pulmonary microvascular permeability in severe chronic left heart failure. *Am Heart J* 124:137–142, 1992.
35. Puri S, Baker BL, Oakley CM, et al: Increased alveolar/capillary membrane resistance to gas transfer in patients with chronic heart failure. *Br Heart J* 72:140–144, 1994.
36. Rajfer SI, Nemanich JW, Shurman AJ, Rosen JD: Metabolic responses to exercise in patients with heart failure. *Circulation* (suppl VI)76:VI-46–VI-53, 1987.
37. Clark A, Coats A: Mechanisms of exercise intolerance in cardiac failure: abnormalities of skeletal muscle and pulmonary function. *Curr Opinion Card* 9:305–314, 1994.
38. Clark AL, Swan JW, Volterrani M, et al: Dead space ventilation and carbon dioxide tension on exercise in chronic heart failure (abstr). *Eur Heart J* (suppl)15:322, 1994.
39. Roubin GS, Anderson SD, Shen WF, et al: Hemodynamic and metabolic basis of impaired exercise tolerance in patients with severe left ventricular dysfunction. *J Am Coll Cardiol* 15:986–994, 1990.
40. Hachamovitch R, Brown HV, Rubin SA: Respiratory and circulatory analysis of CO_2 output during exercise in chronic heart failure. *Circulation* 84:605–612, 1991.
41. Moore DP, Weston AR, Hughes JMB, et al: Effects of increased inspired oxygen concentrations on exercise performance in chronic heart failure. *Lancet* 339:850–853, 1992.
42. Barlow CW, Qayyum MS, Davey PP, et al: Effect of physical training on exercise-induced hyperkalemia in chronic heart failure. Relation with ventilation and catecholamines. *Circulation* 89:1144–1152, 1994.
43. Clark AL, Coats AJS: Usefulness of arterial blood gas estimations during exercise in patients with chronic heart failure. *Br Heart J* 71:528–530, 1994.
44. Wilson JR, Fink L, Maris J, et al: Evaluation of energy metabolism in skeletal muscle in patients with heart failure with gated phosphorus-31 nuclear magnetic resonance. *Circulation* 71:57–62, 1985.
45. Massie B, Conway M, Yonge R, et al: Skeletal muscle metabolism in patients with congestive heart failure: relation to clinical severity and blood flow. *Circulation* 76:1009–1019, 1987.
46. Koike A, Hiroe M, Taniguchi K, Marumo F: Respiratory control during exercise in patients with cardiovascular disease. *Am Rev Respir Dis* 147:425–429, 1993.
47. Paterson DJ, Robbins PA, Conway J: Changes in arterial plasma potassium and ventilation during exercise in man. *Respir Physiol* 78:323–330, 1989.

48. Paterson DJ: Potassium and ventilation in exercise. *J Appl Physiol* 72:811–820, 1992.
49. Clark AL, Piepoli M, Coats AJ: Evidence for skeletal muscle metabolic receptors driving ventilation on exercise. *Circulation* 88:I-415, 1993.
50. Piepoli M, Clark AL, Coats AJS: Role of the skeletal muscle ergoreceptors in the ventilatory response to exercise (abstr). *Eur Heart J* (suppl)15:323, 1994.
51. Adams L, Frankl J, Garlick J, et al: The role of spinal cord transmission in the ventilatory response to exercise in man. *J Physiol* (Lond) 355:85–97, 1984.
52. Haouzi P, Huszczuk A, Porszasz J, et al: Femoral vascular occlusion and ventilation during recovery from heavy exercise. *Respir Physiol* 94:137–150, 1993.
53. Sullivan MJ, Green HJ, Cobb FR: Skeletal muscle biochemistry and histology in ambulatory patients with long-term heart failure. *Circulation* 81:518–527, 1990.
54. Drexler H, Riede U, Munzel T, et al: Alterations of skeletal muscle in chronic heart failure. *Circulation* 85:1751–1759, 1992.
55. Mancini DM, Walter G, Reichnek N, et al: Contribution of skeletal muscle atrophy to exercise intolerance and altered muscle metabolism in heart failure. *Circulation* 85:1364–1373, 1992.
56. Clark AL, Piepoli M, Coats AJS: Muscle bulk and the ventilatory response to exercise (abstr). *Eur Heart J* (suppl)15:582, 1994.
57. Mancini DM, Henson D, La Manca J, et al: Benefit of selective respiratory muscle training on exercise capacity in patients with chronic congestive heart failure. *Circulation* 91:320–329, 1995.
58. Higginbotham MB, Morris KG, Conn EH, et al: Determinants of variable exercise performance among patients with severe left ventricular dysfunction. *Am J Cardiol* 51:52–60, 1983.
59. Szlachcic J, Massie BM, Kramer BL, et al: Correlates and prognostic implication of exercise capacity in chronic congestive heart failure. *Am J Cardiol* 55:1037–1042, 1985.
60. Metra M, Raddino R, Dei Cas L, Visioli 0: Assessment of peak oxygen consumption, lactate and ventilatory threshold and correlation with the resting and exercise hemodynamic data in chronic congestive heart failure. *Am J Cardiol* 65:1127–1133, 1990.
61. Wasserman K, Hansen JE, Sue DY, Whipp BJ, Casaburi R: Calculations, formulae, and examples. In: Wasserman K, Hansen JE, Sue DY, Whipp BJ, Casaburi R, eds. *Principles of Exercise Testing and Interpretation.* Philadelphia: Lea and Febiger, 454–464, 1994.
62. Sullivan MJ, Cobb FR: The anaerobic threshold in chronic heart failure: relation to blood lactate, ventilatory basis, reproducibility, and response to exercise training. *Circulation* (suppl II)81:II-47–II-58, 1989.
63. Lipkin DP, Canepa-Anson R, Stephens MR, Poole-Wilson PA: Factors determining symptoms in heart failure: comparison of fast and slow exercise tests. *Br Heart J* 55:439–445, 1986.
64. Mancini DM, Henson D, LaManca J, Levine S: Respiratory muscle function aud dyspnea in patients with chronic congestive heart failure. *Circulation* 86:909–918, 1992.
65. Cowley AJ, Rowley JM, Stainer K, Hampton JR: The effect of the angiotensin converting enzyme inhibitor, enalapril, on exercise tolerance and abnormalities of limb blood flow and respiratory function in patients with severe heart failure. *Eur Heart J* 14:964–968, 1993.

11

The Role of Increased Dead Space in the Augmented Ventilation of Cardiac Patients

Toshio Kobayashi, MD; Haruki Itoh, MD
Kazuzo Kato, MD

Augmented Ventilation in Cardiac Patients at Rest and During Exercise

Patients with chronic heart failure (CHF) show an augmented ventilatory response to exercise,[1-4] and the magnitude of this augmented ventilation is related to the severity of CHF.[3,4] However, the pathophysiological mechanisms for this augmented ventilation have not yet been fully understood. It was also reported that patients with CHF showed elevated ventilation even at rest.[5]

One of the main mechanisms of exercise hyperpnea in patients with heart failure has been reported to be increased dead space ventilation due to an altered breathing pattern, namely rapid and shallow breathing.[3,6-8] It has been suggested that elevation of pulmonary capillary pressure during exercise reduces lung compliance through accumulation of interstitial fluid.[9,10] Studies in patients with valvular heart disease suggested that the elevated pulmonary capillary wedge pressure during exercise plays an important role in causing dyspnea by decreasing lung compliance.[2,7] This may have resulted from stimulating pulmonary juxtacapillary receptors leading to hyperventilation.[6,8]

From Wasserman, K (ed): *Exercise Gas Exchange in Heart Disease.* Armonk, NY: Futura Publishing Company, Inc., © 1996.

An additional mechanism of this hyperpnea is suggested to be the increased physiological dead space secondary to a ventilation/perfusion mismatch.[5,11–13] Increased pulmonary capillary pressure in patients with heart failure may produce interstitial pulmonary edema that could increase perivascular pressure and lead to maldistribution of pulmonary blood flow.[14] It is reported that maximal cardiac output was inversely related to the ratio of total dead space to tidal volume (V_D/V_T), which suggested that reduced lung perfusion during exercise may accentuate ventilation/perfusion mismatching and increase pulmonary dead space.[5]

Another mechanism which would cause increased ventilation in chronic heart failure is the early appearance of lactic acidosis during exercise.[3,15,16] It is reported that the onset of anaerobic metabolism during exercise is related to the functional capacity of cardiac patients.[16] A higher lactic acid production might lead to increased carbon dioxide output ($\dot{V}CO_2$) since lactic acid buffering by bicarbonate generates additional carbon dioxide, and also lactic acid production might lead to hydrogen ion stimulation of the peripheral chemoreceptors.[17] Possible pathophysiological mechanisms explaining the augmented ventilation in patients with heart failure are illustrated in Figure 1.

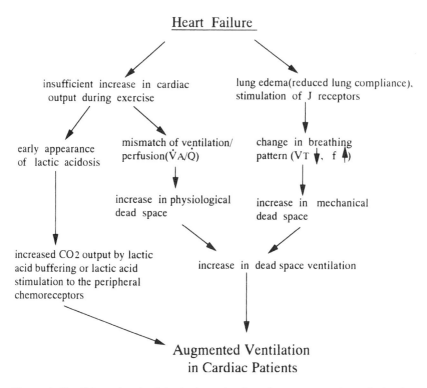

Figure 1. Possible pathophysiological mechanisms for augmented ventilation in cardiac patients.

Exercise Testing with a Face Mask Using a Cycle Ergometer

In Japan, a face mask is preferred to collect the expired gas because this avoids problems of excessive salivation induced by use of a mouthpiece, discomfort of applying a nose clip, and stimulation of the gingiva, which might affect the magnitude and pattern of ventilation. We usually use a face mask with a mechanical dead space of about 0.2 l, and this relatively large dead space of apparatus might affect the magnitude and pattern of ventilation at rest and during exercise, especially in the cardiac patient.

We used 14 patients with CHF and 9 healthy volunteers. According to the functional classification proposed by the New York Heart Association, 6 patients were in class II and 8 in class III. The causes of heart failure were mitral valve regurgitation in 10 patients, and mitral and aortic valve regurgitation in 4 patients. Percent vital capacity (%VC) and forced expiratory volume at 1 second ($FEV_{1.0}\%$) of the patient group were 86.5 $\pm$ 23.0% and 76.7 $\pm$ 12.2% of the predicted values, respectively.

Symptom-limited ramp exercise testing was performed using an upright, electromagnetically-controlled cycle ergometer. After a 4-minute rest period while sitting on the ergometer and 4 minutes of warm-up exercise at a work rate of 20 watts, the subject performed a ramp exercise with an incremental loading rate of 1 watt per 6 seconds up to exhaustion.

The anaerobic threshold (*AT*) was determined by V-slope method, detecting the turning point of the $\dot{V}CO_2$ versus $\dot{V}O_2$ curve.[18] A catheter was placed in the brachial artery for sampling arterial blood. Arterial oxygen, carbon dioxide tensions (PaO_2, $PaCO_2$), and pH were measured by a blood gas analyzer. Cardiac output at rest, during warm up, and every other minute during ramp exercise was measured by dye dilution method with indocyanine green[19] using an ear photometric transducer and a computer.

The ratio of total dead space to tidal volume (V_D/V_T), and effective alveolar ventilation ($\dot{V}_A$) were derived from the following equations: $V_D/V_T = (PaCO_2 - 2\ PECO_2)/PaCO_2$: Bohr equation
$$\dot{V}_A = \dot{V}_E \times (1 - V_D/V_T)$$

Instrument dead space in the system was 0.2 l. Minute ventilation for mechanical dead space ($\dot{V}_D(m)$) and for physiological dead space ($\dot{V}_D(p)$) were calculated by the following equations:

$$\dot{V}_D(m) = 0.2 \times f$$
$$\dot{V}_D(p) = \dot{V}_E - (\dot{V}_A + \dot{V}_D(m))$$

Volume parameters such as $\dot{V}_E$, $\dot{V}_A$, $\dot{V}_D(m)$, $\dot{V}_D(p)$ and cardiac output were corrected for BSA.

Influence of Added External Dead Space on Arterial Blood Gas Tension During Exercise Testing

In patients with CHF, many studies demonstrate normal $PaCO_2$ and PaO_2 during exercise,[5,11,20,21] which suggest that neural and chemoreflex ventilatory control mechanisms are kept intact in cardiac patients. We used a face mask with a mechanical dead space of 0.2 l, and also found that $PaCO_2$ and PaO_2 were within normal range for sea-level subjects in both patients and control subjects at rest and during exercise (Figures 2A, 2B). A previous study confirmed that alveolar PCO_2 could apparently be maintained at the control level while breathing through an external dead space up to 0.35 l at rest and during moderate exercise.[22] Ward et al[23] reported in normal subjects that the control mechanism of exercise hyperpnea to regulate $PaCO_2$ was not impaired by the additional anatomic dead space.

Role of Lactic Acidosis for Augmented Ventilation in Cardiac Patients

Several reports suggested that the early appearance of lactic acidosis would contribute to the increased ventilation in patients with heart failure during exercise.[3,15,16] Hachamovitch et al[24] reported that such patients showed hyperventilation with arterial hypocapnia during constant-load exercise. On the other hand, cardiac patients without respiratory disorders were reported to maintain normal arterial blood gas tension both at rest and during exercise.[5,11,20,21] We used a ramp exercise protocol with an increasing work rate of 1 W/6 sec and found an earlier appearance of AT (32 ± 10 versus 64 ± 9 W) and an earlier pH decrease (Figure 3) in the patient group than in the control group. Minute ventilation per body surface area ($\dot{V}E/BSA$) and ventilation/carbon dioxide production ratio ($\dot{V}E/\dot{V}CO_2$) were significantly higher in the patient group both at rest and during exercise compared with the control group ($p < 0.01$, Figure 4, Figure 5A), while the alveolar ventilation/carbon dioxide production ratio ($\dot{V}A/\dot{V}CO_2$) was not different and was almost constant at rest and during submaximal exercise in the two groups (Figure 5B). Both at rest and during exercise, the $\dot{V}A/BSA$ or $\dot{V}A/\dot{V}CO_2$ values of the patients did not differ from those of the control group at least up to submaximal exercise, which revealed that augmented ventilation in the patients was mainly caused by the increased dead space. This result indicated that the increased ventilation in the patient group could be ascribed to an appropriate response to the increased dead space to maintain $PaCO_2$ within a normal range. However, at peak exercise,

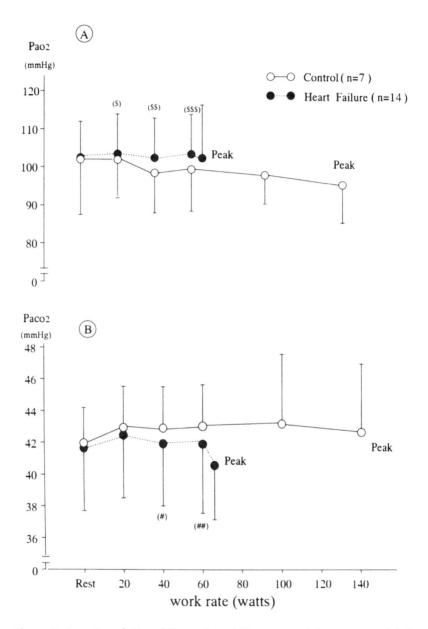

Figure 2. PaO_2 (**panel A**) and $PaCO_2$ (**panel B**) at rest and time course of their changes during exercise. Values are mean ± SD; no significant difference is seen between the two groups. ($) n = 10, ($$) n = 9, ($$$) n = 7, (#) n = 13, (##) n = 7

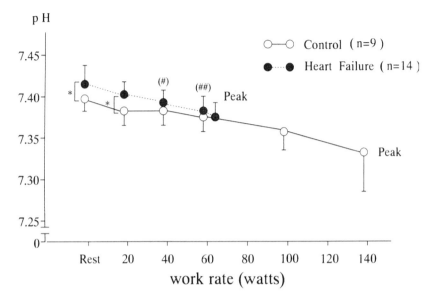

Figure 3. Arterial pH at rest and its change during exercise. Higher pH is shown in the patient group, probably elicited by administration of loop diuretics. Values are mean ± SD; * p < 0.05; (#) n = 13, (##) n = 7.

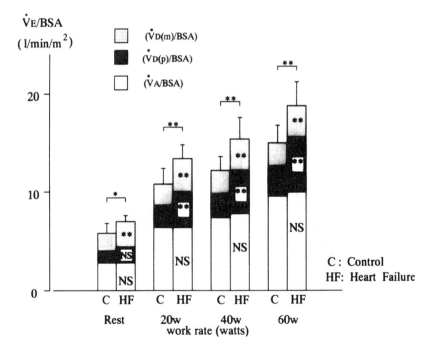

Figure 4. Alveolar ventilation (V̇A/BSA), physiological dead space (V̇D(p)/BSA) and mechanical dead space (V̇D(m)/BSA) ventilation at rest and their changes during exercise. NS, not significant; * p < 0.05; ** p < 0.01; comparison between control and heart failure in V̇A/BSA, V̇D(p)/BSA, V̇D(m)/BSA, and total V̇E/BSA, respectively.

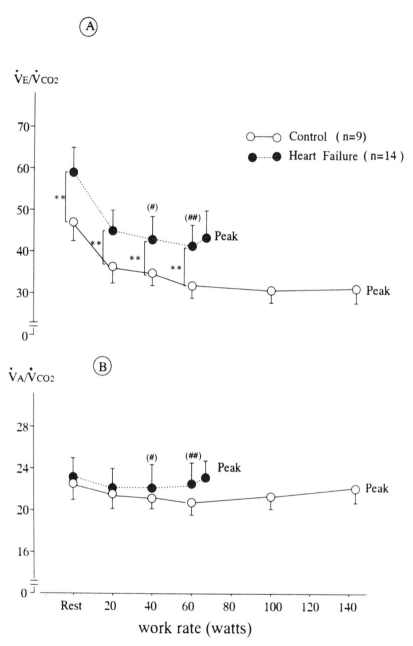

Figure 5. Ventilatory equivalent for carbon dioxide ($\dot{V}_E/\dot{V}_{CO_2}$) (**panel A**) and alveolar ventilatory equivalent for carbon dioxide ($\dot{V}_A/\dot{V}_{CO_2}$) (**panel B**) at rest and their changes during exercise. Values are mean ± SD; * $p < 0.05$, ** $p < 0.01$, (#) n = 13, (##) n = 7.

$PaCO_2$, $\dot{V}E/\dot{V}CO_2$, and $\dot{V}A/\dot{V}CO_2$ tended to be larger in the patient group, which suggested that some other factors such as lactic acidosis resulted in acute hyperventilation in the patients.

Role of Mechanical Dead Space for Augmented Ventilation in Cardiac Patients

Weber et al[3] reported that the main cause of the increased ventilatory response of patients was an increased dead space ventilation due to an altered pattern of rapid and shallow breathing. In our study, such an altered breathing pattern in the patient group was also noted both at rest and during exercise (Figure 6). It was reported[8,25] that rapid and shallow breathing during exercise in patients with mitral stenosis was due to reduced vital capacity, and possibly due to stimulation of the juxtacapillary (J) receptors caused by pulmonary congestion and interstitial edema.

Increased ventilation in patients with CHF at rest was studied by Sullivan et al.[5] Our data also showed that resting mechanical dead space ventilation ($\dot{V}D(m)/BSA$) in the patient group was greater than that of the control group (p < 0.01, Figure 4), and the ratio of mechanical dead space ventilation to the total ventilation ($\dot{V}D(m)/\dot{V}E$) at rest was larger in the patient group (37.3 ± 5.8 versus 30.8 ± 4.4%, p < 0.05, (Figure 7A). These results revealed that a substantial portion of

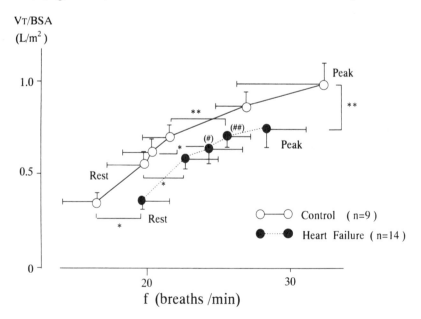

Figure 6. Relationship between tidal volume (VT/BSA) and respiratory frequency (f) at rest and its change during exercise. Values are mean ± SD; * p < 0.05, ** p < 0.01, (#) n = 13, (##) n = 7.

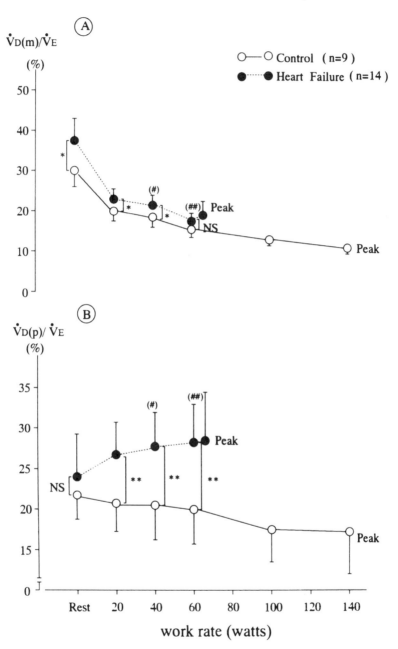

Figure 7. The ratio of mechanical dead space ventilation to the total ventilation ($\dot{V}_D(m)/\dot{V}_E$) (**panel A**) and physiological dead space ventilation to the total ventilation ($\dot{V}_D(p)/\dot{V}_E$) (**panel B**) at rest and their changes during exercise. Values are mean ± SD; NS, not signicant; * p < 0.05, ** p < 0.01, (#) n = 13, (##) n = 7.

resting hyperpnea was caused by the mechanical dead space ventilation. On the other hand, the $\dot{V}_D(m)/\dot{V}_E$ ratio became smaller during exercise than at rest and showed no significant difference between the two groups at 60 watts exercise (15.8 ± 1.6 versus 17.4 ± 1.8%)(Figure 7A).

Role of Physiological Dead Space for Augmented Ventilation in Cardiac Patients

It was suggested that one of the main factors responsible for hyperpnea is the increased physiological dead space secondary to a ventilation/perfusion mismatch.[5,11–13] In our study, $\dot{V}_D(p)/BSA$ at rest was not different between the two groups (Figure 4). However, during exercise, $\dot{V}_D(p)/BSA$ in the patient group increased with increasing exercise intensity. In the patient group, the ratio of $\dot{V}_D(p)$ to $\dot{V}_E$ ($\dot{V}_D(p)/\dot{V}_E$) increased significantly from 24.0 ± 5.0% at rest to 28.5 ± 4.6% at 60 watts exercise (Figure 7B). On the other hand, $\dot{V}_D(p)/\dot{V}_E$ ratio decreased from 22.0 ± 3.9% to 20.0 ± 4.2% in the control group. We found that the increase of cardiac index in the patient group was less than that in the control group for the same work-rate increase, reflecting a rapid widening of arterial-mixed venous oxygen difference. Since Pa_{CO_2} was well regulated, $\dot{V}_A$ increased in proportion to the increase in $\dot{V}_{CO_2}$. Consequently, overall $\dot{V}_A/\dot{Q}$ became significantly greater during exercise in the patient as compared to the control group at low work rates, although it was not significantly different at maximal exercise (Figure 8).

Summary

The pathophysiological mechanisms for the augmented ventilation at rest and during exercise in patients with CHF have not yet been clearly defined. Several mechanisms have been suggested, such as an abnormal respiratory pattern with rapid and shallow breathing, an increased physiological dead space secondary to ventilation/perfusion mismatch, and early lactic acidosis during exercise. We examined patients with CHF and healthy subjects to clarify the mechanisms for augmented ventilation at rest and during exercise. Ventilatory parameters including mechanical dead space ventilation due to added volume of the face mask (0.2 l), arterial blood gas tensions, and pH were measured during symptom-limited ramp exercise testing with a cycle ergometer.

In heart failure patients, minute ventilation ($\dot{V}_E/BSA$), ventilatory equivalent for carbon dioxide ($\dot{V}_E/\dot{V}_{CO_2}$), and respiratory frequency were increased while tidal volume was lower than that for normal subjects both at rest and during exercise. Alveolar ventilation ($\dot{V}_A/BSA$)

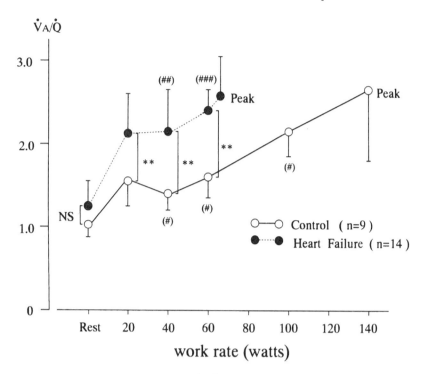

Figure 8. Ventilation/perfusion ratio ($\dot{V}_A/\dot{Q}$) at rest and during exercise. Values are mean ± SD; NS, not significant; ** $p < 0.01$, (#) $n = 8$, (##) $n = 13$, (###) $n = 7$.

and arterial P_{CO_2} (Pa_{CO_2}) were not significantly different between the two groups. The overall ventilation/perfusion ratio ($\dot{V}_A/\dot{Q}$) became significantly larger in the patient group during low work-rate exercise because of an insufficient increase of cardiac output.

References

1. Harrison TR, Pilcher C: Studies in congestive heart failure. II. The respiratory exchange during and after exercise. *J Clin Invest* 8:291–304, 1930.
2. Gazetpoulos N, Davies H, Oliver C, et al: Ventilation and haemodynamics in heart disease. *Br Heart J* 28:1–15, 1966.
3. Weber KT, Kinasewitz GT, Janicki JS, et al: Oxygen utilization and ventilation during exercise in patients with chronic cardiac failure. *Circulation* 65: 1213–1223, 1982.
4. Fink LI, Wilson JR, Ferraro N: Exercise ventilation and pulmonary artery wedge pressure in chronic stable congestive heart failure. *Am J Cardiol* 57: 249–253, 1986.
5. Sullivan MJ, Higginbotham MB, Cobb FR: Increased exercise ventilation in patients with chronic heart failure: intact ventilatory control despite hemodynamic and pulmonary abnormalities. *Circulation* 77:552–559, 1988.

6. Paintal AS: Mechanism of stimulation of type J pulmonary receptors. *J Physiol* 203:511–532, 1969.
7. Ingram RH, McFadden ER: Respiratory changes during exercise in patients with pulmonary venous hypertension. *Prog Cardiovasc Dis* 19:109–115, 1976.
8. Reed JW, Ablett M, Cotes JE: Ventilatory responses to exercise and to carbon dioxide in mitral stenosis before and after valvulotomy: causes of tachypnoea. *Clin Sci Mol Med* 54:9–16, 1978.
9. Brown CC Jr, Fry DL, Ebert RV: The mechanics of pulmonary ventilation in patients with heart disease. *Am J Med* 17:438–446, 1954.
10. Cook CD, Mead J, Schreiner GL, et al: Pulmonary mechanics during induced pulmonary edema in anesthetized dogs. *J Appl Physiol* 14:177–186, 1959.
11. Rubin SA, Brown HV, Swan HJC: Arterial oxygenation and arterial oxygen transport in chronic myocardial failure at rest, during exercise and after hydralazine treatment. *Circulation* 66:143–148, 1982.
12. Rubin SA, Nemerovski M, Brown HV, et al: Mechanisms of dyspnea on exertion in severe, chronic heart failure (abstr). *Clin Res* 29: 237A, 1981.
13. Buller NP, Poole-Wilson PA: Mechanism of the increased ventilatory response to exercise in patients with chronic heart failure. *Br Heart J* 63:281–283, 1990.
14. Hughes JMB, Glazier JB, Maloney JE, et al: Effect of interstitial pressure on pulmonary blood flow. *Lancet* 1:192–193, 1967.
15. Donald KW, Gloster J, Harris EA, et al: The production of lactic acid during exercise in normal subjects and in patients with rheumatic heart disease. *Am Heart J* 62:494–510, 1961.
16. Itoh H, Taniguchi K, Koike A, et al: Evaluation of severity of heart failure using ventilatory gas analysis. *Circulation* (suppl.ll)81 1131–1137, 1990.
17. Casaburi R, Wasserman K, Patessio A, et al: A new perspective in pulmonary rehabilitation: anaerobic threshold as a discriminant in training. *Eur Respir J* (suppl)7:618–623, 1989.
18. Beaver WL, Wasserman K, Whipp BJ: A new method for detecting anaerobic threshold by gas exchange. *J Appl Physiol* 60:2020–2027, 1986.
19. Kinsman, JM, Moore, JW, Hamilton, WF: Studies on the circulation: Injection method: physical and mathematical consideration. *Am J Physiol* 89:322–330, 1929.
20. Franciosa JA, Leddy CL, Wilen M: Relation between hemodynamic and ventilatory responses in determining exercise capacity in severe congestive heart failure. *Am J Cardiol* 53:127–134, 1983.
21. Wilson JR, Ferraro N: Exercise intolerance in patients with chronic left heart failure: relation to oxygen transport and ventilatory abnormalities. *Am J Cardiol* 51:1358–1363, 1983.
22. Stannard JN, Russ EM: Estimation of critical dead space in respiratory protective devices. *J Appl Physiol* 1:326–332, 1948.
23. Ward SA, Whipp BJ: Ventilatory control during exercise with increased external dead space. *J Appl Physiol* 48:225–231, 1980.
24. Hachamovitch R, Brown HV, Rubin SA: Respiratory and circulatory analysis of CO_2 output during exercise in chronic heart failure. *Circulation* 84:605–612, 1991.
25. Ingram RH, McFadden ER: Respiratory changes during exercise in patients with pulmonary venous hypertension. *Prog Cardiovasc Dis* 19:109–115, 1976.

Section 4

Peripheral Mechanisms Determining Exercise Capacity

12

Critical Capillary PO$_2$, Net Lactate Production, and Oxyhemoglobin Dissociation: Effects on Exercise Gas Exchange

Karlman Wasserman, MD, PhD
William W. Stringer, MD

Introduction

The relationship between lactate concentration increase and anaerobiosis during exercise has been disputed based on studies showing that muscle releases lactate despite the mean myocyte partial pressure of oxygen (PO$_2$) being above that which would predict muscle anaerobiosis.[1] Yet levels of exercise which are relatively easy for the subject to perform are not associated with an arterial lactate concentration increase, and conditions which reduce arterial oxygen content or delivery to the exercising muscles induce lactate concentration increases when the work rate is above the lactic acidosis threshold (*LAT*).[2]

Despite many studies which implicate a major role for oxygen in the mechanism for lactate increase during exercise, the mechanism for the lactic acidosis of exercise has spawned major disputes in physiology.[3] The major problem which has nurtured this debate is the equating of the mechanism of lactate turnover, as measured with isotopically labelled lactate, with that of blood lactate **concentration** increase. There has been considerable controversy regarding the technical aspects of the use of isotopically labelled lactate for the purpose of measuring the rate of lactate production.[4] The controversy has pri-

From Wasserman, K (ed): *Exercise Gas Exchange in Heart Disease.* Armonk, NY: Futura Publishing Company, Inc., © 1996.

marily focused on the correct site of isotopically labelled lactate infusion and sampling,[4] but perhaps even more cogent is the fact that the carbon label of lactate is rapidly equilibrated with its precursor, pyruvate.[5,6] As demonstrated by Wolfe et al,[6] measurement of lactate turnover reflects the rate of pyruvate turnover. Since pyruvate is the major substrate for mitochondrial respiration, and the lactate tracer is diluted in the pyruvate pool, lactate tracer will be consumed in proportion to pyruvate consumption and therefore oxygen consumption. Thus, increasing oxygen uptake ($\dot{V}O_2$) should result in a proportional increase in lactate tracer removal and calculated increase in lactate turnover, but which is in fact pyruvate turnover. However, this has little bearing on the mechanism of the increase in blood lactate concentration during exercise.

We now recognize that lactate and pyruvate are a redox couple and that changes in the cell redox state affect the concentration of lactate relative to pyruvate.[2] When the lactate/pyruvate (L/P) ratio increases during exercise, net lactate production increases resulting in an increase in lactate concentration. The increase in L/P ratio indicates that the cell redox state ($NADH+H^+/NAD^+$) has changed in the direction predicted if there were a proportionate increase in anaerobic glycolysis, i.e., mitochondria unable to maintain the cytosolic redox state.[2]

The literature is replete with studies demonstrating an oxygen dependence for the blood lactate concentration increase for work rates above the LAT.[2] Experimental conditions which reduce the oxygen available for mitochondrial respiration, such as hypoxic hypoxia, anemic hypoxia, stagnant (ischemic) hypoxia, and histotoxic hypoxia, increase lactate concentration during heavy exercise. In contrast, conditions which increase oxygen supply in the same work-rate domain reduce the lactate concentration. Similarly, other mechanisms have been suggested as having an important role in the lactate concentration increase during exercise, such as the action of catecholamines, increased aerobic glycolysis with "spillover" of lactate from pyruvate (mass action effect), or enhanced activity of pyruvate dehydrogenase. These mechanisms, however, have been shown experimentally to have no or questionably little effect during exercise in man (see section "Factors affecting lactate concentration increase" in Reference 2 for a more detailed review).

In this chapter, we point out that the capillary PO_2 is heterogeneous, ranging from high values at the arterial to low values at the venous end of the capillary bed, even when the muscle blood flow/metabolic rate ratios ($\dot{Q}m/\dot{V}O_2m$) for individual capillary beds in the muscle are homogeneous (Figure 1). Therefore, measurements of "mean" capillary PO_2, often used to define if there is tissue hypoxia, cannot reveal the absence of anaerobiosis since it will always be above the "critical" capillary PO_2, i.e., the minimum PO_2 in the capillary bed that allows oxygen to diffuse into the myocyte at a rate sufficient to

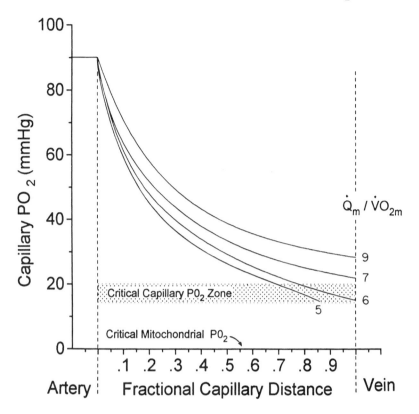

Figure 1. Model of muscle capillary bed oxygen partial pressure (PO_2) as blood travels from artery to vein. The model assumes hemoglobin concentration of 15 g/dL, arterial PO_2 of 90 mm Hg and a linear oxygen consumption along the capillary. The rate of fall of capillary PO_2 depends on the muscle blood flow ($\dot{Q}m$)/muscle $\dot{V}O_2$ ($\dot{V}O_2m$) ratio. The **curves** include a Bohr effect due to a respiratory carbon dioxide production. The capillary PO_2 is heterogeneous along the capillary bed even with a homogeneous $\dot{Q}m/\dot{V}O_2m$. The end-capillary PO_2 cannot decrease below the critical capillary PO_2. See text for application of model. (Reproduced with permission from Reference 2.)

meet the rate of oxygen consumption needed to regenerate ATP, aerobically. Rather than the mean capillary PO_2, we must ask: what is the lowest capillary PO_2 compatible with the myocyte receiving oxygen at the **rate** required to support its **rate** of aerobic metabolism and how does this value relate to the release of lactate during exercise?

Capillary PO_2: Theory

As blood transits through the capillary bed, PO_2 decreases from an arterial to a venous value at a rate depending on the oxygen consumption, oxygen delivery (blood flow x oxygen concentration), and the shape of the oxyhemoglobin dissociation curve (Figure 1). In an organ such as skeletal muscle, where the metabolic rate can markedly increase and exceed the increase in blood flow, the end-capillary PO_2 will progressively decrease as the metabolic rate increases. At very high metabolic rates, the capillary PO_2 must reach a critically low value whereby PO_2 cannot decrease further.[2] This is the PO_2 needed to overcome the diffusive resistance between the capillary and mitochondria to achieve the oxygen flow required to regenerate high energy phosphate in the myocyte, aerobically. The diffusive resistance is determined by the medium for diffusion and the physical distance between the red cells in the muscle capillary (oxygen source) and the mitochondria or myoglobin (oxygen sink).

From the arterial PO_2, the concentration of hemoglobin, the shape of the oxyhemoglobin dissociation curve, and the Bohr effect resulting from the production of respiratory acid (CO_2) from aerobic metabolism, the fall in capillary PO_2 through the muscle capillary bed can be predicted for various blood flow/metabolic rate ratios ($\dot{Q}$ m/$\dot{V}O_2$m). This is illustrated in Figure 1, assuming the rate of oxygen consumption along the capillary bed to be constant. The $\dot{Q}$ m/$\dot{V}O_2$m needed to perform work totally aerobically should be determined by the critical capillary PO_2, i.e., the lowest PO_2 which would sustain the diffusion pressure to satisfy the muscle oxygen requirement. The model calculations demonstrate that for a hemoglobin concentration of 15 gm/dL with full oxygen saturation, a $\dot{Q}$ m/$\dot{V}O_2$m of 5 would result in complete extraction of oxygen from the blood if the critical capillary PO_2 fell to zero; of course this is impossible. Since the critical capillary PO_2 must be above the mitochondrial PO_2 for oxygen to diffuse from capillary to cell, a $\dot{Q}$ m/$\dot{V}O_2$m=5 must result in anaerobic metabolism and a net increase in lactic acid production in cells toward the venous end of the capillary bed. Yet the **average** PO_2 in the tissue perfused by this capillary bed would be relatively high and cannot reveal if there is tissue hypoxia. A $\dot{Q}$ m/$\dot{V}O_2$m=6 would be required to sustain muscle aerobic metabolism during exercise for the capillary PO_2 to remain at or above the critical capillary PO_2 of 15 to 20 mm Hg estimated by Wittenberg and Wittenberg.[7]

Femoral Vein (End-Capillary) PO_2 and Lactate Increase During Exercise in Normal Subjects: Is There a Functional Relationship?

To determine the end-capillary PO_2 and its relationship to the lactic acidosis of exercise, 10 normal subjects[8] were studied during progressively increasing and constant work-rate leg cycling exercise while femoral vein Po$_2$, Pco$_2$, pH, oxyhemoglobin saturation, and lactate were measured at a sampling rate of every 5 seconds for the first 2 minutes, then every 30 seconds for the next 4 minutes of constant work rate, and every minute during progressively increasing work-rate exercise tests. Each subject had a 10 cm, 8 Fr catheter inserted, percutaneously into the femoral vein in the right groin, under sterile conditions, 2 cm below the inguinal ligament with the tip positioned about 4 cm above the inguinal ligament. Arterial blood was sampled every 30 seconds from a brachial artery catheter placed percutaneously. Blood gas and pH measurements were made with a blood gas machine (Model 1306, Instrumentation Laboratories, Lexington, MA). Oxyhemoglobin saturation was measured with a co-oximeter (Model 482, Instrumentation Laboratories, Lexington, MA). Blood lactate concentration was measured with a YSI lactate analyzer (Model 2300, Yellow Springs Instruments, Yellow Springs, OH).

End-Capillary and Critical Capillary Po$_2$ Determined from Femoral Vein Blood

Femoral vein blood Po$_2$ reached a floor or lowest value in the middle of the subjects' work capacities and before lactate concentration started to increase (Figure 2). To further explore the constancy and similarity of femoral vein Po$_2$ during sustained exercise of very different metabolic rates, constant work-rate tests were done with a high sampling density of femoral vein blood (every 5 seconds during the first 2 minutes and then every 30 seconds for 4 minutes) during two 6-minute constant work tests in five different subjects. The low work rate studied was calculated to be at 80% of the *LAT* or moderate work intensity (avg=113 W, $\dot{V}O_2$=1.76 L/min). The high work rate studied was calculated to be at the *LAT* plus 75% of the difference between the *LAT* and $\dot{V}O_2$max or heavy work intensity (avg=265 W, $\dot{V}O_2$=3.36 L/min). The results of these studies are shown in Figure 3.

For the average of the five subjects studied, femoral vein Po$_2$ decreased to the same "floor" value at 30 seconds to 60 seconds after the start of exercise for both the moderate and heavy work intensities (Figure 3A). This value remained the same over the remaining 5 to 5 1/2 minutes despite the well-recognized increase in $\dot{V}O_2$ taking place over the same period. In contrast to Po$_2$, oxyhemoglobin saturation continued to decrease past the time when the end-capillary Po$_2$ (as evidenced from the femoral vein measurements) became constant (middle panels of Figures 2 and 3). The pH decrease (Figure 3C) completely accounted for the further oxyhemoglobin desaturation that took place after the capillary Po$_2$ reached its minimal or critical value.

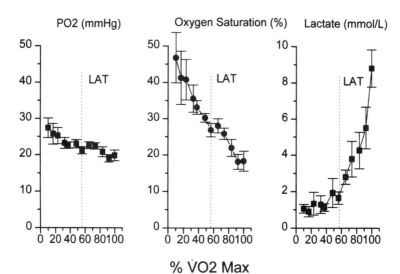

Figure 2. Average (five normal subjects) femoral vein oxygen tension (PO_2) (**left panel**), oxyhemoglobin saturation (O_2Hb saturation) (**middle panel**), and lactate concentration (**right panel**) during increasing work-rate exercise in ramp pattern to the maximal $\dot{V}O_2$. **Vertical dashed line** indicates the average lactic acidosis threshold (*LAT*) determined by gas exchange using the V-slope method.[38] **Vertical bars** indicate standard errors. There is no significant difference between the PO_2 values from the *LAT* to $\dot{V}O_2$max, but the O_2Hb saturation decreased significantly above the *LAT*. (Modified from data reported in Reference 8.)

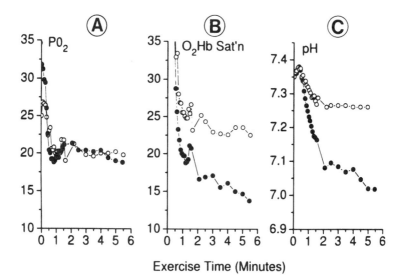

Figure 3. Femoral venous PO_2, oxyhemoglobin saturation (O_2Hb saturation), and pH as related to time of exercise for 2 constant work-rate tests, 1 below (○) and 1 above (●) *LAT*. Data are averages of five normal subjects (different from those shown in Figure 2). Below- and above-LAT work rates averaged 113 and 265 W, respectively. (Reproduced with permission from Reference 8.)

For the work rates selected to be below the *LAT*, oxyhemoglobin dissociation decreased rapidly for the first minute and then more slowly for the next 1 to 2 minutes before oxyhemoglobin saturation reached a constant value. The change after 1 minute followed the decrease in pH. For the work rate above the *LAT*, the decrease in oxyhemoglobin desaturation was much more marked and continued for the entire 6 minutes of exercise. The femoral vein desaturation which was not accounted for by the Po$_2$ decrease could be completely accounted for by the pH decrease, which of course was much more marked for the work rate above the *LAT* (Figure 3C). To illustrate this in a more conventional way, the data shown in Figure 3 were replotted with femoral vein oxyhemoglobin saturations against the independently measured femoral vein Po$_2$ values (Figure 4). The lower part of the oxyhemoglobin dissociation curves for various physiological pH values were overlaid on these data. Two very important points should be noted: 1) the decrease in oxyhemoglobin saturation not accounted for by a decrease in Po$_2$ can be accounted for completely by the decrease in measured pH (Figure 4B); 2) the decrease in oxyhemoglobin satura-

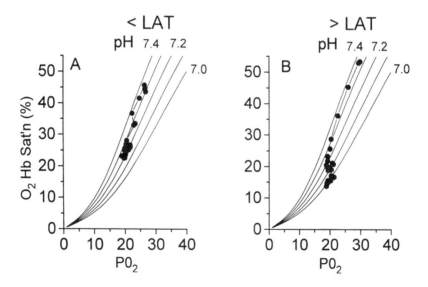

Figure 4. Changing femoral vein oxyhemoglobin saturation (O$_2$Hb saturation; see Figure 3B) as a function of femoral vein Po$_2$ (Figure 3A) for the 6-minute constant work-rate exercise tests shown in Figure 3. Superimposed are the lower part of oxyhemoglobin dissociation curves for pH values of 7.0–7.4. **Panel A:** data for below *LAT*. **Panel B:** data for above *LAT* exercise. Start of exercise is where O$_2$Hb saturation is highest. Femoral vein oxyhemoglobin saturation progressively decreases as exercise is continued, as shown in Figure 3. Oxyhemoglobin saturations fall on pH isopleths in agreement with measured pH (Figure 3C). This indicates that the entire decrease in O$_2$Hb saturation that takes place after Po$_2$ reaches its lowest value can be accounted for by Bohr effect. (Reproduced with permission from Reference 8.)

tion from 25% to 13% is completely accounted for by the Bohr effect (acidification of the capillary blood). While the acidification appears to be the only mechanism for oxyhemoglobin dissociation for work above the *LAT,* it obviously contributes to oxyhemoglobin dissociation below the *LAT,* along with the decrease in PO_2.

Femoral Vein PO_2 and Lactate Increase During Exercise

Because it was evident that femoral vein and therefore end-capillary PO_2 decreased to its lowest value, not at the highest work rate but in the middle range of work rates, when lactate concentration started to increase, we considered that a causal relationship might exist between end-capillary blood reaching a "floor" or "critical" value and lactate concentration increase. Therefore, we plotted the femoral vein blood lactate concentration against the simultaneous femoral vein PO_2 for both the progressively increasing and constant work-rate tests for each subject (Figure 5). These studies show that femoral vein lactate

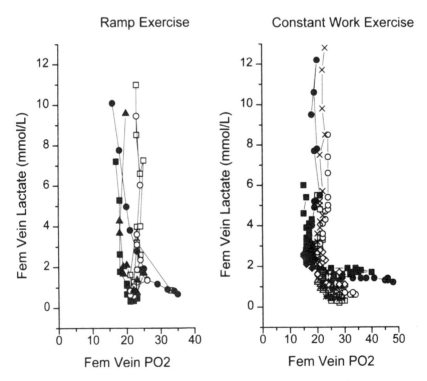

Figure 5. Femoral vein lactate as function of femoral vein PO_2 for increasing (ramp) exercise in five normal subjects (**left panel**) and 10 constant work-rate exercise tests (five below and five above the *LAT*) in five additional normal subjects (**right panel**). The highest PO_2 values are where exercise starts. Different symbols represent different subjects. (Reproduced with permission from Reference 8.)

concentration did not increase until the femoral vein and therefore the end-capillary Po$_2$ reached its lowest value. Thereafter, femoral vein lactate increased without a further fall in femoral vein Po$_2$. It is important to note that femoral vein lactate increased before arterial lactate increased in these studies, and lactate remained higher in the femoral venous than the arterial blood for the entire 6 minutes of the work rate above the *LAT*. This is in agreement with prior studies on lactate balance across the exercising extremity.[9–11]

Lactic Acidosis Facilitation of Oxyhemoglobin Dissociation

In contrast to femoral vein Po$_2$, oxyhemoglobin saturation continued to decrease for the entire 6 minutes of the heavy work rate (above the *LAT*), but became constant for the moderate work rate (below the *LAT*) by 3 minutes of exercise (Figure 3B). The further decrease in oxyhemoglobin saturation observed during heavy work-rate exercise was completely accounted for by the Bohr effect (Figure 4) for which the H$^+$ produced with lactate was essential.[8] These findings are similar to those of Hartley et al[12] who also found that femoral vein Po$_2$ reached a nadir during moderate work and that the increased oxygen extraction from the capillary blood at higher work rates was due to blood acidification.

Since the net increase in lactic acid production during exercise is buffered by intracellular HCO$_3^-$, additional carbon dioxide over that expected from aerobic metabolism is produced as HCO$_3^-$ dissociates. This results in an increase in end-capillary Pco$_2$ without a further fall in Po$_2$ (Figure 6). Simultaneously, the decrease in intracellular HCO$_3^-$ is reflected in a decrease in extracellular HCO$_3^-$ which has been found to be approximately stoichiometric with the increase in arterial blood lactate.[13] Both the carbon dioxide generated from intracellular HCO$_3^-$ and the consumption of extracellular HCO$_3^-$ by the cells (Figure 7) serve to acidify the capillary blood of the myocytes producing lactate.[2] The lactic acidosis of exercise thereby facilitates oxyhemoglobin dissociation and is likely to be an essential mechanism to achieve maximal oxygen extraction. For work rates demanding more oxygen than that consumed at the *LAT*, the further extraction of oxygen (dissociation of oxyhemoglobin) is H$^+$ concentration dependent.

The finding that the lactic acidosis of exercise does not take place until after the critical capillary Po$_2$ is reached supports the concept that lactic acid accumulation in the active muscle takes place when the muscle oxygen supply becomes critical. Thus the anaerobic threshold (*AT*), measured by arterial lactate increase, arterial HCO$_3^-$ decrease or the carbon dioxide generated from the HCO$_3^-$ buffering of lactic acid,[2] describes a V̇o$_2$ at which the critical capillary Po$_2$ had been reached for

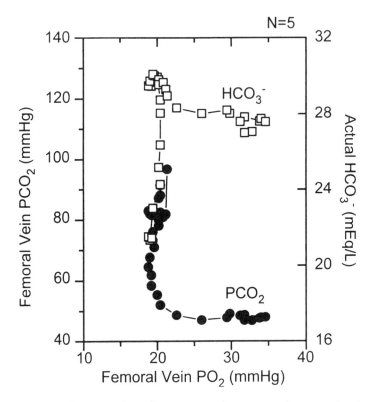

Figure 6. Femoral vein (end-capillary) PCO_2 and HCO_3^- as a function of end-capillary PO_2 during constant work-rate heavy exercise. Values are the average for the five normal subjects whose data are shown in Figure 3. Values at the start of exercise are at the right and move leftward as $\dot{V}O_2$ increases.

a given work task. The further finding that the PO_2 decreased to its lowest or critical value before lactate concentration started to increase in femoral vein blood also lends support to the concept that the lactate increase during exercise is tissue oxygen supply dependent.

In support of the concept that the lactic acidosis of exercise results from tissue hypoxia is the observation that the muscle lactate/pyruvate ratio,[14–16] a measure of the cell redox state (changes in proportion to the cytosolic $NADH+H^+/NAD^+$ ratio), increases at the lactate threshold. This same phenomenon has been observed in the arterial blood of man.[17] The cytosolic $NADH+H^+/NAD^+$ ratio is regulated by the mitochondrial redox state through the mitochondrial membrane shuttles (glycerol 3-phosphate and malate-aspartate). These feed electrons and protons directly to mitochondrial coenzymes as illustrated in Figure 8. Only mechanisms which limit the reoxida-

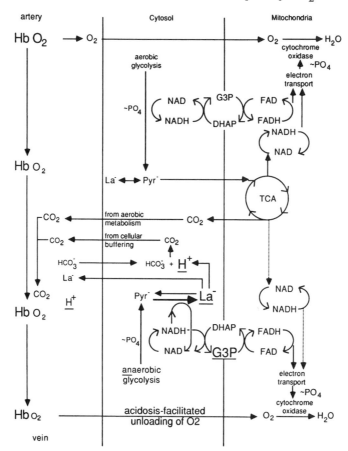

Figure 7. Scheme of changing capillary oxyhemoglobin (O$_2$Hb) saturation during blood transit from artery to vein during heavy intensity exercise. At arterial end of capillary, O$_2$Hb dissociates primarily due to decrease in Po$_2$. Glycolysis proceeds aerobically, without an increase in lactate (La$^-$), since mitochondrial membrane redox shuttles (e.g., dihydroxyacetone phosphate, DHAP) regulate cystolic redox state (NADH+H$^+$/NAD$^+$, abbreviated NADH/NAD). Primary substrate for tricarboxylic acid (TCA) cycle is pyruvate (pyr$^-$). As pyt- is decarboxylated and oxidized, electrons and protons reduce mitochondrial NAD to NADH, the latter being reoxidized by the electron transport chain and O$_2$ produced aerobically from this process reduces pH (and Bohr effect). As blood reaches the venous end of the capillary where Po$_2$ becomes critically low, mitochondrial membrane redox shuttle fails to reoxidize NADH to NAD at an adequate rate. Thus NADH/NAD increases. Accordingly, pyr- is converted to La- and DHAP is converted to glycerol 3-phosphate (G3P)[25] in proportion to the change in cell redox state. The effect is an increase in cell La- with a stoichiometric increase in H$^+$. The latter is buffered by the HCO$_3^-$ in the cell. Decreasing cellular HCO$_3^-$ and increasing cellular La- result in intracellular-extracellular La- and HCO$_3^-$ exchange. Simultaneously, CO$_2$ formed during intracellular buffering leaves the cell. Aerobically and anaerobically produced CO$_2$ and decreasing HCO$_3$ acidify the capillary blood toward the venous end of the capillary, enhancing dissociation of O$_2$Hb. This acidosis-facilitated dissociation allows aerobic metabolism to proceed without further reduction in capillary Po$_2$. FAD = coenzyme flavine adenine dinucleotide; FADH-reduced FAD. (Modified from Reference 2.)

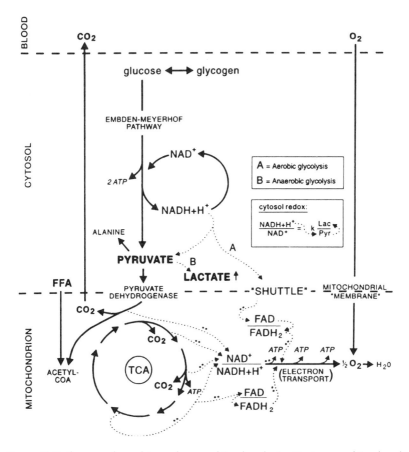

Figure 8. Pathways of aerobic and anaerobic glycolysis. During aerobic glycolysis (**pathway A**), cytosolic NADH+H+ is reoxidized by mitochondrial membrane shuttles, mitochondrial coenzymes, the electron transport chain, and oxygen. During anaerobic glycolysis (**pathway B**), pyruvate reoxidizes cytosolic NADH+H+ to NAD+ with production of lactate. Since lactate does not accumulate for exercise below the lactic acidosis threshold (*LAT*), glycolysis takes place aerobically. Above *LAT* work rates, lactate concentration increases relative to pyruvate, indicating a change in cytosolic redox state and an increase in NADH+H+/NAD+ ratio. FFA, free fatty acid; Lac, lactate; Pyr, pyruvate; TCA, tricarboxylic acid; K, equilibrium coefficient. (Reproduced with permission from Reference 2.)

tion of these mitochondrial coenzymes would result in increases in cytosolic NADH+H+/NAD+ and lactate/pyruvate ratios. The reoxidation of these mitochondrial coenzymes is oxygen supply dependent. As would be predicted, however, patients with a deficiency in the mitochondrial NADH+H+-coenzyme Q reductase, an enzyme which catalyzes the transfer of electrons and protons to the electron transport chain, develop a lactic acidosis at inappropriately low work rates similar to that found in patients with heart failure.[18]

Role of the Lactic Acidosis in the Respiratory Adaptation to Heavy Work

$\dot{V}_{O_2}$ kinetics are slowed only for work rates above the *AT* due to the development of a slow component in the $\dot{V}_{O_2}$ response to heavy exercise.[19,20] This slow component has been shown in a number of studies to correlate with the increase in lactate.[20–24] Lactate concentration in response to exercise can be reduced by exercise training[21] and increased by reducing the oxygen content without reducing arterial P_{O_2} by raising the carboxyhemoglobin concentration in the blood of normal subjects.[22] In these studies, the slow component in $\dot{V}_{O_2}$ kinetics changed in proportion to the lactate change.

Figure 9 illustrates the pattern of $\dot{V}_{O_2}$ increase for work rates with and without a lactic acidosis. We observed that the slow rise in $\dot{V}_{O_2}$ takes place during exercise only for work rates above the *LAT*. $\dot{V}_{O_2}$ increases more slowly the higher the blood lactate concentration increase, as previously reported.[20–24] To facilitate quantitation of this delay in $\dot{V}_{O_2}$ reaching a steady state, Whipp and Wasserman[20] suggested subtracting the 3-minute $\dot{V}_{O_2}$ value from the 6-minute value, as illustrated in Figure 9. Wasserman hypothesized that the slow component in $\dot{V}_{O_2}$ kinetics is due to the facilitated release of oxygen from hemoglobin under conditions of tissue hypoxia.[2] This would explain why the increase in blood lactate consistently accompanies, quantitatively, the slow increase in $\dot{V}_{O_2}$ after 3 minutes of exercise, the time at which $\dot{V}_{O_2}$ is in a steady state if exercise is performed without a lactic acidosis. Thus, the lactic acidosis makes more oxygen available for oxidative metabolism, thereby serving as an adaptive mechanism to facilitate aerobic metabolism.[2] The electron source for the electron transport chain to account for the increase in $\dot{V}_{O_2}$ may be glycerol 3-phosphate. Katz and Sahlin[25] measured increases in intracellular glycerol 3-phosphate in proportion to the increase in intracellular lactate during heavy exercise. Since this compound is the component of the mitochondrial proton shuttle to flavine adenine dinucleotide (FAD) shown in Figure 8, by means of its increase in concentration, it might diffuse to sites within the muscle which have sufficient oxygen to support oxidative metabolism.

The adaptive mechanism which allows $\dot{V}_{O_2}$ to increase during the slow component is postulated to operate through the Bohr effect under conditions of cellular hypoxia, with the H^+ accompanying the lactate increase promoting oxyhemoglobin dissociation as shown in

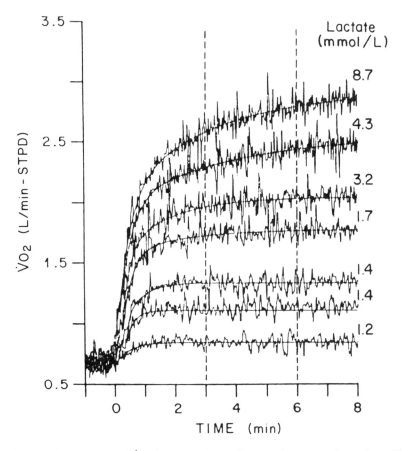

Figure 9. Time course of $\dot{V}O_2$ for seven leg cycling work rates performed on different days in a single subject. Each **curve** is second-by-second average of four to eight replicate studies. End-exercise (1 minute post-exercise) antecubital venous lactate concentrations are shown to right of $\dot{V}O_2$ measurements for each work rate. The three lowest work rates were designed to be below the subject's anaerobic threshold and the four remaining work rates were designed to be at progressively higher work levels. (Modified from Reference 39.)

Figure 4. This mechanism enables oxygen extraction by the exercising muscle to increase without a decrease in capillary P_{O_2}. At a given work rate, this increase in oxygen supply to the anaerobic, lactic acid-producing myocytes should allow $\dot{V}_{O_2}$ to increase, partially correcting the anaerobic state as diagramed in Figure 7. In support of this hypothesis, the rate of lactate rise has been found to slow in proportion to the slowing of the $\dot{V}_{O_2}$ rise.[26]

The slow increase in $\dot{V}_{O_2}$ during constant work-rate exercise may therefore represent a respiratory adaptation for performing heavy intensity exercise. The exercise lactic acidosis plays an essential role in this adaptation. In this respect, it is of interest that patients with myophosphorylase[27] and phosphofructokinase[28] deficiencies, conditions in which lactate does not increase in response to exercise, do not have a normal increase in arterial-venous oxygen difference at their maximal $\dot{V}_{O_2}$. In contrast to patients with myophosphorylase and phosphofructokinase deficiencies, the arterial-venous oxygen difference is not abnormally low in patients with carnitine palmotoyl transferase deficiency, another muscle enzyme defect, but without impairment in development of an exercise lactic acidosis.[28] This is consistent with the hypothesis that it is necessary to develop a metabolic acidosis in order to achieve the large oxygen extraction required to perform heavy intensity exercise.[29]

Femoral Vein P_{O_2} and Lactate Concentration Increase in Heart Disease Patients: Is There a Functional Relationship?

The data shown in this section come from the report of Koike et al.[30] The group of 10 subjects with heart failure performed three exercise protocols, a progressively increasing work-rate test in ramp pattern, a moderate intensity exercise test (80% of *LAT*), and a heavy intensity exercise test (the *LAT* plus 50% of the difference between the *LAT* and $\dot{V}_{O_2}$max). Femoral vein P_{O_2} fell to a low value in the middle and not at the highest $\dot{V}_{O_2}$ of the subjects' aerobic capacities (Figure 10). In five subjects, the P_{O_2} actually increased as $\dot{V}_{O_2}$ increased (Figure 10, right column). While this seems paradoxical, the reproducibility of the phenomenon in a given subject attests to the reliability of the phenomenon. The remaining five subjects decreased their femoral vein P_{O_2} to a constant level similar to that of the normal subjects (Figure 10, left column). The failure for the femoral vein P_{O_2} to decrease further, despite an increase in $\dot{V}_{O_2}$, suggests that the end-capillary P_{O_2} had reached its lowest

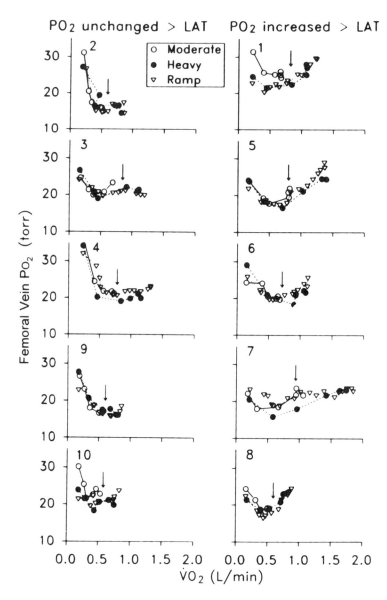

Figure 10. Femoral vein oxygen partial pressure (PO_2) plotted as a function of oxygen uptake ($\dot{V}O_2$) during two constant work-rate tests of moderate and heavy intensity and an incremental (ramp) exercise test for 10 patients with chronic heart failure. **Numbers** correspond to patients described in the original report. Femoral vein PO_2 rapidly decreased toward a minimal value with increasing $\dot{V}O_2$. After the femoral vein PO_2 reached its nadir, it increased in five patients despite increasing $\dot{V}O_2$ (**right column**), but was unchanged for the other five patients (**left column**). **Arrows** show the lactic acidosis threshold (*LAT*) determined noninvasively by the V-slope method[38] during the incremental exercise test. (Reproduced with permission from Reference 30.)

value, and that the critical capillary Po$_2$ had been reached at a submaximal work rate. The lowest or critical capillary Po$_2$ was found to be highly reproducible in the three protocols for each of the 10 subjects (Figure 10).

The femoral vein blood lactate concentration was plotted against its respective Po$_2$ value for each exercise protocol for each subject to estimate the end-capillary Po$_2$ at which femoral vein lactate concentration increased in each patient. As for the normal subjects, lactate concentration did not increase until the lowest Po$_2$ had been reached in the femoral vein (Figure 11). This suggests that the lactate concentration increase occurred after the critical capillary Po$_2$ was reached. The finding that femoral vein Po$_2$ increased in 5 of the 10 patients as work rate and lactate increased is best accounted for by an inhomogeneity in the $\dot{Q}m/\dot{V}O_2m$ ratios of the exercising muscle, as suggested by Koike et al.[30] This is modeled below. This finding should caution against the interpretation that because a femoral vein blood sample is drawn at the subject's highest $\dot{V}O_2$ that it is necessarily the lowest Po$_2$ of the muscle capillary bed during exercise. A single measurement has limited meaning with respect to the critical capillary Po$_2$. Finding a constant femoral vein Po$_2$ as work rate and $\dot{V}O_2$ increased would suggest homogeneity in $\dot{Q}m/\dot{V}O_2m$ ratios and that the end capillary Po$_2$ had reached its lowest (critical) value.

The Critical Capillary Po$_2$ in Heart Failure and Normal Subjects: Factors Limiting Exercise in Heart Failure

The critical capillary Po$_2$ ranged between 16 to 22 mm Hg for the normal subjects and 14 to 20 mm Hg for the patient group (Figure 12). It was positively correlated with the peak $\dot{V}O_2$/kg in the patient group and negatively correlated in the normal subjects. From Fick's law of Diffusion,* this finding suggests that those patients who reach their critical capillary Po$_2$ at a lower work rate have a lower maximal $\dot{V}O_2$. It also illustrates that the critical capillary Po$_2$ can be at a lower level if the mass flow of oxygen is reduced, as predicted from the Fick equation for diffusion. Increased maximal $\dot{V}O_2$ in normal fit subjects, in contrast, is accompanied by a lower critical capillary Po$_2$. This is possible only if there is an increase in capillary diffusion area and/or shorter diffusion path for oxygen. Obviously a correlation with only five subjects in the normal group must be interpreted cautiously. The different direction of the regressions for the patients and the physically fit subjects, however, suggests that different factors determine the maximal aerobic capacity in the two groups.

One of the pressing questions in heart failure research is whether the

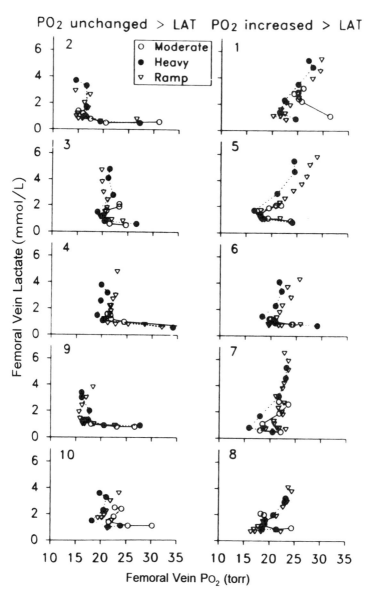

Figure 11. Relationship between femoral vein lactate and oxygen partial pressure (PO_2) for each exercise test for each patient shown in Figure 10. Each patient performed three tests, a progressively increasing work-rate test in "ramp" pattern, and moderate and heavy intensity constant work-rate tests. The highest PO_2 values are where exercise starts. Femoral vein lactate increased after femoral vein PO_2 reached its lowest value. After reaching the minimum value, PO_2 was unchanged in five and increased in five patients. (Reproduced with permission from Reference 30.)

exercise limitation in heart failure patients is due to failure to transport oxygen[17] or a bioenergetic defect in the muscle cells resulting from a critical reduction in aerobic enzymes.[31,32] Many studies have demonstrated that lactate increases in the blood of heart failure patients at exceptionally low work or metabolic rates.[10,11,24,33-36] This could be due to either the failure of the cardiovascular system to transport sufficient oxygen to the muscles to support mitochondrial respiration or the failure to utilize the oxygen delivered to the muscles. Because a defect in the aerobic enzymes of the tricarboxylic acid cycle would impair production of electrons needed for the electron transport chain and utilization of oxygen by the mitochondria, this defect should result in an abnormally high P_{O_2} at the end of the muscle capillary bed. We observed that patients with heart

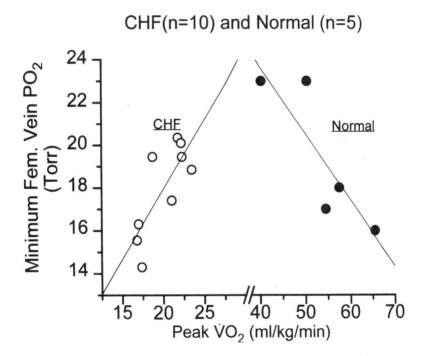

Figure 12. Lowest femoral vein P_{O_2} (critical capillary P_{O_2}) versus peak $\dot{V}_{O_2}$ in patients with cardiac disease (CHF) and fit normal subjects. Linear regression lines were separately calculated for each group. For the patients, the r=0.70 (P=0.01). For the normal subjects, r=0.86 (P=0.06). (Data taken from References 30 and 8, respectively.)

---

*DO_2=kxP(cap-mito)O_2xA/L, where DO_2=the rate of O_2 molecular diffusion per unit time, k=diffusion coefficient for O_2 in the tissue fluid, P(cap-mito)=the partial pressure gradient of O_2 between the capillary and mitochondria, A=diffusion surface area, and L=the path length for O_2 diffusion.

failure do not have abnormally elevated end-capillary PO_2 levels when lactate starts to increase and their estimated critical capillary PO_2 is in the same narrow range as that for normal subjects (Figure 12). This is consistent with the concept that oxygen transport is a major factor accounting for the reduced exercise tolerance in heart failure patients.

A further point relating to the bioenergetic limitation during exercise in heart failure patients is the pattern of change in lactate and lactate/pyruvate ratio. As illustrated in Figure 8, the increase in lactate should take place without an increase in $NADH+H^+/NAD^+$ and lactate/pyruvate ratio if the aerobic enzymes of the tricarboxylic acid cycle were deficient and accounted for the exercise limitation. That is, pyruvate should increase and, by mass action, cause lactate to increase without an increase in lactate/pyruvate ratio. If lactate increases with an increase in lactate/pyruvate ratio in heart failure patients, the electron transport of oxygen must be the limiting factor and not an inadequacy in aerobic enzymes. If the rate of high energy phosphate regeneration were inadequate, a muscle cannot sustain its contraction, i.e., muscle fatigue. The finding that $\dot{V}O_2$ is reduced and lactate is increased for the fatiguing work rate in patients with heart failure,[11] suggests that the failure to produce high energy phosphate, aerobically, limits exercise in these patients.

Critique of Femoral Vein Blood Sampling as a Measure of Critical Capillary PO_2

The femoral vein blood drains multiple capillary beds of the lower extremity. During leg cycling exercise, the only practical way of discovering the lowest PO_2 found in the muscle capillary bed (critical capillary PO_2) is by sampling the effluent blood from the muscle, the deep femoral vein being the most accessible. However, the results obtained are influenced by the uniformity of the muscle blood flow relative to the muscle oxygen consumption ($\dot{Q}m/\dot{V}O_2m$ ratio) in the exercising muscles and other tissues of the exercising extremity. Capillary beds with a low $\dot{Q}m/\dot{V}O_2m$ ratio contribute blood with a low PO_2 to the femoral vein, and blood with a relatively high $\dot{Q}m/\dot{V}O_2m$ ratio contribute blood with a high end-capillary PO_2 to the femoral vein (Figure 1). Nonnutritive blood flow would, of course, result in no decrease in end-capillary PO_2.

The more uniform the $\dot{Q}m/\dot{V}O_2m$ ratios, the closer the femoral vein PO_2 will be to the lowest capillary PO_2 since it will receive less contamination from high $\dot{Q}m/\dot{V}O_2m$ ratio muscle capillary beds. Also, the more uniform the $\dot{Q}m/\dot{V}O_2m$ ratio of the muscle capillary beds, the less likely that femoral vein PO_2 will change as $\dot{V}O_2$ increases, after the critical capillary PO_2 of the lowest $\dot{Q}m/\dot{V}O_2$ muscle capillary bed is reached. Based on modeling studies illustrated in Figure 1, the following patterns of change in femoral vein PO_2 as $\dot{V}O_2$ increases could be expected during exercise:

1. Continuously Decreasing Femoral Vein PO_2

If the critical capillary PO_2 is not reached in the capillary beds contributing to the femoral vein flow, PO_2 will continue to decrease until the subject reaches his maximally tolerated work rate. Alternatively, femoral vein PO_2 may continue to decrease if there were uneven $\dot{Q}m/\dot{V}O_2m$ ratio capillary beds with high $\dot{Q}m/\dot{V}O_2m$ units dominating at low $\dot{V}O_2$ values.

2. Femoral Vein PO_2 Decreasing to a Constant Value at Submaximal Exercise

The femoral vein PO_2 would become constant at submaximal work rates if the critical capillary PO_2 was reached in the capillary beds contributing to femoral vein flow before maximal $\dot{V}O_2$ was reached and the distribution of $\dot{Q}m/\dot{V}O_2m$ ratios remained constant (or uniform) as $\dot{V}O_2$ increased.

3. Femoral Vein Decreasing to a Nadir at Submaximal Work and Then Increasing

If there were uneven $\dot{Q}m/\dot{V}O_2m$ ratio muscle capillary beds, the PO_2 in the femoral vein could reflect the PO_2 in the capillary bed with the lowest $\dot{Q}m/\dot{V}O_2m$ ratio, i.e., the bed with the highest oxygen extraction. When the lowest $\dot{Q}m/\dot{V}O_2m$ ratio capillary bed reaches its critical value, by definition it cannot decrease further and increasing work rate beyond that level presumably would result in a lactic acidosis in that muscle region. The muscle units with a higher $\dot{Q}m/\dot{V}O_2m$, or increasing contamination from skin blood flow, could contribute to the femoral vein flow more prominently as work rate increases thereby causing the femoral vein PO_2 to increase. A second scenario for this phenomenon is to attribute the increase in femoral vein PO_2 to a failure in muscle mitochondrial respiration ($\dot{V}O_2$) to keep pace with the increase in work rate and blood flow, thereby failing to utilize oxygen by the muscles. This mechanism, while accounting for the increase in femoral vein PO_2, would not account for the increase in $\dot{V}O_2$ observed while femoral vein PO_2 increases. A third possibility is that the lactic acidosis causes a rightward shift in the oxyhemoglobin dissociation curve and the muscle simultaneously has saturated its oxygen utilizing capacity.

4. Femoral Vein PO_2 Increasing as $\dot{V}O_2$ Increases

The phenomenon of femoral vein PO_2 increasing as $\dot{V}O_2$ increases can only take place if $\dot{Q}m/\dot{V}O_2m$ increases. The phenomenon of capillary blood flow increasing faster than metabolic rate is not described in rapid sampling of mixed venous or femoral vein blood in response to exercise. Defects in mitochondrial respiration or tissue edema could result in a failure to utilize oxygen. While this mechanism would explain a relatively high end-capillary PO_2, it would prevent $\dot{V}O_2$ from increasing, and thereby would not explain the experimental observations shown in Figures 2, 3 and 10.

In this study, we have obtained results consistent with the model of femoral vein PO_2 decreasing to a constant level at submaximal exercise in the normal subjects and half of the patients, and femoral vein PO_2 decreasing to a nadir at submaximal work and then increasing in the remaining patients with cardiovascular disease.

Physiological Interaction Between Exercise Lactic Acidosis and Muscle Respiration

We conclude that a critical capillary PO_2 is reached in exercising muscle in the middle work-rate range and not at $\dot{V}O_2$max as previously suggested.[37] The critical capillary PO_2 is reached before the lactic acidosis develops. The lactic acidosis then serves as an essential mechanism in promoting oxyhemoglobin dissociation without reducing the PO_2 (Bohr effect). This allows $\dot{V}O_2$ to increase as lactate increases when heavy exercise is performed. In this way, the lactic acidosis, itself brought on by tissue anaerobiosis, serves as a respiratory adaptation which allows $\dot{V}O_2$ to increase, partially alleviating the anaerobic state. During heavy exercise, this is reflected in slowing of $\dot{V}O_2$ kinetics in proportion to the lactate increase.

We found that femoral vein (end-capillary) lactate did not increase until after the capillary PO_2 had fallen to its critical (lowest) value in both the healthy subjects and patients with heart disease. When the critical capillary PO_2 was reached, lactate increased without a further fall in PO_2. However, this does not mean that the maximum metabolic rate ($\dot{V}O_2$) had been reached. If more oxygen were unloaded from hemoglobin by the increase in H^+ concentration (Bohr effect), $\dot{V}O_2$ could continue to increase in the tissue, despite no further reduction in capillary PO_2. The increased H^+ produced with lactate moves the oxyhemoglobin dissociation curve downward, thereby allowing oxygen consumption to increase in the presence of an anaerobically-induced lactic acidosis. This is, functionally, a respiratory adaptation to anaerobiosis and may represent the most important functional role for the exercise lactic acidosis.

Summary

To determine the critical capillary P_{O_2} and its relationship to the lactic acidosis of exercise, normal subjects and patients with heart disease were studied during progressively increasing and constant workrate leg cycling exercise while femoral vein P_{O_2}, P_{CO_2}, pH, and lactate were measured at a high sampling rate (5-second to 60-second intervals). Oxyhemoglobin saturation was also measured in the femoral vein and arterial blood in normal subjects. Femoral vein (end-capillary) P_{O_2} reached a critical (floor or lowest) value in the middle of the subjects' work capacities before lactate started to increase in both the normal subjects and the patients. The critical capillary P_{O_2} ranged from 16 to 22 torr for the normal subjects and 14 to 20 torr for the patients. Remarkably, end-capillary lactate did not increase until after the lowest femoral vein P_{O_2} had been reached. In contrast to P_{O_2}, oxyhemoglobin saturation continued to decrease above the lactate threshold. The further decrease in oxyhemoglobin saturation was completely accounted for by the acidosis (Bohr effect) which became progressively more significant as $\dot{V}_{O_2}$ increased. Since the increase in intracellular lactic acid concentration is buffered by intracellular HCO_3^-, both the carbon dioxide generated from intracellular HCO_3^- and the consumption of extracellular HCO_3^- by the cells serve to acidify the capillary blood of the muscles producing lactate. The lactic acidosis of exercise thereby facilitates oxyhemoglobin dissociation. Importantly, these studies support the concept that the *LAT*, measured by blood lactate or the carbon dioxide generated from the buffering of lactic acid, estimates the $\dot{V}_{O_2}$ at which the critical capillary P_{O_2} had been reached, and above which the further dissociation of oxyhemoglobin is H^+ concentration dependent.

References

1. Connett RJ, Gayeski TEJ, Honig CR: Lactate efflux is unrelated to intracellular P_{O_2} in a working red muscle in situ. *J Appl Physiol* 61:402–408, 1986.
2. Wasserman, K: Coupling of external to cellular respiration during exercise: the wisdom of the body revisited. *Am J Physiol* 266:E519–E539, 1994.
3. Brooks GA: Anaerobic threshold: review of the concept and directions for future research. *Med Sci Sports Exerc* 17:22–31, 1985.

4. Norwich KH, Mazzeo RS, Brooks GA, Katz J: Letters to the Editor. Complexity of lactate kinetics. *J Appl Physiol* 61:2280–2282, 1986.
5. Sahlin, K: Lactate production cannot be measured with tracer techniques. Letters to the Editor. *Am J Physiol* 252:E439–E440, 1987.
6. Wolfe RR, Jahoor F, Miyoshi H: Evaluation of the isotopic equilibration between lactate and pyruvate. *Am J Physiol* 254:E532–E535, 1988.
7. Wittenberg BA, Wittenberg JB: Transport of oxygen in muscle. *Ann Rev Physiol* 51:857–878, 1989.
8. Stringer WW, Wasserman K, Casaburi R, Porszasz J, Maehara K, French W: Lactic acidosis as a facilitator of oxyhemoglobin dissociation during exercise. *J Appl Physiol* 76:1462–1467, 1994.
9. Andersen P, Saltin B: Maximal perfusion of skeletal muscle in man. *J Physiol* 366:233–249, 1985.
10. Donald KW, Gloster J, Harris AE, Reeves J, Harris, P: The production of lactic acid during exercise in normal subjects and in patients with rheumatic heart disease. *Am Heart J* 62:273–293, 1961.
11. Sullivan MJ, Knight D, Higginbotham MB, Cobb FR: Relation between central and peripheral hemodynamics during exercise in patients with chronic heart failure. *Circulation* 80:769–781, 1989.
12. Hartley LH, Vogel JA, Landowne M: Central, femoral, and brachial circulation during exercise in hypoxia. *J Appl Physiol* 34: 87–90, 1973.
13. Stringer WW, Casaburi R, Wasserman K: Acid-base regulation during exercise and recovery in man. *J Appl Physiol* 72:954–961, 1992.
14. Bylund-Fellenius A-C, Walker PM, Lander A, Hold S, Hold J, Schersten T: Energy metabolism in relation to oxygen partial pressure in human skeletal muscle during exercise. *Biochem J* 200:247–255, 1981.
15. Karlsson J: Pyruvate and lactate ratios in muscle tissue and blood during exercise in man. *Acta Physiol Scand* 81:455–458, 1971.
16. Sahlin K, Katz A, Henriksson J: Redox state and lactate accumulation in human skeletal muscle during dynamic exercise. *Biochem J* 245:551–556, 1987.
17. Wasserman K, Beaver WL, Whipp BJ: Gas exchange theory and the lactic acidosis (anaerobic) threshold. *Circulation* (suppl II)81:II14–II30, 1990.
18. Bogaard JM, Scholte HR, Busch FM, Stam H, Versprille A: Anaerobic threshold as detected from ventilatory and metabolic exercise responses in patients with mitochondrial respiratory chain defect. In: Tavassi L, DiPrampero PE, eds. *Advances in Cardiology. The Anaerobic Threshold: Physiological and Clinical Significance.* Basel: Karger Press, 135–145, 1986.
19. Barstow TJ, Casaburi R, Wasserman K: Oxygen uptake kinetics and the O_2 deficit as related to exercise intensity and blood lactate. *J Appl Physiol* 75: 755–762, 1993.
20. Whipp BJ, Wasserman K: Oxygen uptake kinetics for various intensities of constant-load work. *J Appl Physiol* 33:351–356, 1972.
21. Casaburi, R, Storer TW, Ben-Dov I, Wasserman K: Effect of endurance training on possible determinants of $\dot{V}O_2$ during heavy exercise. *J Appl Physiol* 62:199–207, 1987.
22. Koike A, Wasserman K, McKenzie DK, Zanconato S, Weiler-Ravell, D: Evidence that diffusion limitation determines oxygen uptake kinetics during exercise in humans. *J Clin Invest* 86:1698–1706, 1990.
23. Roston WL, Whipp BJ, Davis JA, Effros RM, Wasserman K: Oxygen uptake kinetics and lactate concentration during exercise in humans. *Am Rev Respir Dis* 135:1080–1084, 1987.
24. Zhang Y-Y, Wasserman K, Sietsema KE, Barstow, TJ, Mizumoto G, Sullivan CS: O_2 uptake kinetics in response to exercise: a measure of tissue anaerobiosis in heart failure. *Chest* 103:735–741, 1993.

25. Katz A, Sahlin K: Effect of decreased oxygen availability on NADH and lactate contents in human skeletal muscle during exercise. *Acta Physiol Scand* 131:119–127, 1987.

26. Wasserman K, Casaburi R, Beaver WL, Roston WL, Whipp BJ: Assessing the adequacy of tissue oxygenation during exercise. In: Bryan-Brown C, Ayers SM, eds. *New Horizons*. Fullerton, CA: Social Critical Care Medicine, 109–144, 1987.

27. Lewis SF, Haller RG: The pathophysiology of McArdle's disease: clues to regulation in exercise and fatigue. *J Appl Physiol* 61:391–401, 1986.

28. Lewis SF, Vora S, Haller RG: Abnormal oxidative metabolism and O$_2$ transport in muscle phosphofructokinase deficiency. *J Appl Physiol* 70: 391–398, 1991.

29. Wasserman K, Hansen JE, Sue DY: Facilitation of oxygen consumption by lactic acidosis during exercise. *News in Physiol Sci* 6:29–34, 1991.

30. Koike A, Wasserman K, Taniguchi K, Hiroe M: Critical capillary oxygen partial pressure and lactate threshold in patients with cardiovascular disease. *J Am Coll Cardiol* 23:1644–1650, 1994.

31. Drexler H, Riede U, Munzel T, Konig H, Funke E, Just H: Alterations of skeletal muscle in chronic heart failure. *Circulation* 85:1751–1759, 1992.

32. Sullivan MJ, Green HJ, Cobb FR: Altered skeletal muscle metabolic response to exercise in chronic heart failure. *Circulation* 84:1597–1607, 1991.

33. Weber KT, Janicki JS: Lactate production during maximal and submaximal exercise in patients with chronic heart failure. *J Am Coll Cardiol* 6:717–724, 1985.

34. Lipkin DP, Perrins J, Poole-Wilson PA: Respiratory gas exchange in the assessment of patients with impaired ventricular function. *Br Heart J* 54: 321–328, 1985.

35. Matsumura N, Nishijima H, Kojima S, Hashimoto F, Minami M, Yasuda H: Determination of anaerobic threshold for assessment of functional state in patients with chronic heart failure. *Circulation* 68:360–367, 1983.

36. Wilson JR, Ferraro N, Weber KT: Respiratory gas analysis during exercise as a noninvasive measure of lactate concentration in chronic congestive heart failure. *Am J Cardiol* 51:1639–1643, 1983.

37. Connett RJ, Honig CR, Gayeski TE, Brooks GA: Defining hypoxia: a systems view of O$_2$, glycolysis, energetics, and intracellular Po$_2$. *J Appl Physiol* 68:833–842, 1990.

38. Beaver WL, Wasserman K, Whipp BJ: A new method for detecting the anaerobic threshold by gas exchange. *J Appl Physiol* 60:2020–2027, 1986.

39. Casaburi R, Barstow TJ, Robinson T, Wasserman K: Influence of work rate on ventilatory and gas exchange kinetics. *J Appl Physiol* 67:547–555, 1989.

13

Peripheral and Central Oxygen Extraction in Chronic Heart Failure

Hiroshi Yamabe, MD
Mitsuhiro Yokoyama, MD

Introduction

Exercise intolerance is not only a characteristic manifestation of chronic heart failure (CHF), but it also reflects the severity of heart failure[1] and is related to its prognosis.[2] However, the physiological basis of exercise intolerance is complex.[3,4] In normal humans, both central mechanisms and peripheral mechanisms[5,6] have been debated as important determinants of maximal oxygen uptake ($\dot{V}O_2$max), and this controversy has not been entirely resolved. Recently, muscle oxygenation has been studied to examine the mechanisms related to $\dot{V}O_2$max in healthy subjects.[7-10] In patients with CHF, the factors speculated to affect exercise capacity include those related to oxygen transport capacity,[11-16] skeletal muscle anatomy and metabolic function,[17,18] abnormal ventilation,[19] and severity of symptoms.[20] Oxygen extraction is a function of oxygen transport and oxygen consumption. Since patients with CHF have both reduced oxygen supply and reduced oxygen demand, measurement of oxygen extraction is useful to determine which of these factors is an actual feature of exercise intolerance. Here we present the results of our analysis of the oxygen kinetics during exercise, and discuss the mechanism of exercise intolerance in CHF from the viewpoint of peripheral oxygen utilization.

From Wasserman, K (ed): *Exercise Gas Exchange in Heart Disease.* Armonk, NY: Futura Publishing Company, Inc., © 1996.

Subjects

Fifty-nine patients with stable CHF were studied. Their average age was 55 ± 9 years, and average body weight and height was 61.5 ± 8.8 kg and 163 ± 6.7 cm, respectively. The New York Heart Association (NYHA) functional classification was class I in 25 patients, class II in 21, and class III in 13. The clinical diagnosis was myocardial infarction in 34 patients, idiopathic dilated cardiomyopathy in 8, and valvular heart disease in 17, the last consisting of mitral stenosis in 9 patients, mitral regurgitation in 5, and aortic regurgitation in 3. Patients with angina pectoris, pulmonary disease, anemia, or obstructive peripheral vascular disease were excluded from this study. The study protocol was approved by the Institutional Research Committee of the Kobe University School of Medicine. The risks of the study were explained fully to the patients and informed written consent for participation was obtained.

Study Design

All patients underwent a multistage symptom-limited exercise test with an electronically braked bicycle ergometer (Siemens Elema 380B). The workload was increased by 25 watts every 3 minutes, and the end point of exercise was severe fatigue or dyspnea. The patients practiced exercising before the study to become accustomed to the apparatus. Before and during exercise, the expired gases, the right-side cardiac pressures, the arterial pressure, the arterial, mixed, and leg venous blood gases, blood hemoglobin concentration, and the leg blood flow (LBF) were measured.

Statistical analysis was conducted using one-way analysis of variance (ANOVA) and paired t test. Values are given as means $\pm$ standard deviation. P values less than 0.05 were considered to indicate statistical significance.

Measurement of Oxygen Uptake, Oxygen Delivery, and Oxygen Extraction

The apparatus used for expired gas analysis with breath-by-breath technique was a Minato RM-300 system (Osaka, Japan) with a hot wire flow meter. The oxygen uptake ($\dot{V}O_2$ mL/min) was averaged for 30-second period. A polyethylene catheter was inserted into the radial artery to measure arterial pressure. A 5-lumen 7.5-F Swan-Ganz catheter was inserted from the cubital vein and positioned in the pulmonary artery to measure right-side heart pressures. A 5-Fr thermodilution catheter was inserted into the external iliac vein to measure LBF. The reliability of this system is described in a previous report.[21] Blood samples were withdrawn from the radial artery, the pulmonary artery, and the leg vein. The partial oxygen pressure (PO_2) was measured using a 1312 Blood Gas Manager (Instrumentation Laboratory), and the oxygen saturation of hemoglobin (SO_2) was measured using a Co-Oximeter 482 (Instrumentation Laboratory). The formulas of calculated variables are as follows: blood oxygen content (vol%) = 1.39 × (hemoglobin concentration) × SO_2/100 + 0.003 × PO_2; arteriovenous oxygen difference $(C(a-v)O_2)$ = arterial oxygen content − mixed venous oxygen content; leg $C(a-v)O_2$ = arterial oxygen content − leg venous oxygen content); cardiac output (L/min) = $\dot{V}O_2$/$C(a-v)O_2$; leg oxygen uptake (leg $\dot{V}O_2$ = LBF × $C(a-v)O_2$; systemic oxygen delivery (L/min) = (arterial oxygen content × cardiac output; leg oxygen delivery (L/min) = (arterial oxygen content) × LBF; systemic oxygen extraction ratio (%) = $\dot{V}O_2$/(oxygen delivery) × 100; and leg oxygen extraction ratio (%) = leg$\dot{V}O_2$/(leg oxygen delivery) × 100. The values at the end of exercise were used as the peak values.

Severity of Chronic Heart Failure and Oxygen Extraction

Figure 1 shows the peak systemic oxygen extraction ratio and leg oxygen extraction ratio in the patients of each NYHA functional classification. There were significant differences among the three groups in both systemic and leg oxygen extraction ratio, with progressive increase with class from I to III being observed for systemic oxygen extraction ratio (58.6±5.6%, 61.2±6.0%, and 66.4±7.5%, respectively, p<0.01) and for leg oxygen extraction ratio (73.3±6.2%, 75.1±6.7%, and 80.2±7.0%, respectively, p<0.05). It is obvious that the patients with severe CHF did not show deteriorated function of oxygen extraction compared to those with less severe CHF.

Relation Between Oxygen Delivery and Exercise Tolerance

A strong linear correlation was found between peak systemic oxygen delivery and peak $\dot{V}O_2$ (Figure 2; r=0.95, p<0.001) and between peak leg oxygen delivery and peak leg$\dot{V}O_2$ (Figure 3; r=0.97, p<0.001). The finding suggests that the close link is present between metabolic rate and oxygen transport at peak exercise in CHF.

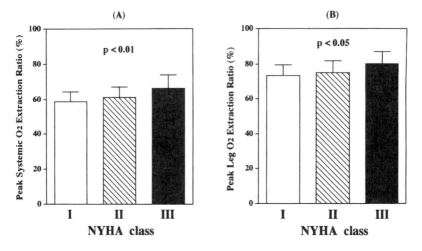

Figure 1. Systemic O_2 extraction ratio (**side A**) and leg O_2 extraction ratio (**side B**) at peak exercise. Both measurements significantly increased, the higher the NYHA functional class.

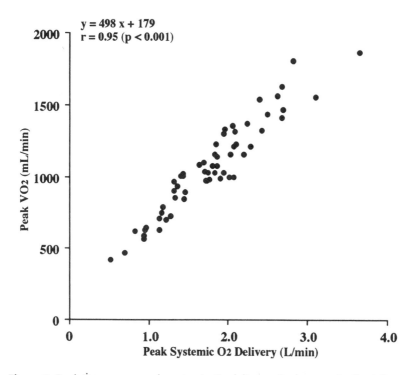

Figure 2. Peak $\dot{V}O_2$ versus peak systemic O_2 delivery. Peak systemic O_2 delivery strongly correlated with peak $\dot{V}O_2$ (y=498x+179, r=0.95, p<0.001).

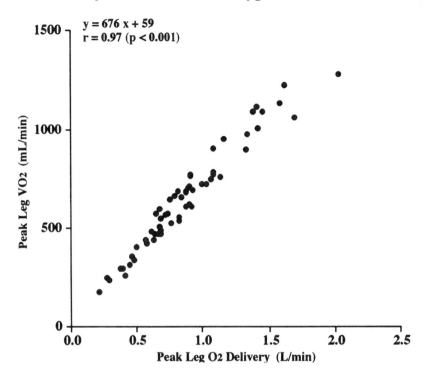

Figure 3. Peak leg $\dot{V}O_2$ versus peak leg O_2 delivery. The correlation between peak leg O_2 delivery and peak leg $\dot{V}O_2$ (y=676x+59, r=0.97, p<0.001) was as strong as that for the whole body. The results of Figures 2 and 3 support a tight link between O_2 transport capacity and exercise intolerance in chronic heart failure.

Relation Between Oxygen Extraction Ratio and $\dot{V}O_2$

The average oxygen extraction ratio at peak exercise was 61.2±6.8% for the whole body and 75.5±7.0% for the working leg. The latter was significantly larger than the former (p<0.001). The delivered oxygen was more efficiently utilized in working muscles than in the remainder of the body. There was a significant negative correlation between peak $\dot{V}O_2$ and peak systemic oxygen extraction ratio (Figure 4; r=0.31, p<0.05), and also between peak $\dot{V}O_2$ and peak leg oxygen extraction ratio (Figure 5; r=0.26, p<0.05). Similar analyses revealed no significant correlations between peak $\dot{V}O_2$ and peak $A\dot{V}O_2D$ or peak leg$\dot{V}O_2D$. The poor exercise tolerance in CHF was, thus, not due to the skeletal muscle incapacity to extract oxygen. However, the variations of both the systemic and leg oxygen extraction ratios were rather large in our total subjects.

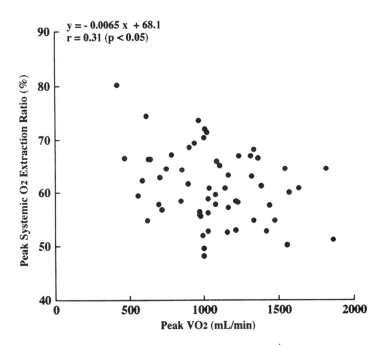

Figure 4. Peak systemic O_2 extraction ratio versus peak $\dot{V}O_2$. There was a significant negative correlation between peak $\dot{V}O_2$ and systemic O_2 extraction ratio ($y=-0.0065x+68.1$, $r=0.31$, $p<0.05$).

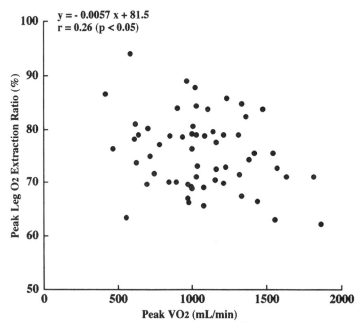

Figure 5. Peak leg O_2 extraction ratio versus peak $\dot{V}O_2$. There was a significant negative correlation between peak $\dot{V}O_2$ and peak leg O_2 extraction ratio ($y=-0.0057x+81.5$, $r=0.26$, $p<0.05$).

Leg Venous PO_2 at Peak Exercise

The Table shows the measured values of $\dot{V}O_2$, systemic oxygen delivery, leg$\dot{V}O_2$, leg oxygen delivery, leg venous pH, PCO_2, PO_2, and SO_2 at rest and at peak exercise. Compared to the value at rest, pH, PO_2, and SO_2 all showed significant reductions at peak exercise, while PCO_2 values were significantly increased. The leg venous PO_2 at peak exercise, which reflects the oxygen diffusion pressure of the working muscle, showed a mean value of 21.4±3.5 mm Hg, but ranged widely from 11 to 30 mm Hg. Peak leg oxygen delivery was significantly correlated with leg venous PO_2 at peak exercise (Figure 6; r=0.36, p<0.01), which may be a result of relatively insufficient oxygen delivery to the oxygen demand or the altered blood flow distribution among the muscle fibers according to oxidative function. There was a significant positive correlation between peak leg venous PO_2 and peak $\dot{V}O_2$ (Figure 7; r=0.37, p<0.01). The average leg venous SO_2 was 23.7±6.4%. This value was lower than the calculated value (36%) at standard condition for the given PO_2 level. Thus, the Bohr effect due to decreased pH and increased PCO_2 was operative for SO_2 reduction at peak exercise.

Summary of the Results

This study showed that the peak oxygen extraction ratio of the working leg was higher in CHF patients with more severe symptoms. It was also shown that strong linear correlations existed between peak $\dot{V}O_2$ and peak oxygen delivery both systemically and in the leg, and

Table

Findings at Rest and at Peak Exercise in Multistage Exercise Test

		Rest	Peak exercise	p
$\dot{V}O_2$	(mL/min)	213±42	1072±319	<0.001
Leg $\dot{V}O_2$	(mL/min)	23±10	649±262	<0.001
Sys O_2 delivery	(mL/min)	815±237	1775±616	<0.001
Leg O_2 delivery	(mL/min)	80±29	872±378	<0.001
Leg venous pH		7.37±0.03	7.18±0.06	<0.001
Leg venous PCO_2	(mmHg)	44.6±4.0	68.8±8.9	<0.001
Leg venous PO_2	(mmHg)	37.3±7.4	21.4±3.5	<0.001
Leg venous SO_2	(%)	66.3±13.4	23.7±6.4	<0.001

$\dot{V}O_2$=oxygen uptake, Sys=systemic, O_2=oxygen, PCO_2=partial carbon dioxide pressure, PO_2=partial oxygen pressure, SO_2=oxygen saturation.

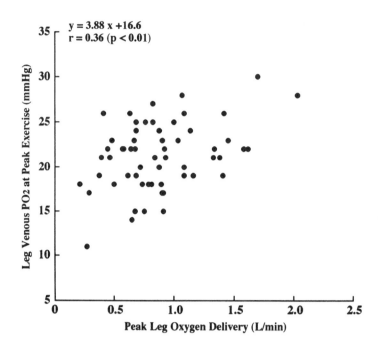

Figure 6. Leg venous PO_2 at peak exercise versus peak leg O_2 delivery. Leg venous PO_2 at peak exercise was significantly correlated with peak leg O_2 delivery (y=3.88x+17.6, r=0.36, p<0.01).

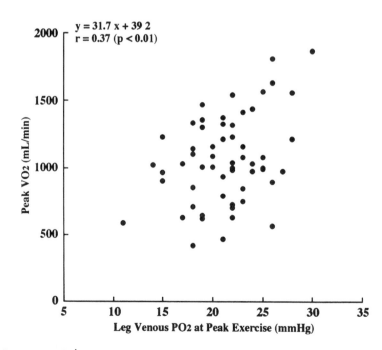

Figure 7. Peak $\dot{V}O_2$ versus leg venous PO_2 at peak exercise. A significant positive correlation was found between peak leg venous PO_2 and peak $\dot{V}O_2$ (y=31.7x+392, r=0.37, p<0.01).

that the leg venous PO_2 at peak exercise significantly correlated with exercise intolerance.

Physiological Basis of Exercise Capacity and Critical Capillary PO_2

The physiological basis of exercise capacity in normal subjects is controversial.[22] Two mechanisms of determination of $\dot{V}O_2$max have been considered: the central theory proposes that the upper limit of oxygen transport determines the $\dot{V}O_2$max, while the peripheral theory asserts that it is the capacity for oxidative metabolism of skeletal muscle. Several recent studies in healthy subjects[7–9] have suggested that the oxygen transport is rather important. DiPrampero[7] calculated the percent contribution of each factor in a review of several reports of hemodynamic and histochemical studies, and concluded that the oxygen transport capacity accounted for 75% of the change in $\dot{V}O_2$max induced by exercise training. Roca et al[8] measured the leg venous PO_2 and compared it with the change in $\dot{V}O_2$max under normoxic and hypoxic conditions in normal subjects. They found that the mean decrease in leg venous PO_2 at peak exercise (from 16.8±5.6 mm Hg to 14.4±5.2 mm Hg and to 12.0±5.0 mm Hg) paralleled the mean reduction in $\dot{V}O_2$max (from 4462±587 mL/min to 3530±428 mL/min and to 2790±542 mL/min). Knight et al[9] found similar results. The results of these studies are consistent with the "critical capillary PO_2" hypothesis that there exists a minimal capillary PO_2 level to maintain an increase in $\dot{V}O_2$ during exercise. However, Pirnary et al[10] observed that leg venous PO_2 under the control condition (16.6±2.4 mm Hg) decreased to 12.9±2.3 mm Hg after administration of beta-blocker without a significant reduction of $\dot{V}O_2$max. They concluded that normal subjects cannot attain the critical capillary PO_2 under normal conditions. Thus, the controversy has not been entirely resolved.

The leg venous PO_2 observed at peak exercise in our study was 21.4±3.5 mm Hg. This value positioned at almost midpoint among several values reported in healthy subjects: 16.5±1.3 mm Hg,[9] 16.6±2.4 mm Hg,[10] 16.8±5.6 mm Hg,[8] 19.8±3.3 mm Hg,[23] 21.7±3.18 mm Hg,[24] 24.0±1.0 mm Hg[25] and 24.9±4.3 mm Hg.[26] On the other hand, the available data in patients with cardiac disease are very limited. Rubin et al[25] reported it 17±1 mm Hg in patients with CHF. Koike et al[27] reported it 23.0±4.4 mm Hg in patients with cardiovascular disease, while they found that leg venous PO_2 attained the minimal level (18.2±2.0 mm Hg) before peak exercise. These results and our own indicate that patients with CHF can attain capillary PO_2 levels similar to those of normal subjects even though factors such as a decreased muscle capillary density or perivascular edema may cause critical capillary PO_2 to be elevated.[15,19]

Pathophysiology of Exercise Intolerance in Chronic Heart Failure

In patients with CHF, as well as in normal subjects, both central and peripheral mechanisms may affect the exercise intolerance, since patients with CHF have impaired oxygen transport capacity and abnormal skeletal muscle function. There has been increasing evidence that the factors related to oxygen transport capacity such as cardiac output response,[11–13] heart rate response,[12,13] pulmonary hemodynamics,[14] and muscle blood flow[15,16] are important in exercise intolerance in CHF. On the other hand, it has been observed that left ventricular function is not significantly correlated with exercise capacity in patients with left ventricular disease.[28] Several recent studies have focused on the skeletal muscle dysfunction as a modifying factor affecting exercise intolerance in CHF.[17,18,29–33] A magnetic resonance spectroscopy study[34] suggested that abnormal oxidative energy production during exercise is independent of the blood supply to the muscles in CHF. Histochemical studies[29,30,31] have also demonstrated the presence of atrophic oxidative muscle fibers and decreased activity of the oxidative enzymes in CHF.

Mechanism of Peak $\dot{V}O_2$ and Peak Oxygen Delivery Coupling

We found strong linear correlations between peak oxygen delivery and peak $\dot{V}O_2$ for both the whole body and the leg. This suggests that the metabolic rate is closely linked to the oxygen delivery at peak exercise. A possible explanation for this relationship is that peak $\dot{V}O_2$ is limited by oxygen transport capacity. In this situation, delivered oxygen would be extracted extensively. However, it also seems possible that patients with poor exercise capacity could not perform exercise efficiently due to skeletal muscle dysfunction. This could also result in a linear relationship between peak $\dot{V}O_2$ and peak oxygen delivery. In this situation, however, insufficient oxygen extraction would still be observed and muscle venous PO_2 would be expected to be higher, the more severe the exercise limitation. Thus, the analyses of leg venous PO_2 and oxygen extraction ratio are useful measurements to answer this question as described below. Our results are quite opposite to this speculation.

Oxygen Extraction and Exercise Tolerance in Chronic Heart Failure

Reduced oxidative function of skeletal muscles may impair the efficient extraction of oxygen, even when sufficient oxygen is provided. This condition would result in elevated muscle capillary PO_2 and reduced oxygen extraction during exercise in patients with poor exercise capacity. However, our results are not in accord with this hypothesis. Specifically, large oxygen extraction ratios were found in both whole body and working leg in the severe CHF group. In addition, significant negative correlations were also observed between the peak $\dot{V}O_2$ and peak oxygen extraction ratios for the whole body and the leg. The increased systemic oxygen extraction shown by patients with poor exercise tolerance is consistent with the description reported by Wilson et al.[15] We consider that the factors involved in increased systemic oxygen extraction are relatively reduced cardiac output for the oxygen demand and the enhanced shift of blood flow to the working leg from inactive organs.[35] The finding of a significant positive correlation between leg venous PO_2 at peak exercise and peak $\dot{V}O_2$ is also important. This is similar to the result reported by Koike et al,[27] although they used the minimal leg venous PO_2 and a small number of patients. This finding could indicate either that the low oxygen diffusion pressure lessens the supply of consumable oxygen to muscle mitochondria or that the shunt blood flow of the leg is increased in patients with good exercise capacity. The finding that peak leg oxygen delivery was significantly correlated with leg PO_2 at peak exercise seems to support the first mechanism. Thus, we consider that the major determinant of peak $\dot{V}O_2$ in CHF is oxygen transport capacity.

Limitations of the Study

The peak $\dot{V}O_2$ as measured in our study is not necessarily $\dot{V}O_2$max. $\dot{V}O_2$max is defined as the $\dot{V}O_2$ plateau despite an increase in workload. We did not analyze whether the $\dot{V}O_2$ plateau was attained. It remains controversial whether patients with CHF can reach the $\dot{V}O_2$ plateau or not.[36–38] Myers et al[39] reported that the variability in $\dot{V}O_2$ during exercise was too large to detect the $\dot{V}O_2$ plateau. Confirmation of whether the $\dot{V}O_2$ plateau has been reached may require that patients continue exercising for several minutes while maximal workload is exceeded, which is very difficult for patients with CHF. We believe that peak $\dot{V}O_2$ is very close to $\dot{V}O_2$max even though peak $\dot{V}O_2$ is somewhat smaller than $\dot{V}O_2$max. Another limitation of our study is that leg venous PO_2 is not quite identical to muscle end-capillary PO_2. In the leg venous blood, shunt blood may contaminate the muscle capillary blood. However, shunt blood in the leg blood flow should be a small part especially during exercise. The choice of bicycle ergometer may be a problem, when one expects that $\dot{V}O_2$max could be more easily measured on a treadmill.[40] However, Franciosa et al[41] reported that the peak $\dot{V}O_2$ measured during exercise on an ergometer did not differ from that measured during treadmill exercise in the identical patients with CHF. It is, therefore, unclear whether the use of an ergometer for exercise affected our results.

Conclusion

The close link between peak $\dot{V}O_2$ and peak oxygen delivery for both the whole body and the working leg, and the positive correlation between peak $\dot{V}O_2$ and the leg venous PO_2, support the concept that the reduced oxygen transport capacity is a major determinant of exercise intolerance in CHF.

Summary

Fifty-nine patients with chronic heart failure (CHF) underwent exercise tolerance testing with measurement of expiratory gases, leg blood flow, and arterial and venous blood gases. Strong correlations were found between peak systemic oxygen delivery and peak $\dot{V}O_2$ (r=0.95, p<0.001) and between peak leg oxygen delivery and peak leg $\dot{V}O_2$ (r=0.97, p<0.001). The peak oxygen extraction ratio showed a significant negative correlation with peak oxygen delivery, for both the whole body (r=0.31, p<0.05) and the leg (r=0.26, p<0.05). These results suggest that the major determinant of exercise intolerance in CHF is the reduced oxygen transport capacity. The leg venous PO_2 at peak exercise (average, 21.4±3.5 mm Hg) showed a significant positive correlation with peak $\dot{V}O_2$ (r=0.37, p<0.01) and with peak leg oxygen delivery (r=0.36, p<0.01), suggesting that the decreased oxygen diffusion pressure depressed peak $\dot{V}O_2$, and also that the oxygen diffusion pressure is affected by the capacity for oxygen transport to the muscles. It is concluded that the oxygen transport system is important in exercise tolerance in patients with CHF.

References

1. Patterson JA, Naughton J, Gunnar RM: Treadmill exercise in assessment of the functional capacity of patients with cardiac disease. *Am J Cardiol* 30:757–762, 1972.
2. Szlachcic J, Massie BM, Kramer BL, et al: Correlates and prognostic implication of exercise capacity in chronic heart failure. *Am J Cardiol* 55:1037–1042, 1985.
3. Lipkin DP, Poole Wilson PA: Symptom limiting exercise in chronic heart failure. *Br Med J* 292:1030–1031, 1986.
4. Flowler MB: Exercise intolerance in heart failure. *J Am Coll Cardiol* 17:1073–1074, 1991.
5. Shephard RJ: *Physiology and Biochemistry of Exercise*. New York: Praeger Publishers, 60, 1982.
6. Kaijser L: Limiting factors for aerobic muscle performance. *Acta Physiol Scand* (suppl)346:1–96, 1970C-1.

7. DiPrampero PE: Metabolic and circulatory limitations to $\dot{V}O_2$max at the whole animal level. *J Exp Biol* 115:319–331, 1985.
8. Roca J, Hogan MC, Story D, et al: Evidence for tissue diffusion limitation of $\dot{V}O_2$max in normal humans. *Am Physiol Society* 291–299,1989.
9. Knight DR, Schaffartzik W, Poole DC: Effects of hypoxia on maximal leg O_2 supply and utilization in men. *Am Physiol Society* 2586–2594, 1993.
10. Pirnary F, Lamy M, Petit JM, et al: Analysis of femoral venous blood during maximum muscular exercise. *J Appl Physiol* 33:289–292, 1972.
11. Franciosa JA, Leddy CL, Wilen M, et al: Relation between hemodynamic and ventilatory responses in determining exercise capacity in severe congestive heart failure. *Am J Cardiol* 53:127–134, 1984.
12. Steffen E, Meiler MD, Ashoton MS, et al: An analysis of the determinants of exercise performance in congestive heart failure. *Am Heart J* 113:1207–1217, 1987.
13. Higginbotham MB, Morris KG, Conn EH, et al: Determinants of variable exercise performance among patients with severe left ventricular dysfunction. *Am J Cardiol* 51:52–60, 1983.
14. Franciosa JA, Baker BJ, Seth L: Pulmonary versus systemic hemodynamics in determining exercise capacity of patients with chronic left ventricular failure. *Am Heart J* 110:807–813, 1985.
15. Wilson JR, Martin JL, Schwartz D, et al: Exercise intolerance in patients with chronic heart failure: role of impaired nutritive flow to skeletal muscle. *Circulation* 69:1079–1087, 1984.
16. Wilson JR, Ferraro N: Exercise intolerance in patients with chronic heart failure: relation to oxygen transport and ventilatory abnormalities. *Am J Cardiol* 51:1358–1363, 1983.
17. Massie BM: Exercise tolerance in congestive heart failure: role of cardiac function, peripheral blood flow, and muscle metabolism and effects of treatment. *Am J Med* (suppl 3A)84:75–82, 1988.
18. Sullivan MJ, Green HJ, Cobb FR: Altered skeletal muscle metabolic response to exercise in chronic heart failure: relation to skeletal muscle aerobic enzymatic activity. *Circulation* 84:1597–1607, 1991.
19. Franciosa JA, Leddy CL, Schwartz DE, et al: Relation between hemodynamic and ventilatory responses in determining exercise capacity in severe congestive heart failure. *Am J Cardiol* 53:127–134, 1984.
20. Engler R, Ray R, Hissins CB, et al: Clinical assessment and follow-up of functional capacity in patients with chronic congestive cardiomyopathy. *Am J Cardiol* 49:1832–1837, 1982.
21. Yamabe H, Takata T, Yokoyama M, et al: Lactate threshold is not an onset of insufficient oxygen supply to the working muscle in patients with chronic heart failure. *Clin Cardiol* 17:391–394, 1994.
22. Shephard RJ: *Physiology and Biochemistry of Exercise*. New York: Praeger Publishers, 63–66, 1982.
23. Stringer W, Wasserman K, Casaburi R, et al: Lactic acidosis as a facilitator of oxyhemoglobin dissociation during exercise. *J Appl Physiol* 76:1462–1467, 1994.
24. Doll E, Keul J, Maiwald C: Oxygen tension and acid-base equilibria in venous blood of working muscle. *Am J Physiol* 215:23–29, 1968.
25. Roubin GS, Anderson SD, Shen WF, et al: Hemodynamic and metabolic basis of impaired exercise tolerance in patients with severe left ventricular dysfunction. *J Am Coll Cardiol* 15:986–994, 1990.
26. Roca J, Agusti AGN, Alonso A, et al: Effects of training on muscle O_2 transport at $\dot{V}O_2$max. *J Appl Physiol* 73:1067–1076, 1992.

27. Koike A, Wasserman K, Taniguchi K, et al: Critical capillary oxygen pressure and lactate threshold in patients with cardiovascular disease. *J Am Coll Cardiol* 23:1644–1650, 1994.
28. Franciosa JA, Park M, Levine TB: Lack of correlation between exercise capacity and indexes of resting left ventricular performance in heart failure. *Am J Cardiol* 47:33–39, 1981.
29. Lipkin D, Jones D, Round J, et al: Abnormalities of skeletal muscle in patients with chronic heart failure. *Int J Med* 18:184–195, 1988.
30. Sullivan MJ, Green HJ, Cobb FR: Skeletal muscle biochemistry and histology in ambulatory patients with long-term heart failure. *Circulation* 81:518–527, 1990.
31. Drexler H, Riede U, Munzel T, et al: Alterations of skeletal muscle in chronic heart failure. *Circulation* 85:1751–1759, 1992.
32. Massie BM: Exercise intolerance in congestive heart failure: role of cardiac function, peripheral blood flow and muscle metabolism and effects of treatment. *Am J Med* (suppl 3A)84:75–82, 1988.
33. Mancini DM, Coyle E, Coggan A, et al: Contribution of intrinsic skeletal muscle change to P-31 NMR skeletal muscle metabolic abnormalities in patients with chronic heart failure. *Circulation* 80:1338–1346, 1989.
34. Massie B, Conway M, Rajagoropalan B, et al: Skeletal muscle metabolism during exercise under ischemic conditions in congestive heart failure: evidence for abnormalities unrelated to blood flow. *Circulation* 78:320–326, 1988.
35. Yamabe H, Itoh K, Yokoyama M, et al: The role of cardiac output response on blood flow distribution during exercise in patients with chronic heart failure. *Eur Heart J* (In press.)
36. Wilson JR, Fink LI, Ferraro N, et al: Use of maximal bicycle exercise testing with respiratory gas analysis to assess exercise performance in patients with congestive heart failure secondary to coronary artery disease or to idiopathic dilated cardiomyopathy. *Am J Cardiol* 58:601–606, 1986.
37. Eldridge JE, Ramsey-Green CL, Hossack KF: Effects of the limiting symptom on the achievement of maximal oxygen consumption in patients with coronary artery disease. *Am J Cardiol* 57:513–517, 1986.
38. Ehsani AA, Biello D, Seals DR, et al: The effect of left ventricular systolic function on maximal aerobic exercise capacity in asymptomatic patients with coronary artery disease. *Circulation* 70:552–560, 1984.
39. Myers J, Walsh D, Froelicher V, et al: Effect of sampling on variability and plateau in oxygen uptake. *J Appl Physiol* 68:404–410, 1990.
40. Bruce RA: Exercise testing for evaluation of ventricular capacity in man. *N Engl J Med* 296:671–674, 1977.
41. Franciosa JA, Ziesche S, Wilen M: Functional capacity of patients with chronic left ventricular failure: relationship of bicycle exercise performance to clinical and hemodynamic catheterization. *Am J Med* 67:460–466, 1979.

14

Peripheral Arterial Disease:
Pathophysiology, Exercise Performance, and Effect of Exercise Training on Gas Exchange and Muscle Metabolism

William R. Hiatt, MD; Eugene E. Wolfel, MD
Judith G. Regensteiner, PhD

Introduction

Patients with peripheral arterial disease (PAD) develop atherosclerotic occlusions in the major arteries supplying their lower extremities. During walking activity (and other forms of lower extremity exercise), the restricted blood flow is not able to meet the metabolic demand of the muscles in the lower extremity. This results in muscle ischemia and the symptom of intermittent claudication. Thus, patients with claudication are only able to walk short distances before they must stop and rest to relieve their ischemic calf muscle pain. Patients with claudication also have a marked limitation in peak exercise performance when tested on the treadmill, as compared to age-matched normal subjects.[1,2] The claudication-limited exercise performance and walking impairment are associated with disability in persons who are unable to carry out their normal personal, social, and occupational activities.[3] Patients with other forms of cardiovascular disease (congestive heart failure and coronary artery disease) also have severe lim-

From Wasserman, K (ed): *Exercise Gas Exchange in Heart Disease.* Armonk, NY: Futura Publishing Company, Inc., © 1996.

Table 1

Peak Exercise Performance in Healthy Individuals and
Patients with Cardiovascular Disease.

	Healthy	CHF	CAD	PAD
Number	23	9	7	15
Age	54 ± 8	49 ± 2	60 ± 3	60 ± 12
Sex (%male)	100%	78%	57%	100%
Peak $\dot{V}O_2$	29.4 ± 5.0	$18.6 \pm 1.4^*$	$17.5 \pm 0.7^*$	$12.7 \pm 1.8^{*+}$

Peak exercise performance was determined with graded treadmill testing. Subjects were tested who were healthy, and age-matched to the patient groups. Patients with congestive heart failure (CHF) had ischemic cardiomyopathy (N=6), idiopathic dilated cardiomyopathy (N=2), or post-viral cardiomyopathy (N=1). Their left ventricular ejection fraction was 16.7 ± 2.3%. Patients with coronary artery disease (CAD) had documentation of their disease by cardiac catheterization or thallium treadmill testing. All of these patients stopped exercise because of angina or ST segment depression. Patients with peripheral arterial disease (PAD) had disease documented by the ankle-brachial index, with disease defined as a ratio less than 0.90. Peak $\dot{V}O_2$ is in ml/lg/min.

itations in exercise performance. The exercise impairment in these groups is related to decreased cardiac output and/or anginal pain during exercise. However, patients with PAD evaluated in our laboratory have greater limitations in peak exercise performance than do patients with other forms of cardiovascular disease undergoing exercise testing (Table 1). Although patients with different cardiovascular diseases have a wide variation in functional disease severity, limited arterial flow to the lower extremities is associated with a highly restricted exercise capacity and limited walking ability.

The pathophysiology of claudication is primarily related to the restricted muscle blood flow. However, additional factors further limit exercise performance such as inactivity with deconditioning, muscle denervation, and alterations in muscle oxidative and glycolytic metabolism. Despite the multifactorial nature of the exercise impairment, these patients can be reliably assessed with graded treadmill testing. Importantly, patients experience large improvements in peak exercise performance and community-based walking ability with a supervised exercise training program. A detailed discussion of these concepts, and potential mechanisms of the training response, are the focus of this chapter.

Pathophysiology of Claudication

Hemodynamic Changes with PAD

When an arterial stenosis reaches a critical level (generally greater than 60% to 70%) there is decrease in both pressure and flow across the stenosis. In patients with claudication, a single high grade proximal stenosis or occlusion usually produces no symptoms at rest because collateral blood flow is adequate to meet the low metabolic demand of the extremity. Only with multiple occlusions in series does resting arterial flow fall below a critical level and patients develop ischemic pain at rest (with progression to ulceration and gangrene if the extremity is not re-vascularized).

With exercise, there is a marked increase in the metabolic demand of the leg muscles, resulting in arteriolar vasodilation and a fall in peripheral resistance. In healthy subjects, an increase in cardiac output and systemic blood pressure maintains skeletal muscle blood flow during exercise. In contrast, patients with PAD typically have a 40% reduction in arterial flow as compared to values in healthy subjects at comparable work rates.[4] With exercise, pressure within the artery decreases distal to the stenosis in proportion to the decrease in peripheral resistance because of the limited arterial flow.[5] In addition to decreased pressure and flow within the artery distal to the stenosis, the force of each muscle contraction during walking exercise exceeds the intra-arterial pressure resulting in a further compromise to flow.[6] The net effect of all of these factors during exercise is a marked decrease in oxygen delivery to skeletal muscle distal to the arterial stenosis.[7]

Effect of PAD on Muscle Histology and Function

Several abnormalities have been described in ischemic skeletal muscle in patients with PAD. Patients with claudication have a selective loss of type II glycolytic fibers relative to type I oxidative fibers in the gastrocnemius muscle of their affected legs.[8,9] This altered fiber type distribution was associated with muscle weakness.[9] In addition, a chronic denervation occurs in ischemic skeletal muscle that was also correlated with muscle weakness and dysfunction.[9,10] The denervation and changes in muscle fiber composition not only result in muscle dysfunction, but also may adversely affect muscle metabolism as discussed below.

Effect of PAD on Muscle Metabolism

In patients with PAD, exercise to the point of muscle ischemia is associated with a marked depletion in muscle phosphocreatine content as compared to control subjects at similar work rates.[7,11] The limitation in the oxidative production of high energy phosphates is associated with an increase in femoral vein lactate concentration and an increase in the lactate/pyruvate ratio in the ischemic muscle as compared to resting values.[7,12] The amount of lactate released during exercise may be greater in PAD patients as compared to control subjects at the same normalized work rate.[13,14] However, other investigators have observed a similar increase in muscle lactate content in both patients and controls, despite more muscle work performed by the control subjects.[15] Also during exercise, the muscle lactate/pyruvate ratio was lower in PAD subjects as compared to controls when normalized to muscle oxygen tension.[7] In contrast to the above findings in chronic leg ischemia, when normal subjects exercised during acute ischemic conditions induced by an occluding cuff, the ischemic leg venous lactate concentration and leg lactate release was twice that of the non-ischemic leg at the same work rate.[16] Thus, patients with chronic arterial occlusive disease may have a *relative* impairment in muscle lactate production during ischemic exercise. Furthermore, patients with PAD have only a modest increase in arterial (systemic) lactate concentration during maximal claudication-limited exercise.[12,17] This blunted increment in blood lactate concentration with exercise may be due to the reduced type II fiber population, poor wash out of lactate from ischemic muscle, or because the patient stops exercise at a low work rate that is below their systemic lactate threshold.

In addition to alterations in muscle lactate metabolism, patients with PAD have other metabolic abnormalities associated with their disease. An increase in muscle oxidative enzyme activities has been postulated as an adaptive response to decreased oxygen delivery.[18,19] However, in a number of studies of PAD patients there was no change or decrease in the activities of several oxidative enzymes, with no correlation between the enzyme activity and exercise performance.[9,20,21] The lack of an increase in muscle oxidative enzymes in these patients may be due to inactivity and deconditioning (claudication pain limits activity), or is related to the denervation of skeletal muscle.[22]

In contrast to the lack of consistent changes in muscle enzyme activities, PAD patients have changes in muscle intermediary metabolism that are of functional significance. For example, carnitine interacts with the acyl-CoA pool (intermediates in the oxidation of fuel substrates) through the reversible transfer of acyl groups from acyl-CoA's to form the corresponding acylcarnitines. This reaction provides unesterified CoA for other metabolic reactions,[23] and the resultant formation of short-chain acylcarnitines may serve to modulate changes in the acyl-CoA pool under conditions of acute metabolic stress. Thus, changes in the relationship between unesterified carnitine and acylcarnitines provides an index of changes in cellular oxidative metabolism.[24]

Consistent with the concepts presented above, patients with claudication accumulate short-chain acylcarnitines in ischemic skeletal muscle at rest.[25,26] Importantly, there was an inverse correlation between muscle short-chain acylcarnitine content in the diseased legs at rest and peak exercise performance. This correlation indicated that the greater the degree of chronic disruption of oxidative metabolism in patients with claudication (as reflected by acylcarnitine accumulation), the worse the exercise performance. Thus, the accumulation of acylcarnitines serves as a marker of the functional disease severity in patients with PAD.

The changes in carnitine metabolism, and the lack of a consistent increase in muscle oxidative enzymes in PAD, is consistent with the concept that these patients have an acquired mitochondrial defect in oxidative metabolism. Evidence for this concept comes from the relationship between the muscle adenosine diphosphate (ADP) concentration at the end of exercise and the phosphocreatine resynthesis rate during recovery. With decreased oxygen delivery (as in heart failure), ADP accumulates during exercise to a similar degree as in normal subjects at the same work rate. However, the rates of phosphocreatine resynthesis and adenosine triphosphate (ATP) production are reduced as compared to healthy controls.[27] In contrast, patients with PAD have both an exaggerated accumulation of ADP at the end of exercise and a decrease in phosphocreatine resynthesis rate during recovery as compared to control subjects.[27] These observations suggest a mixed metabolic disorder in PAD, with tissue hypoxia accounting for the decrease in phosphocreatine resynthesis rate. In addition, there may be an abnormality in the K_m of ADP in the regulation of mitochondrial ATP synthesis, a finding consistent with a mitochondrial myopathy. Thus, while the initial disease process of PAD is a reduced blood and oxygen delivery to skeletal muscle, neurologic injury to muscle fibers and metabolic sequelae contribute to the disease pathophysiology and clinical severity.

Exercise Testing and Performance in PAD

Exercise Testing

Treadmill testing is designed to permit the collection of objective data on the exercise capacity of patients with claudication. Several different exercise testing modalities have been used in this patient population, but graded treadmill testing provides the best estimate of peak exercise performance in patients with claudication.[28] The major measurements used with the graded test are the time at which the patient first notices the onset of claudication pain and the claudication-limited maximal exercise duration. The graded treadmill test is highly reproducible, provides consistent results over time, and is well tolerated by all patients with claudication.[17,28] The measurement of oxygen consumption during graded exercise testing provides an additional objective physiologic marker of peak exercise performance and cardiovascular function. Constant-load exercise testing has also been employed to evaluate patients with claudication. Testing patients at a constant external work rate allows for the evaluation of changes in the physiologic and metabolic responses to steady state exercise resulting from specific treatments of claudication. For example, when oxygen consumption is measured during constant-load tests, changes in the metabolic cost of a given work rate (i.e., walking efficiency) can be ascertained.

PAD Exercise Performance

The claudication-limited peak oxygen consumption of PAD patients (measured with the graded treadmill protocol) has been shown to be in the range of 12 to 15 mL/kg/min[2,29] or approximately 40% to 50% of the age predicted maximal oxygen consumption for normal subjects.[2,25,30] Examples of peak ($\dot{V}O_2$) in different groups of patients are presented in Table 1. These were consecutive patients tested in our laboratory with well characterized congestive heart failure, coronary artery disease, and PAD as compared to age-matched healthy subjects. The data demonstrate that PAD patients have a relatively greater impairment in peak $\dot{V}O_2$ than our other cardiovascular-limited patients. At peak exercise (lower absolute work rate than in control subjects), patients with PAD had a peak respiratory exchange ratio (RER) and blood lactate concentration that was less than in control subjects.[2,25] However, the peak heart rate, systolic and diastolic blood pressures, were similar between patients and controls. This finding suggests a similar degree of sympathetic activation at peak exercise in both groups.

Exercise Training for PAD

Exercise rehabilitation is an established and highly effective intervention for the treatment of claudication. Several controlled trials of exercise training have been conducted over the past 30 years. All studies of exercise treatment for claudication have reported an increase in treadmill exercise performance, and pain-free walking time during exercise.[31-34] This consistent finding demonstrates that exercise training programs have a clinically important impact on functional capacity in patients for whom other treatment options are limited, and in whom spontaneous recovery does not occur. In addition, there is virtually no morbidity or mortality from exercise training.

A hospital-based, supervised treadmill exercise program is an effective mode of exercise therapy for patients with claudication. The exercise sessions are typically held 3 times a week for approximately 1 hour each, and 3 to 6 months of training are customary. The beginning training work rate is determined from the graded treadmill test on entry, as the intensity that initially brings on claudication pain. During the exercise sessions, the patient walks on the treadmill until reaching a moderate level of pain, followed by a rest period until the pain abates. The alternation of rest and exercise is repeated throughout each training session. In subsequent visits, the speed or grade of the treadmill is increased if the patient is able to walk for 10 minutes or longer at the lower work rate without achieving moderate claudication pain.

Several studies of exercise training have been conducted in the PAD patient population at the University of Colorado.[29,35] In the most recent study, patients with disabling claudication were randomized to 12 weeks of supervised walking exercise on a treadmill (as described above), strength training (data not shown), or a non-exercising control group.[35]

Subjects were tested on both a graded and constant-load treadmill protocol (conducted on separate days) on entry, and after 12 and 24 weeks. The graded treadmill protocol consisted of an initial work rate of 2 mph, 0% grade for 3 minutes. Subsequent stages increased 3.5% in grade every 3 minutes (with no change in speed) to maximal claudication pain. During exercise, heart rate (by 12-lead EKG) and brachial blood pressure were monitored every minute, and oxygen consumption was monitored continuously. The RER was calculated as carbon dioxide output/oxygen uptake ($\dot{V}CO_2/\dot{V}O_2$). Venous blood for lactate analysis[36] was obtained from the forearm at rest, and every minute during graded treadmill exercise. All subjects (at all evaluations) reached a maximal level of claudication pain that limited exercise during the graded treadmill test.

Subjects were also tested on a constant-load treadmill protocol to determine whether changes in steady state $\dot{V}O_2$ and other metabolic responses occurred as a result of the training programs. The work rate for the constant-load protocol was individually set at the treadmill grade at which claudication pain first began on the graded protocol. The grade of the constant-load test ranged from 0% to 7% with an average of 2% in all subjects. Through the remainder of the study, this work rate was held constant for subsequent evaluations.

The results for the treadmill trained group (n=9) are presented in Table 2. The control group had no change in peak treadmill walking time or $\dot{V}O_2$ during the study period. Patients in the treadmill trained

Table 2

Changes in Treadmill Performance and Metabolism with Treadmill Training.

	Entry	Week 12	Week 24
Walking Time (min)			
Graded	9.6±5.7	14.7±7.3*	17.2±7.3*+
Constant	13.2±10.9	30.5±17.9*	39.2±19.6*+
$\dot{V}O_2$ *(mL/kg/min)*			
Graded	15.0±2.4	16.9±4.8*	17.8±4.7*
Constant	11.9±1.7	10.1±1.9*	9.9±1.3*
RER			
Graded	0.97±0.09	0.97±0.09	1.01±0.09*+
Constant	0.89±0.07	0.82±0.04*	0.83±0.05*
Lactate concentration (mM)			
Graded	2.2±1.2	2.4±1.8	3.1±1.2*
Constant	1.4±0.4	1.0±0.5*	0.9±0.2*

Subjects randomized to the treadmill group were treated with a 24-week supervised exercise training program as previously described.[35] Training consisted of 1 hour sessions of intermittent treadmill exercise, three times a week. Testing was performed with a graded treadmill protocol to maximal, claudication-limited exercise. Constant-load exercise was also performed at a work rate that was associated with the onset of claudication on the entry graded test. Constant-load tests at 12 and 24 weeks were performed at the same work rate as on entry. Measurements of $\dot{V}O_2$, percent peak $\dot{V}O_2$, heart rate, respiratory exchange ratio (RER), and blood lactate concentration are reported for 6 minutes of exercise on the constant-load protocol.

* P <0.05 compared to entry value, and + P<0.05 week 24 compared to week 12. Control subjects had no change in their metabolic parameters, but a decrease in walking time on the constant-load protocol at 12 weeks.

group had an increase in exercise duration with both graded and constant-load treadmill testing after 12 weeks. Importantly, there were further improvements in exercise performance with an additional 12 weeks (total of 24 weeks) of training. With exercise training, patients demonstrated an increase in peak $\dot{V}O_2$, RER, and blood lactate concentration during graded treadmill testing. These data provide further evidence that the trained patients achieved a higher peak exercise intensity as compared to pre-training values.

The constant-load treadmill exercise test was also utilized to evaluate changes in hemodynamics and the metabolic responses to exercise under steady state conditions. All subjects had reached steady state with respect to the ventilatory parameters by 4 minutes, with the ventilatory and lactate measurements reported at 6 minutes of exercise. After 12 weeks of treadmill training, the steady state $\dot{V}O_2$ (6 minute value at the same grade and speed as on entry) was reduced 15% compared to entry values. In addition, heart rate, RER, and blood lactate concentration at 6 minutes of exercise were also reduced as compared to entry values. An additional 12 weeks of treadmill training resulted in a increase in peak walking duration (as compared to the first 12 weeks), but did not further improve the metabolic parameters.

The lower steady state $\dot{V}O_2$ observed with training in PAD patients may be the result of modifications in gait or the biomechanics of walking that allow for less energy expenditure to support a given level of exercise. The decrease in the oxygen cost of walking exercise may allow the activity to be sustained for longer periods of time in the community setting. Further evidence that treadmill training modified the systemic responses to a constant exercise work rate was a 17 beat per minute reduction in heart rate, the reduction in RER (greater reliance on fatty acid oxidation), and the decrease in blood lactate concentration. Similar training responses in heart rate, RER, and blood lactate concentration have been observed with exercise conditioning in both normal subjects, and in patients with coronary artery disease.[37,38]

Previous studies have also evaluated the effects of exercise training in PAD on skeletal muscle blood flow and skeletal muscle metabolism. The majority of studies show no evidence of increased muscle blood flow with training, and no correlation between changes in flow and degree of exercise improvement.[29,39,40] In contrast, evidence that training alters the peripheral physiologic responses to exercise is the observation that femoral vein oxygen saturation is reduced at maximal exercise after training.[39,40] These results suggest that training improves oxygen extraction during exercise. Some studies have also shown that training induces an increase in oxidative enzyme activities, but the findings are not consistent across all studies or for all oxidative enzymes.[19,41] Additional support for an improvement in intermediary metabolism is a decrease in plasma short-chain acylcarnitine concentration with training that was correlated with the increase in exercise performance.[29] As discussed above, accumulations of short-chain acylcarnitines in plasma and muscle serve as a marker of the altered skeletal muscle metabolism seen in PAD. A reduction in plasma acylcarnitine concentration suggests an improvement in metabolism that has functional significance.

Summary

Patients with PAD have a chronic disease that produces a moderate to severe impairment in walking ability. Peak exercise performance is reduced 50%, and claudication pain limits patients to only short walking distances in the community. The causes of the walking impairment are likely to be multifactorial. Arterial occlusive disease, with inadequate skeletal muscle blood flow to meet the metabolic demands of exercise, is the primary pathophysiologic process in the etiology of claudication. However, over time, patients with PAD acquire a distal motor neuropathy and loss of type II muscle fibers which lead to muscle weakness and dysfunction. Altered muscle metabolism, including the accumulation of acylcarnitines in skeletal muscle, are associated with the impairment in exercise performance. Treadmill exercise training results in clinically important improvements in peak exercise performance, and claudication pain severity, allowing patients to perform a greater range of activities. Exercise training is also associated with a decreased metabolic cost of walking exercise and possible improvements in muscle metabolism that allows patients to increase their walking capacity.

References

1. Eldridge JE, Hossack KF: Patterns of oxygen consumption during exercise testing in peripheral vascular disease. *Cardiology* 74:236–240, 1987.
2. Hiatt WR, Nawaz D, Brass EP: Carnitine metabolism during exercise in patients with peripheral vascular disease. *J Appl Physiol* 62:2383–2387, 1987.
3. Regensteiner JG, Steiner JF, Panzer RJ, et al: Evaluation of walking impairment by questionnaire in patients with peripheral arterial disease. *J Vasc Med Biol* 2:142–152, 1990.
4. Lundgren F, Zachrisson H, Emery P, et al: Leg exchange of amino acids during exercise in patients with arterial insufficiency. *Clin Physiol* 8:227–241, 1988.
5. Lundgren F, Bennegard K, Elander A, et al: Substrate exchange in human limb muscle during exercise at reduced blood flow. *Am J Physiol* 255:H1156–H1164, 1988.
6. Coffman JD, Mannick JA: A simple objective test for arteriosclerosis obliterans. *N Engl J Med* 273:1297, 1965.
7. Bylund-Fellenius AC, Walker PM, Elander A, et al: Peripheral vascular disease. *Am Rev Respir Dis* 129:S65–S67, 1984.
8. Makitie J: Peripheral neuromuscular system in peripheral arterial insufficiency. *Scand J Rheumatol* 30(suppl):157–162, 1979.
9. Regensteiner JG, Wolfel EE, Brass EP, et al: Chronic changes in skeletal muscle histology and function in peripheral arterial disease. *Circulation* 87:413–421, 1993.
10. England JD, Regensteiner JG, Ringel SP, et al: Muscle denervation in peripheral arterial disease. *Neurology* 42:994–999, 1992.
11. Hands LJ, Bore PJ, Galloway G, et al: Muscle metabolism in patients with peripheral vascular disease investigated by 31P nuclear magnetic resonance spectroscopy. *Clin Sci* 71:283–290, 1986.
12. Maass U, Alexander K: Lactate and pyruvate changes during treadmill exercise in patients with intermittent claudication. *Z Kardiol* 71:39–43, 1982.
13. Pernow B, Zetterquist S: Metabolic evaluation of the leg blood flow in claudicating patients with arterial obstructions at different levels. *Scand J Clin Lab Invest* 21:277–287, 1968.
14. Sorlie D, Myhre K, Mjos OD: Exercise- and post-exercise metabolism of the lower leg in patients with peripheral arterial insufficiency. *Scand J Clin Lab Invest* 38:635–642, 1978.

15. Bylund-Fellenius AC, Walker PM, Elander A, et al: Energy metabolism in relation to oxygen partial pressure in human skeletal muscle during exercise. *Biochem J* 200:247–255, 1981.
16. Sundberg CJ: Exercise and training during graded leg ischaemia in healthy man with special reference to effects on skeletal muscle. *Acta Physiol Scand* 150(suppl 615):1–50, 1994.
17. Hiatt WR, Nawaz D, Regensteiner JG, et al: The evaluation of exercise performance in patients with peripheral vascular disease. *J Cardiopulmonary Rehabil* 12:525–532, 1988.
18. Jansson E, Johansson J, Sylven C, et al: Calf muscle adaptation in intermittent claudication. Side-differences in muscle metabolic characteristics in patients with unilateral arterial disease. *Clin Physiol* 8:17–29, 1988.
19. Lundgren F, Dahllof AG, Schersten T, et al: Muscle enzyme adaptation in patients with peripheral arterial insufficiency: spontaneous adaptation, effect of different treatments and consequences on walking performance. *Clin Sci* 77:485–493, 1989.
20. Clyne CAC, Mears H, Weller RO, et al: Calf muscle adaptation to peripheral vascular disease. *Cardiovasc Res* 19:507–512, 1985.
21. Henriksson J, Nygaard E, Andersson J, et al: Enzyme activities, fibre types and capillarization in calf muscles of patients with intermittent claudication. *Scand J Clin Lab Invest* 40:361–369, 1980.
22. Wicks KL, Hood DA: Mitochondrial adaptations in denervated muscle: Relationship to muscle performance. *Am J Physiol* 260:C841–C850, 1991.
23. Bieber LL, Emaus R, Valkner K, et al: Possible functions of short-chain and medium-chain carnitine acyltransferases. *Fed Proc* 41:2858–2862, 1982.
24. Shug AL, Thomsen JH, Folts JD, et al: Changes in tissue levels of carnitine and other metabolites during myocardial ischemia and anoxia. *Arch Biochem Biophys* 187:25–33, 1978.
25. Hiatt WR, Wolfel EE, Regensteiner JG, et al: Skeletal muscle carnitine metabolism in patients with unilateral peripheral arterial disease. *J Appl Physiol* 73:346–353, 1992.
26. Brass EP, Hiatt WR: Carnitine metabolism during exercise. *Life Sci* 54:1383–1393, 1994.
27. Kemp GJ, Taylor DJ, Thompson CH, et al: Quantitative analysis by 31P magnetic resonance spectroscopy of abnormal mitochondrial oxidation in skeletal muscle during recovery from exercise. *NMR Biomed* 6:302–310, 1993.
28. Gardner AW, Skinner JS, Cantwell BW, et al: Progressive versus single-stage treadmill tests for evaluation of claudication. *Med Sci Sports Exerc* 23:402–408, 1991.
29. Hiatt WR, Regensteiner JG, Hargarten ME, et al: Benefit of exercise conditioning for patients with peripheral arterial disease. *Circulation* 81:602–609, 1990.
30. Hossack KF, Bruce RA: Maximal cardiac function in sedentary normal men and women: comparison of age-related changes. *J Appl Physiol* 53:799–804, 1982.
31. Mannarino E, Pasqualini L, Menna M, et al: Effects of physical training on peripheral vascular disease: a controlled study. *Angiology* 40:5–10, 1989.
32. Creasy TS, McMillan PJ, Fletcher EWL, et al: Is percutaneous transluminal angioplasty better than exercise for claudication? - Preliminary results from a prospective randomized trial. *Eur J Vasc Surg* 4:135–140, 1990.
33. Dahllof A, Holm J, Schersten T, et al: Peripheral arterial insufficiency. Effect of physical training on walking tolerance, calf blood flow, and blood flow resistance. *Scand J Rehab Med* 8:19–26, 1976.

34. Larsen OA, Lassen NA: Effect of daily muscular exercise in patients with intermittent claudication. *Lancet* 2:1093–1096, 1966.
35. Hiatt WR, Wolfel EE, Meier RH, et al: Superiority of treadmill walking exercise versus strength training for patients with peripheral arterial disease. Implications for the mechanism of the training response. *Circulation* 90:1866–1874, 1994.
36. Rosenberg JD, Rush BF: An enzymatic-spectrophotometric determination of pyruvic and lactic acid in blood. Methodologic aspects. *Clin Chem* 12:299–307, 1966.
37. Poulin MJ, Paterson DH, Govindasamy D, et al: Endurance training of older men: responses to submaximal exercise. *J Appl Physiol* 73:452–457, 1992.
38. Ades PA, Waldmann ML, Poehlman ET, et al: Exercise conditioning in older coronary patients. Submaximal lactate response and endurance capacity. *Circulation* 88:572–577, 1993.
39. Zetterquist S: The effect of active training on the nutritive blood flow in exercising ischemic legs. *Scand J Clin Lab Invest* 25:101–111, 1970.
40. Sorlie D, Myhre K: Effects of physical training in intermittent claudication. *Scand J Clin Lab Invest* 38:217–222, 1978.
41. Dahllof A, Bjorntorp P, Holm J, et al: Metabolic activity of skeletal muscle in patients with peripheral arterial insufficiency. Effect of physical training. *Eur J Clin Invest* 4:9–15, 1974.

15

Peripheral Determinants of Exercise Intolerance in Patients with Chronic Heart Failure

Martin J. Sullivan, MD; Brian D. Duscha, MS
Cris A. Slentz, PhD

Chronic heart failure (CHF) is a major cause of morbidity and mortality in the United States affecting 2 to 3 million people[1] with an estimated 300,000 new cases occurring each year.[2] There are two major causes of symptoms in this disorder: 1) congestion caused by fluid overload, and 2) exercise intolerance, often with disabling dyspnea and fatigue. Although therapy with loop diuretics, digoxin, and vasodilators can often relieve fluid overload and reduce mortality in the majority of ambulatory patients with CHF, many patients remain unable to perform activities of daily life despite maximal medical therapy.

Chronic heart failure research in the past has focused on central hemodynamics. It is now well established that, in CHF patients, the degree of left ventricular systolic dysfunction, as measured by left ventricular ejection fraction, does not correlate with exercise tolerance or symptom status.[3-9] These findings suggest that there is a complex interplay between central hemodynamic factors (systolic and diastolic LV dysfunction, LV and RV filling pressures, cardiac output, and RV function), pulmonary factors (respiratory muscle fatigue, air flow limitations, and hyperpnea), and peripheral factors (skeletal muscle blood

From Wasserman, K (ed): *Exercise Gas Exchange in Heart Disease.* Armonk, NY: Futura Publishing Company, Inc., © 1996.

flow, metabolism, histology/biochemistry, and contractile function) in determining exercise capacity in patients with CHF. This chapter reviews recent studies that examine the peripheral mechanisms of exercise intolerance in CHF.

Blood Flow Changes in Chronic Heart Failure

Several studies have shown that CHF patients have reduced skeletal muscle blood flow and increased vascular resistance at rest and during submaximal exercise (Figure 1, A&B).[10-13] Patients with CHF compensate for this reduced blood flow with an increased arteriovenous oxygen difference (Figure 1C), such that resting and low-level submaximal oxygen uptake ($\dot{V}O_2$) are similar to that of normals[10] (Figure 1D). In patients, femoral venous oxygen content and oxygen saturation are lower at rest and during submaximal exercise, but are similar to normal subjects at maximal exercise (Figure 1E&F). It is important to note, however, that the major difference in blood flow between normals and CHF patients is the greatly reduced peak blood flow to exercising skeletal muscle.[10] This is shown in Figure 1A which reveals peak leg blood flows that are three times higher in normals when compared with CHF patients. The reduced peak $\dot{V}O_2$ in CHF is accompanied by a normal maximal leg arteriovenous difference,[10] suggesting that a low peak oxygen delivery plays a primary role in reducing peak oxygen consumption in this disease. Additional support for this idea comes from studies by Wilson et al[11-16] and from our laboratory[10] which have demonstrated strong correlations between leg blood flow at peak exercise and peak $\dot{V}O_2$. It is likely that the reduced peak blood flow in working skeletal muscle is due primarily to reduced peak cardiac output, although peripheral factors may also play a role independent of central hemodynamic abnormalities.

Studies by Zelis et al[17,18] have demonstrated that in addition to the reduced blood flow and increased vascular resistance, CHF patients also have a decreased vasodilator response to adrenergic blockade, ischemia, and direct arterial vasodilators. Studies have shown that cardiac output and leg blood flow are reduced both at rest and during exercise in CHF patients.[10] In addition, increased leg vascular resistance at rest and during exercise occur in these patients while arterial blood pressure and flow to nonexercising tissues are maintained, suggesting that increased skeletal muscle vasomotor tone is an autoregulatory mechanism which prevents hypotension or hypoperfusion of vital organs in the face of a decreased cardiac output.[10] Although increased vasoconstriction, due to neurohumoral activation,[19,20] or decreased endogenous vasodilation[21-24] likely contribute to this response, these results suggest that increased "vascular stiffness" may also be a

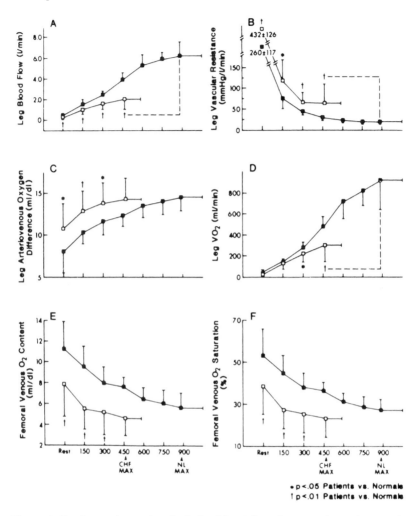

Figure 1. Resting and exercise single leg blood flow, leg vascular resistance, leg arteriovenous oxygen difference, single leg $\dot{V}O_2$, femoral venous oxygen content, and femoral venous oxygen saturation in **patients** with chronic heart failure (n=30) (□) and **normal subjects** (n=12) (■); *p<0.05, +p<0.01 patients versus normal subjects. **Dashed lines** indicate intergroup comparisons of maximal data. (Reprinted with permission from Reference 10.)

factor in the increased vasomotor tone in CHF. This is supported by the findings that 1) capillary basement membranes could be thickened in CHF,[25] 2) diuresis restores about 30% of vasomotor responsiveness,[26] and 3) "vascular stiffness" reverses slowly after cardiac transplantation.[27]

Improvement in endurance exercise performance in normal subjects after exercise training is accompanied by changes in both skeletal muscle oxidative capacity and changes in peak muscle blood flow (secondary to increased cardiac output and/or reduced vascular resistance to the exercising muscle). The finding that increases in peak blood flow and oxygen extraction occur concomitant with increases in exercise tolerance with either long-term angiotensin converting enzyme (ACE) inhibitor therapy[28,29] or exercise training[30,31] suggests that, in CHF patients, both are likely limiting factors in exercise capacity. Drexler et al,[29] in a placebo controlled trial, examined leg blood flow, peak $\dot{V}O_2$, metabolism, and central hemodynamics before and after acute and chronic (4 months) ACE inhibitor therapy in patients with CHF. This study demonstrated an improvement in peak $\dot{V}O_2$ with long-term, but not short-term ACE inhibitor therapy and was accompanied by increased peak exercise leg blood flow, leg $\dot{V}O_2$ and an increase in femoral venous oxygen extraction. Importantly, they suggest that some of these benefits may be due to increased exercise training effects. Mancini et al[28] have also found peak leg blood flow increases in patients who improve exercise tolerance after ACE inhibitor therapy.

Skeletal Muscle Changes in Patients with Chronic Heart Failure

Prior to the 1980's, it was believed that abnormalities in cardiac output and pulmonary capillary wedge pressures were the sole mechanisms responsible for exercise intolerance in CHF. Although hemodynamic factors such as decreases in cardiac output and limb blood flow (Figure 2) are closely related to peak $\dot{V}O_2$, several lines of evidence suggest that these are not the only factors limiting exercise in CHF patients.[32–35] Peak pulmonary capillary wedge pressures[34–36] show no relationship to peak $\dot{V}O_2$ or to symptoms of exertional fatigue versus dyspnea (Figure 3). Several other studies have demonstrated that anaerobic metabolism in skeletal muscle during exercise in patients with CHF is not totally due to decreased perfusion. These studies demonstrate that 1) acutely increasing skeletal muscle blood flow with vasodilators and inotropic agents does not improve exercise capacity or decrease skeletal muscle lactate production in CHF patients, despite increasing cardiac output[12,14,15,37]; 2) some patients with CHF have normal leg blood flow during exercise and yet have early lactate production and decreased peak $\dot{V}O_2$[13]; 3) patients with CHF demonstrate decreases in phosphocreatine (PCr) and pH with normal forearm blood flow[42,43]; 4) during one-leg exercise, leg blood flow to the single leg is increased at a given work rate compared to two-legged exercise with no change in blood lactate.[38] These observations have been con-

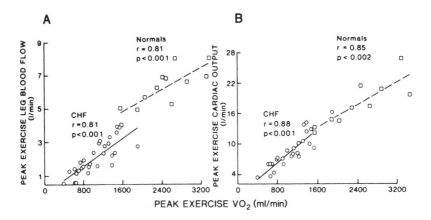

Figure 2. Plots of relations of peak exercise V̇O₂ to single leg blood flow (**panel A**) and cardiac output (**panel B**) in patients with chronic heart failure due to systolic left ventricular (LV) dysfunction (**open circle,** solid predicted regression lines) and normal subjects (**open box,** dashed predicted regression lines); r=correction coefficient. (Reprinted with permission from Reference 10.)

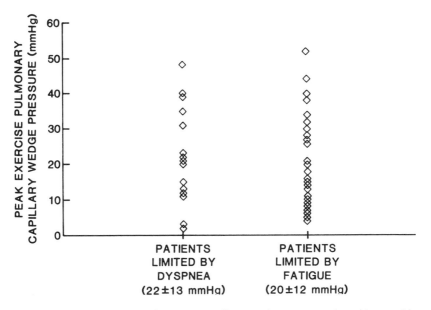

Figure 3. Peak exercise pulmonary capillary wedge pressure in patients with chronic heart failure grouped according to primary limiting symptom during bicycle exercise. Mean values are shown in parentheses under each column of data points. (Reproduced with permission from Reference 35.)

firmed by ^{31}P-NMR studies showing early anaerobic metabolism in CHF when compared with normals even after occlusion of skeletal muscle blood flow.[32,39] These results support the concept that in addition to oxygen delivery, histologic and biochemical changes in skeletal muscle play an important role in determining skeletal muscle alterations that contribute to early acidosis, fatigue, and exercise intolerance in patients with CHF.

Changes in Skeletal Muscle Metabolism in Chronic Heart Failure

A growing body of literature suggests that skeletal muscle metabolism is altered in patients with CHF.[39-46] Previous studies examining skeletal metabolism during forearm[34-36] and leg exercises[45] via phosphorus magnetic resonance imaging (^{31}P-MRI) have confirmed that patients with CHF often exhibit increased glycolytic metabolism and impaired oxidative phosphorylation in exercising skeletal muscle. Patients with CHF demonstrate reductions in pH and increases in Pi/PCr during submaximal exercise when compared to normals. Studies by Wilson et al[42] and Massie et al[43] demonstrated that pH and inorganic phosphate/phosphocreatine (Pi/PCr) were reduced at a given work rate when compared to normals even when forearm blood flow was normal in CHF patients. Patients also demonstrated an excessive decrease in pH for a given decrease in Pi/PCr suggesting heightened glycolytic metabolism. Analysis of rest and exercise biopsies of the vastus lateralis in patients with CHF and normal subjects support this concept[45] by demonstrating a prominent rise in lactate, glucose, and glucose-6-PO_4 in skeletal muscle during low-level exercise.

Although it is likely that early anaerobic metabolism plays an important role in skeletal muscle fatigue and exercise intolerance, several lines of evidence suggest that this is not the sole factor mediating skeletal muscle fatigue in this disorder: 1) Wilson et al[47] have markedly reduced lactate concentration during exercise by administering dichloroacetate to CHF patients that yielded no improvements in exercise tolerance or symptoms, 2) studies have not demonstrated reduced anaerobic metabolism during submaximal exercise after successful vasodilation therapy,[48] 3) blood lactate levels at peak exercise are consistently lower in patients versus normals[10,49] without an alteration in the blood to skeletal muscle lactate gradient,[45] and 4) during peak exercise (as indicated by nearly complete femoral venous oxygen extraction, high femoral venous PCO_2 levels, respiratory exchange ratio (RER) levels of 1.37 ± 0.14, and high subjective leg fatigue) CHF patients exhibit less PCr depletion and lactate accumulation in skeletal muscle versus normals.[45] These data suggest that there are additional physiological mechanisms other than intramuscular lactate accumulation and the depletion of high energy phosphates that contribute to skeletal muscle fatigue in CHF patients. Other metabolic pathways that may play important roles in early skeletal muscle fatigue include calcium uptake and sarcoplasmic reticulum function in muscle during contraction.[50,51] It is possible that a reduced $Na^+ - K^+$ or Ca^{++} ATPase activity contributes to contractile dysfunction in skeletal muscle in CHF. Drexler[52] and Norgaard[53] have raised the possibility that an increased calcium turnover may cause CHF skeletal muscle metabolism to change. Norgaard suggests that intracellular accumulation of calcium and hydrogen ions would compromise mitochondrial function, resulting in a decreased pH and early fatigue.

Histologic and Biochemical Changes in Skeletal Muscle in Chronic Heart Failure

Histologic characteristics have important ramifications to substrate use in exercising skeletal muscle. Histologic analysis from skeletal muscle biopsies in CHF patients have shown decreases in the percent composition of slow-twitch type I fibers which have a high potential for aerobic oxidation, and an increase in fast-twitch type IIb fibers when compared to normals.[46,52,54] (Figure 4). Evidence from cross-sectional population studies suggests that alteration of type I

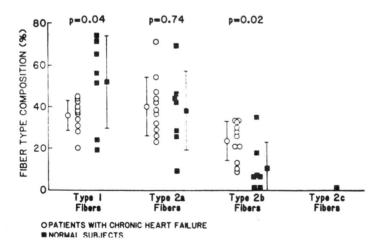

Figure 4. Graphic plotting of relative fiber type composition of the vastus lateralis in patients with long-term heart failure and in normal subjects. (Reproduced with permission from Reference 54.)

fiber composition might occur as the result of years of inactivity.[55] However, the magnitude of change in CHF patients exceeds exercise deconditioning patterns seen in normal subjects.[54] In addition, individual muscle fibers appear to be smaller and capillaries per fiber are reduced in CHF patients. Drexler et al[52] have demonstrated reduced surface area and volume density of mitochondria, and reduced capillary length density in skeletal muscle in CHF. Drexler has also demonstrated that the mitochondria volume density changes are related to peak $\dot{V}O_2$ (Figure 5). In support of these histologic analyses, Sullivan et al[56] have found evidence of decreases in myosin heavy chain type I isoforms and increases in type IIa and IIb isoform content in patients with CHF.[57]

Several laboratories have demonstrated decreases in aerobic enzyme activity in skeletal muscle in patients with CHF.[45,52,54,60] Enzymes showing a reduction in activity include hexokinase, citrate synthetase, succinate dehydrogenase, and 3-hydroxyacyl-CoA dehydrogenase (Figure 6). These alterations have been previously shown to be a potent stimulus for early anaerobic metabolism in normal humans.[55] It is possible that this shift in fiber typing may be in part responsible for a de-

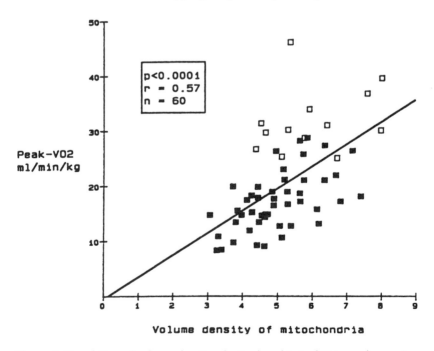

Figure 5. Correlation of volume density of mitochondria (vol%) to peak exercise $\dot{V}O_2$. **Filled squares** denote patients with heart failure, **open squares** denote normal individuals (r=0.59, p<0.001 for patients with heart failure only; n=47). (Reproduced with permission from Reference 52.)

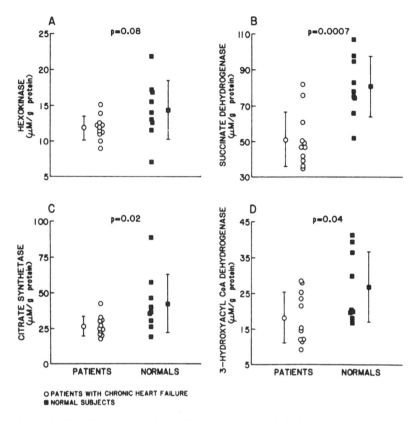

Figure 6. Graphic plotting of hexokinase, succinate dehydrogenase, citrate synthetase, and 3-hydroxyacyl-CoA dehydrogenase in mixed skeletal muscle samples in patients with long-term heart failure and in normal subjects. (Reproduced with permission from Reference 54.)

crease in aerobic enzyme activity. Previous studies have confirmed that glycolysis and glycogenolysis are accelerated in CHF in response to exercise.[10,11,33,39,55,57] Sullivan et al[45] have found inverse relationships between oxidative enzyme activity and blood lactate accumulation during submaximal exercise. Both Sullivan[45] and Mancini[46] found a reduced activity in the enzyme 3-hydroxycyl-CoA dehydrogenase, a mitochondrial enzyme reflective of fat oxidation. Drexler et al[52] have demonstrated a reduced activity level for cytochrome oxidase in skeletal muscle mitochondria, indicating a reduced oxidative capacity of exercising muscle. These changes would be expected to induce early anaerobic metabolism, leading to increased lactate concentrations.

When viewed together, these studies demonstrate that the heart failure state is associated with major changes in skeletal muscle histology and biochemistry. These changes include decreases in oxidative enzyme content, and relative composition in highly oxidative type I fibers with an increase in type IIb fibers. Similar biochemical and histologic changes have been previously reported after exercise deconditioning, and are associated with the acceleration of lactate production during exercise.[55] Thus, the alterations of skeletal muscle seen in CHF patients may play a role in exercise intolerance.

Skeletal Muscle Contractile Function in Chronic Heart Failure

In addition to metabolic, histologic, and biochemical abnormalities, Minotti et al[58] have reported evidence of skeletal muscle contractile dysfunction in CHF. These investigators compared static and dynamic isokinetic endurance between patients with CHF and normal subjects. They demonstrated that static endurance, defined as the time it takes for force to decline to 60% of maximum during a maximal voluntary isometric contraction, was reduced in patients versus normals (40 ± 14 versus 77 ± 29, p<0.02). This is important because isometric contraction of >60% MVC generally occludes arterial inflow. Dynamic endurance, defined as the decline in peak torque during 15 successive contractions, was reduced in CHF patients even after occlusion of arterial inflow. A finding which provides a strong link between skeletal muscle performance and symptoms was that the dynamic endurance was closely related to peak $\dot{V}O_2$ in CHF patients (Figure 7). These results provide strong evidence that skeletal muscle contractile dysfunction occurs independent of reduced perfusion and plays an important role in determining exercise performance in CHF.

Skeletal muscle atrophy has been a consistent finding in patients with CHF[59–61] which may contribute to exertional fatigue. Lipkin et al[62] have found a 55% reduction in isometric tension of the quadriceps femoris in CHF patients when compared to normal subjects, although skeletal muscle size was not measured in this study. The cross-sectional area of the knee extensors in CHF patients has been shown to be significantly smaller when compared to age-matched sedentary controls.[59] However, the relationship between strength and cross-sectional area is similar in CHF patients and controls. Based on this finding, it can be concluded that muscle size and not force per cross-sectional area is responsible for the decreased isometric strength in CHF patients. It is important to note that body mass index was similar between the CHF patients and the normals, thus, eliminating differences in body size as a possible factor. In an insightful study, Mancini et al[60] examined calf muscle volume and 24-hour urinary creatine ex-

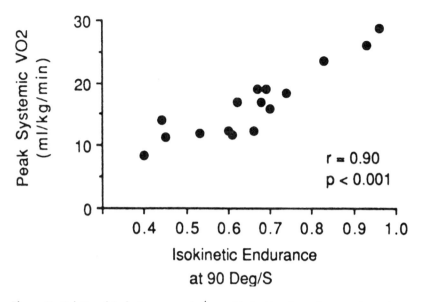

Figure 7. Relationship between peak $\dot{V}O_2$ with isokinetic endurance in patients with chronic heart failure. 90 Deg/S = angular velocity of isokinetic in degrees per second. (Reproduced with permission from Reference 58.)

cretion in patients with CHF. There was a reduction in the creatine-to-height ratio in 68% of CHF patients suggesting reduced skeletal muscle mass. Calf muscle volume was reduced in the patients and was weakly related to work slope (r=0.42, p<0.05), suggesting that skeletal muscle atrophy contributes to exercise intolerance in this disorder (Figure 8).

However, skeletal muscle atrophy does not appear to explain all of the reductions in exercise tolerance in CHF. Sullivan[63] has examined metabolism using ^{31}P-MRI of the quadriceps during knee extensor exercise in normal subjects and patients with CHF that were matched for quadriceps femoris muscle mass. Peak $\dot{V}O_2$ was significantly reduced in patients versus normals, and PCr/Pi decreased faster in CHF subjects during exercise. These results indicate that exercise intolerance accompanied by altered skeletal muscle metabolism can occur in the absence of skeletal muscle atrophy. Because oxidative metabolism is not highly correlated with muscle mass, it suggests that muscle atrophy is not solely responsible for a decrease in oxidative metabolism. Other studies by Mancini et al[60] which compare muscle size and peak oxygen consumption support this hypothesis.

Several mechanisms may cause skeletal muscle alterations in CHF patients. Exercise deconditioning in normals increases lactate production at submaximal levels of exercise, decreases aerobic oxidative en-

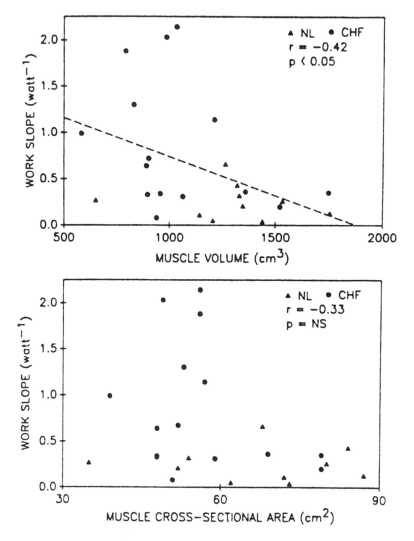

Figure 8. Scatter plots showing correlations between work slope and calf muscle volume, and work slope and the largest muscle cross-sectional area in normal subjects (NL) and patients with heart failure (CHF). Work slope = (Pi/PCr)/watts. (Reproduced with permission from Reference 60.)

zymes, mitochondrial volume density, and decreases fiber size.[55,64,65] Although many of these changes are also found in CHF patients, the magnitude exceeds what is generally seen with exercise deconditioning in normal subjects. Some changes found in CHF patients that are not found in deconditioned normals include alterations in fiber type composition, relative myosin heavy chain expression, or decreases in the number of capillaries per fiber. These findings suggest that in addition to deconditioning, other factors such as circulating proteolytic factors like TNF, neurohumoral activation, or changes in neural activation may contribute to alterations in skeletal muscle in CHF. Although these are the most widely studied in altering skeletal muscle in CHF, other hormones such as IGF-1 or insulin may play key roles. Recent studies by Kraus et al[66] have found increases in mRNA coding for proteins of glycolytic metabolism and decreases in mitochondrial mRNA in skeletal muscle in CHF. Similar findings have been reported in animals with heart failure,[67–70] which suggest that changes in mRNA and not proteolysis are responsible for changes in skeletal muscle in CHF. Additional research needs to be done in humans to determine the causes of changes in skeletal muscle metabolism in CHF.

Exercise Training in Chronic Heart Failure

Studies examining exercise training in patients with CHF and severe systolic LV dysfunction have provided important information on the mechanisms of exercise intolerance in CHF. Although exercise has previously been felt to be contraindicated in patients with CHF, at least 10 studies have now shown that training improves peak $\dot{V}O_2$ and symptoms of CHF.[30,31,71–79] Exercise training represents an important therapy in CHF which likely acts primarily through effects in skeletal muscle. Studies have shown that after 4 to 6 months of cardiac rehabilitation, patients improved peak $\dot{V}O_2$ by 23%, developed a training bradycardia, and increased peak arteriovenous oxygen difference without significant changes in exercise cardiac output.[30,80] This was accompanied during submaximal exercise by a marked decrease in arterial and femoral venous lactate accumulation without a change in leg blood flow or femoral venous oxygen saturation. Patients demonstrated an increase in the $\dot{V}O_2$ at the anaerobic threshold (AT), improved symptoms, and a marked increase in endurance time at a fixed submaximal work rate. Coats et al,[31,72] in a randomized crossover trial, also demonstrated improved peak $\dot{V}O_2$ with training which was accompanied by an improved quality of life. An important finding in this study was that adrenergic activation, assessed by ^{3}H-norepinephrine spillover and by spectral analysis of heart rate variability, was decreased in patients after training. This has important consequences because therapies like exercise training which reduce neurohumoral activation in CHF generally confer long-term morbidity and mortality benefits in CHF. Resistance training or weightlifting have also been shown to improve functional capacity in these patients.[71] Studies by Davies et al have shown that exercise training reduces hyperkalemia during exercise in patients with CHF which may lead to decreased fatigue during low-level exercise. A recent study by Kavanagh et al[76] found an increase in peak $\dot{V}O_2$ after training in patients with severe CHF (peak $\dot{V}O_2 < 15$ mL/kg/min). In this study, changes in peak $\dot{V}O_2$ were closely related to improvements in quality of life. These studies indicate that exercise training improves peak $\dot{V}O_2$ and symptoms to a degree that is similar to the effects of vasodilator therapy. It appears that exercise training improves exercise tolerance in CHF mainly through effects on skeletal muscle without major improvement in central hemodynamics. These results support the concept that peripheral factors play an important role in determining the response to therapy in this disorder.

Summary

Although abnormal heart function is the primary initiation event in the syndrome of CHF, there is now clear evidence that peripheral abnormalities play a role in exercise intolerance in CHF. This is underscored by the finding that exercise training can improve functional class and maximal exercise intolerance. Submaximal exercise intolerance also improves without alterations in cardiac output, ejection fraction, LV filling pressures, or leg blood flow. Numerous studies have also shown that vasodilator therapy which has immediate salutary hemodynamic benefits does not improve symptoms or peak $\dot{V}O_2$ for weeks to months after initiating treatment. In addition to alterations in vasomotor tone and increased vascular stiffness in peripheral vessels in CHF which may act to further decrease perfusion, a growing body of literature has demonstrated significant alterations in skeletal muscle biochemistry, histology, contractile function, and size which appear to have an important effect on exercise tolerance in CHF. These studies suggest that exercise intolerance in CHF is due to a complex interaction of abnormalities in central hemodynamics leading to decreased cardiac output, pulmonary functions, peripheral blood flow, and skeletal muscle composition and function which must all be taken into consideration when evaluating new therapies in this disorder.

References

1. Schocken DD, Arrieta MI, Leverton PE, Ross EA: Prevalence and mortality rate of congestive heart failure in the United States. *J Am Coll Cardiol* 20:301–306, 1992.
2. Smith WM: Epidemiology of congestive heart failure. *Am J Cardiol* 55:3A-8A, 1985.
3. Benge W, Litchfield RL, Marcus ML: Exercise capacity in patients with severe left ventricular dysfunction. *Circulation* 61:955–959, 1980.

4. Higginbotham MB, Morris KG, Conn EH, et al: Determinants of variable exercise performance among patients with severe left ventricular dysfunction. *Am J Cardiol* 51:52–60, 1983.
5. Franciosa JA, Park M, Levine TB: Lack of correlation between exercise capacity and indexes of resting left ventricular performance in heart failure. *Am J Cardiol* 47:33–39, 1981.
6. Weber KT, Kinasewitz GT, Janicki JS, et al: Oxygen utilization and ventilation during exercise in patients with chronic cardiac failure. *Circulation* 65:1213–1223, 1982.
7. Szlachcic J, Massie BM, Kramer BL, et al: Correlates and prognostic implication of exercise capacity in chronic congestive heart failure. *Am J Cardiol* 55:1037–1042, 1985.
8. Metra M, Raddino R, Dei Cas L, et al: Assessment of peak oxygen consumption, lactate and ventilatory thresholds and correlation with resting and exercise hemodynamic data in chronic congestive heart failure. *Am J Cardiol* 65:1127–1133, 1990.
9. Marantz PR, Tobin JN, Wassertheil-Smoller S, et al: The relationship between left ventricular systolic function and congestive heart failure diagnosed by clinical criteria. *Circulation* 77(3):607–612, 1988.
10. Sullivan MJ, Knight JD, Higginbotham MB, Cobb FR: Relation between central and peripheral hemodynamics during exercise in patients with chronic heart failure: muscle blood flow is reduced with maintenance of arterial perfusion pressure. *Circulation* 80:769–781, 1989.
11. Wilson JR, Martin JL, Schwartz D, et al: Exercise intolerance in patients with chronic heart failure: role of impaired nutritive flow to skeletal muscle. *Circulation* 69:1079–1087, 1984.
12. Wilson JR, Martin JL, Ferraro N: Impaired skeletal muscle nutritive flow during exercise in patients with heart failure: role of cardiac pump dysfunction as determined by effect of dobutamine. *Am J Cardiol* 54:1308–1315, 1984.
13. Wilson JR, Mancini DH, Dunkman: Exertional fatigue due to skeletal muscle dysfunction in patients with heart failure. *Circulation* 87:470–475, 1993.
14. Wilson JR, Ferraro N: Effect of the Renin-Angiotensin System on limb circulation and metabolism during exercise in patients with heart failure. *J Am Coll Cardiol* 6(3):555–556, 1985.
15. Wilson JR, Martin JL, Ferraro N, Weber KT: Effect of hydralazine on perfusion and metabolism in the leg during upright bicycle exercise in patients with heart failure(abstr). *Therapy and Prevention, Congestive Heart Failure* 68(2):425–432, 1983.
16. Wilson JR, Ferraro N, Wiener DH: Effect of the sympathetic nervous system on limb circulation and metabolism during exercise in heart failure. *Circulation* 72:72–81, 1985.
17. Zelis R, Flaim SF: Alterations in vasomotor tone in congestive heart failure. *Prog in Cardiovasc Dis* XXIV(#6):437–459, 1982.
18. Zelis R, Mason DT, Braunwald E: A comparison of the effects of vasodilator stimuli on peripheral resistance vessels in normal subjects and in patients with congestive heart failure. *J Clin Invest* 47:960–970, 1968.
19. Zelis R, David D: The sympathetic nervous system in congestive heart failure. *Heart Failure* 2:21–32, 1986.
20. Wilson JR, Frey MJ, Mancini DM, Ferraro N, Jones R: Sympathetic vasoconstriction during exercise in ambulatory patients with left ventricular failure. *Circulation* 79(5):1021–1027, 1989.

21. Katz SD, Biasucci L, Sabba C, et al: Impaired endothelium-mediated vasodilation in the peripheral vasculature of patients with congestive heart failure. *J Am Coll Cardiol* 19(5):918–925, 1992.
22. Katz S, Schwarz M, Yuen J, et al: Impaired acetyl-choline-mediated vasodilation in patients with congestive heart failure: role of endothelium-derived vasodilating and vasconstricting factors. *Circulation* 88:55–61, 1993.
23. Treasure CB, Vita JA, Cox DA, et al: Endothelium-dependent dilation of the coronary microvasculature is impaired in dilated cardiomyopathy. *Circulation* 81(3):772–779, 1990.
24. Kaiser L, Spickard RC, Olivier NB: Heart failure depresses endothelium-dependent responses in canine femoral artery. *Am J Physiol* 256(4 Pt 2): H962-H967, 1989.
25. Longhurst J, Capone RJ, Zelis R: Evaluation of skeletal muscle capillary basement membrane thickness in congestive heart failure. *Chest* 67:195–198, 1975.
26. Sinoway L, Minotti J, Musch T, et al: Enhanced metabolic vasodilation secondary to diuretic therapy in decompensated congestive heart failure secondary to coronary artery disease. *Am J Cardiol* 60(1):107–111, 1987.
27. Sinoway LI, Minotti JR, David D, et al: Delayed reversal of impaired vasodilation in congestive heart failure after heart transplantation. *Am J Cardiol* 61(13):1076–1079, 1988.
28. Mancini DM, Davis L, Wexler JP, et al: Dependence of enhanced maximal exercise performance on increased peak skeletal muscle perfusion during long-term captopril therapy in heart failure. *J Am Coll Cardiol* 10(4):845–850, 1987.
29. Drexler H, Banhardt U, Meinertz T, et al: Contrasting peripheral short-term and long-term effects of converting enzyme inhibition in patients with congestive heart failure: double-blind, placebo-controlled trial. *Circulation* 79(3)491–502, 1989.
30. Sullivan MJ, Higginbotham MB, Cobb FR: Exercise training in patients with left ventricular dysfunction: central and peripheral hemodynamic effects. *Circulation* 78:506–515, 1988.
31. Coats AJS, Adanopoulos S, Radaelli A, et al: Controlled trial of physical training in chronic heart failure. *Circulation* 85:2119–2131, 1992.
32. Weiner DH, Fink LI, Maris J, Jones RA, Chance B, Wilson JR: Abnormal skeletal muscle bioenergetics during exercise in patients with heart failure: role of reduced muscle blood flow. *Circulation* 73:1127–1136, 1986.
33. Massie BM, Conway M, Yonge R, et al: Skeletal muscle metabolism in patients with congestive heart failure: relation to clinical severity and blood flow. *Circulation* 76:1009–1019, 1987.
34. Fink LI, Wilson JR, Ferraro N: Exercise ventilation and pulmonary artery wedge pressure in chronic stable congestive heart failure. *Am J Cardiol* 57: 249–253, 1986.
35. Sullivan MJ, Higginbotham MB, Cobb FR: Increased exercise ventilation in patients with chronic heart failure: intact ventilatory control despite hemodynamic and pulmonary abnormalities. *Circulation* 77:552–559, 1988.
36. Massie BM: Exercise tolerance in congestive heart failure: role of cardiac function, peripheral blood flow, and muscle metabolism and effect of treatment. *Am J Med* (suppl 3A)84:75–82, 1988.
37. Mancini DM, Schwarz M, Ferraro N, et al: Effect of dobutamine ion skeletal muscle metabolism in patients with congestive heart failure. *Am J Cardiol* 65:1121–1146, 1990.

38. Sullivan MJ, Cobb FR: Dynamic regulation of leg vasomotor tone in patients with chronic heart failure. *J Appl Physiol* 71(3):1070–1075, 1991.

39. Massie BM, Conway M, Rajagopalan B, et al: Skeletal muscle metabolism during exercise under ischemic conditions in congestive heart failure: evidence for abnormalities unrelated to blood flow. *Circulation* 78:320–326, 1988.

40. Minotti JR, Christoph I, Massie BM: Skeletal muscle function, morphology, and metabolism in patients with congestive heart failure. *Chest* (5 suppl)101: 333S-339S, 1992.

41. Zannad F, Chait Z: Skeletal muscle metabolic, morpho-histologic, and biochemical abnormalities in congestive heart failure. *Heart Failure* 10(2): 58–66, 1994.

42. Wilson JR, Fink L, Maris J, et al: Evaluation of energy metabolism in skeletal muscle of patients with heart failure with gated phosphorus-31 nuclear magnetic resonance. *Circulation* 71:57–62, 1985.

43. Massie BM, Conway M, Yonge R, et al: 31p nuclear magnetic resonance evidence of abnormal skeletal metabolism in patients with congestive heart failure. *Am J Cardiol* 60:309–315, 1987.

44. Mancini DM, Ferraro N, Tuchler M, et al: Detection of abnormal calf muscle metabolism in patients with heart failure using phosphorus-31 nuclear magnetic resonance. *Am J Cardiol* 62:1234–1240, 1988.

45. Sullivan MJ, Green HJ, Cobb FR: Altered skeletal muscle metabolic response to exercise in chronic heart failure: relation to skeletal muscle aerobic enzyme activity. *Circulation* 84:1597–1607, 1991.

46. Mancini DM, Clyle E, Coggan A, et al: Constriction of intrinsic skeletal muscle changes in 31p NMR: skeletal muscle metabolic abnormalities in patients with chronic heart failure. *Circulation* 80:1338–1346, 1989.

47. Wilson JR, Mancini DM, Ferraro N, Egler J: Effect of dichloroacetate on the exercise performance of patients with heart failure. *J Am Coll Cardiol* 12: 1464–1469, 1988.

48. Drexler H, Banhardt U, Meinertz T, Wollschlager H, Lehmann M, Just H: Contrasting peripheral short-term and long-term effects of converting enzyme inhibition in patients with congestive heart failure. *Circulation* 79: 491–502, 1989.

49. Weber K, Kinasewitz G, Janicki J, Fishman A: Oxygen utilization and ventilation during exercise in patients with chronic heart failure. *Circulation* 65:1213–1223, 1982.

50. Green HJ: Manifestations and sites of neuromuscular fatigue. *Biochem Exerc* VII 21:13–35, 1990.

51. Volpe P, Martini A, Nori A: The sarcoplasmic reticulum of skeletal muscle: a look from inside. In: Frank GB, et al, eds. *Excitation-Contraction Coupling in Skeletal Cardiac and Smooth Muscle.* New York: Plenum Press, 263–275, 1992.

52. Drexler H, Riede U, Munzel T, Konig H, Funke E, Just H: Alterations of skeletal muscle in chronic heart failure. *Circulation* 85(5):1751–1759, 1992.

53. Norgaard A, Bjerregaard P, Baandrup U, Kjeldsen K, Reske-Nielson E, Bloch Thomsen PE: The concentration of the Na, K-pump in skeletal and heart muscle in congestive heart failure. *Int J Cardiol* 26:185–190, 1990.

54. Sullivan MJ, Green HJ, Cobb FR: Skeletal muscle biochemistry and histology in ambulatory patients with long-term heart failure. *Circulation* 81: 518–527, 1990.

55. Saltin B, Gollnick PD: Skeletal muscle adaptability: significance for metabolism and performance. In: Peachey LD, ed. *The Handbook of Physiology:*

The Skeletal Muscle System. Bethesda, MD: American Physiological Society, 555–631, 1992.

56. Sullivan MJ, Klitgaard H, Kraus WE, Duscha BD, Cobb FR, Saltin B: Altered contractile protein expression in skeletal muscle in chronic heart failure: evidence for a novel myopathy. Presented at the 67th Scientific Sessions Nov. 11–12, 1994, Dallas, TX, American Heart Association.
57. Weber KT, Janicki JS: Lactate production during maximal and submaximal exercise in patients with chronic heart failure. *J Am Coll Cardiol* 6:717–724, 1985.
58. Minotti JR, Christoph I, Oka R, et al: Impaired skeletal muscle function in patients with congestive heart failure: relationship to systemic exercise performance. *J Clin Invest* 88:2077–2082, 1991.
59. Minotti JR, Pillay P, Oka R, Wells L, Christoph I, Massie BM: Skeletal muscle size: relationship to muscle function in heart failure. *J Appl Physiol* 75(1): 373–381, 1993.
60. Mancini DM, Walter G, Reichek N, et al: Contribution of skeletal muscle atrophy to exercise intolerance and altered muscle metabolism in heart failure. *Circulation* 85(4):1364–1373, 1992.
61. Magnusson G, Isberg B, Karlberg KE, et al: Skeletal muscle strength and endurance in chronic congestive heart failure secondary to idiopathic dilated cardiomyopathy. *Am J Cardiol* 73:307–309, 1994.
62. Lipkin DP, Jones DA, Round JM, et al: Abnormalities of skeletal muscle in patients with chronic heart failure. *Int J Cardiol* 18:187–195, 1988.
63. Sullivan MJ, Kuhn CM, Charles HC, Negro-Villar, Kennedy JE, Cobb FR: Skeletal muscle adrenergic activation is increased at rest and during exercise in chronic heart failure. *Circulation*(suppl II) 84:II74, 1991.
64. Coyle EF, Martin WH, Sinacore DR, Joyner MJ, Hagberg JM, Holloszy JO: Time course of loss of adaptation after stopping prolonged intense endurance training. *J Appl Physiol* 57:1857–1864, 1984.
65. Larsson L, Ansved T: Effects of long-term physical training and detraining on enzyme histochemical and functional skeletal muscle characteristics in man. *Muscle Nerve* 8:714–722, 1985.
66. Kraus WE, Whellan MD, Campbell ME, et al: Altered gene expression for metabolic proteins in the skeletal muscle of subjects with chronic heart failure. (submitted to *Circulation* 1995.)
67. Sabbah HN, Hansen-Smith F, Sharov VG, et al: Decreased proportion of type I myofibers in skeletal muscle of dogs with chronic heart failure. *Circulation* 87:1729–1737, 1993.
68. Perreault CL, Gonzalez SH, Litwin SE, Sun X, Franzini AC, Morgan JP: Alterations in contractility and intracellular Ca_2+ transients in isolated bundles of skeletal muscle fibers from rats with chronic heart failure. *Circ Res* 73(2):40–412, 1993.
69. Wilson JR, Coyle EF, Osbakken M: Effect of heart failure on skeletal muscle in dogs. *Am J Physiol* 262 (Heart Circ Physiol 31):H993-H998, 1992.
70. Arnold L, Brosnan J, Rajagopalan B, Radda GK: Skeletal muscle metabolism in heart failure in rats. *Am J Physiol (Heart Circ Physiol 30)*:H434-H442, 1991.
71. Douard H, Pate P, Broustet JP: Exercise training in patients with chronic heart failure. *Heart Failure* 10(2):80–87, 1994.
72. Coats AJS, Adamopoulos S, Meyer T, et al: Effects of physical training in chronic heart failure. *Lancet* 335:63–66, 1990.
73. Lee AP, Ice R, Blessey R, et al: Long-term effects of physical training on coronary patients with impaired ventricular function. *Circulation* 15:1519–1526, 1979.

74. Uren NG, Lipkin DP: Exercise training as therapy for chronic heart failure. *Br Heart J* 67:430–433, 1992.
75. Jette M, Heller R, Landry F, et al: Randomized 4-week exercise program in patients with impaired left ventricular function. *Circulation* 84:1561–1567, 1991.
76. Kavanagh T, Myers MG, Baigrie RS, et al: Cardiac respiratory training responses to a 1-year walking program in patients with chronic heart failure (abstr). *Eur Heart J* (suppl)14:415, 1993.
77. Minotti JR, Massie BM: Exercise training in heart failure patients: does reversing the peripheral abnormalities protect the heart? *Circulation* 85:2323–2325, 1992.
78. Minotti JR, Johnson EC, Hudson TL, et al: Skeletal muscle response to training exercise in congestive heart failure. *J Clin Invest* 86:751–758, 1990.
79. Conn EH, Williams RS, Wallace AG: Exercise responses before and after physical conditioning in patients with severely depressed left ventricular function. *Am J Cardiol* 49:296–300, 1982.
80. Sullivan MJ, Higginbotham MB, Cobb FR: Exercise training in patients with chronic heart failure delays ventilatory anaerobic threshold and improves submaximal exercise performance. *Circulation* 79:324–329, 1989.

Section 5

Clinical Applications

16

Short-Term Exercise Training After Cardiac Surgery

Haruki Itoh, MD
Kazuzo Kato, MD

In patients who have undergone cardiac surgery following, for example, acute myocardial infarction, physical training is known to improve exercise capacity,[1] subsequent daily activities, and thus improve quality of life. No established method exists, however, to determine exercise intensity in the early phase of post-cardiac surgery. In order to safely obtain improvement in exercise capacity over a short time, supervised aerobic exercise is performed during early postoperative stages. In this chapter, we propose to show that exercise training at the anaerobic threshold (AT) is safe and effective.

Determination of Exercise Intensity for Physical Training

The level of exercise generally recommended for physical training is at 40% to 85% of predicted maximal heart rate.[2] It is almost impossible to quantify the exercise intensity by this method since the range of training heart rate is very large. Also, the heart rate response to exercise is modified in patients following cardiac surgery as a result of cardiac drugs (e.g., beta adrenoceptor blockade), abnormal hemodynamics, or cardiac rhythm (e.g., atrial fibrillation), etc. Therefore, selecting the training work rate based on the predicted heart rate is not practical in patients in early post-cardiac surgery stages.

The AT was originally developed to detect the work rate at which the oxygen supply to the exercising muscles cannot fully satisfy the re-

From Wasserman, K (ed): *Exercise Gas Exchange in Heart Disease.* Armonk, NY: Futura Publishing Company, Inc., © 1996.

quirement[3]; in other words, *AT* is the upper limit of aerobic exercise. *AT* has recently been used as the exercise intensity during physical training as part of cardiac rehabilitation.[4]

Exercise intensity at the *AT* level has many advantages in cardiac patients. First, systemic acidosis does not develop during exercise below *AT* because lactic acid does not accumlate. Figure 1 shows the change in pH of arterial blood during incremental exercise. Each line represents a subject, with the dotted line below *AT* and solid line above it. Although the exercise capacities of subjects are widely diverse, pH decreases above *AT* in all subjects. Second, catecholamines such as norepinephrine, which is an indicator of sympathetic nerve tone, will not increase excessively. Figure 2 demonstrates the plasma norepinephrine concentration during constant exercise at *AT* and 20% above *AT* in 8 normal volunteers. The norepinephrine level stays relatively low and does not increase during *AT* level exercise, but increases progressively during exercise at 20% above *AT*.[5] Third, the left ventricular ejection fraction does not decrease below *AT* level, but does decrease above the *AT* (Figure 3). We measured left ventricular ejection fraction during ramp exercise using a nuclear stethoscope.[6] Twenty-three patients with ischemic heart disease or valve disease participated in this study. When the work rate exceeds *AT,* the ejection

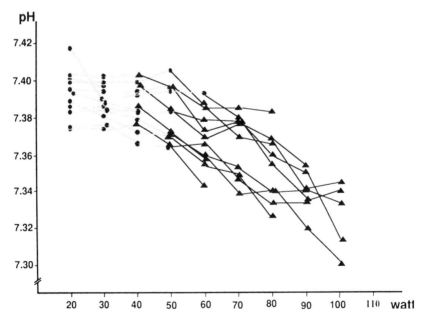

Figure 1. The change in arterial pH during incremental exercise. **Each line** represents a subject. The **dotted line** is for below *AT* and the **solid line** is for above *AT*. The pH decreases above *AT* in all subjects.

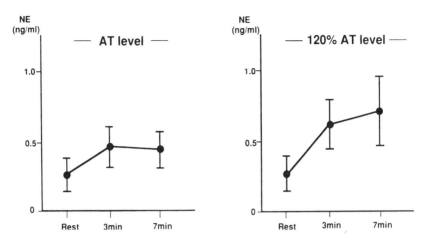

Figure 2. The plasma norepinephrine level during constant work rate exercise at *AT* and 20% above *AT* in 8 normal volunteers. The norepinephrine level stays relatively low and does not increase during *AT* level exercise. In contrast, it increases progressively during exercise at 20% above *AT*. (Data from Reference 5.)

fraction of the left ventricle begins to decrease. Asanoi et al reported that the mechanism for the increase in cardiac output was different above and below *AT* in normal subjects. The increase in stroke volume was primarily mediated by changes in loading conditions during aerobic exercise and by enhanced contractility during anaerobic exercise.[7]

These are important observations for avoiding arrhythmias, hyperpnea, and left ventricular deterioration due to afterload mismatch during exercise in cardiac patients. As long as patients perform exercise at or below *AT* level, oxygen uptake ($\dot{V}O_2$) and other parameters reach steady state within 3 minutes. Thus, exercise at the *AT* enables us to extrapolate the physiological responses of heart rate, minute ventilation ($\dot{V}E$), and $\dot{V}O_2$ to exercise of a much longer duration, thereby providing useful information about the patient's physiological performance and training under cardiovascular, ventilatory, and metabolic stress.

The Indices Used for Evaluation of the Efficacy of Training

Peak $\dot{V}O_2$ and *AT*

Peak $\dot{V}O_2$ is recognized as one of the best parameters of exercise capacity since it represents the maximum work capacity in each subject. It is measured by the rate of oxygen consumption at peak exercise (peak $\dot{V}O_2$) and it depends on the maximum oxygen delivery, i.e., cardiac output.[8] Peak $\dot{V}O_2$ is influenced not only by the subject's motiva-

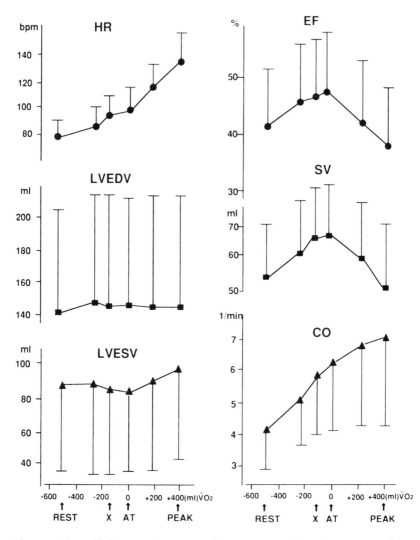

Figure 3. Plots of left ventricular ejection fraction (EF), stroke volume (SV), and cardiac output (CO) during incremental exercise test. EF and SV at the *AT* were significantly higher than those at rest and other levels of work except for the midpoint between 20 watts and *AT* (X). (Reproduced with permission from Reference 5.)

tion, but also by the subjectivity of the personnel supervising the test who decide when the test should be terminated. It is also influenced by the gender and age of the subject.

AT is an objective index obtained from submaximal exercise testing and is not influenced by patient motivation. Since *AT* has a close relationship with endurance performance,[9] it has been used as a measure of endurance capacity. In the field of cardiology, it has been recognized that *AT* is a useful submaximal exercise index in patients with heart disease to evaluate functional capacity.[10]

Peak $\dot{V}O_2$ and *AT* decrease in accordance with the age of the subjects, and are higher in males than females in a normal population.[11] Therefore, to evaluate the efficacy of therapeutic intervention using peak $\dot{V}O_2$ or *AT* in individual subjects, each subject is required to have a baseline cardiopulmonary exercise test. Both of the indices are decreased when functional capacity is severe.

Oxygen Pulse

Oxygen pulse is calculated by dividing the $\dot{V}O_2$ by the heart rate. It is equal to the product of stroke volume and arterial-venous oxygen difference. The oxygen pulse, especially at peak exercise when arterial-venous oxygen difference reaches its maximum in each subject, is closely dependent on the stroke volume. This index, therefore, is useful in evaluating the change in stroke volume and oxygen extraction in peripheral tissue. Thus, it will be reduced when stroke volume is reduced and/or in the presence of anemia, or any other factors which would prevent the normal extraction of oxygen from capillary blood, e.g., high level of carboxy-hemoglobin.

$\Delta\dot{V}O_2/\Delta WR$

$\Delta\dot{V}O_2/\Delta WR$ is measured during ergometer ramp protocol exercise in which work rate is progressively increased to maximum. It is calculated using $\dot{V}O_2$ plots from 60 seconds to 90 seconds after the start of the ramp protocol to just above *AT*. The delay is taken into account in this calculation since $\dot{V}O_2$ increases with a time delay as work rate is increased at the beginning of the ramp protocol. $\Delta\dot{V}O_2/\Delta WR$ might be especially reduced in patients with ischemic heart disease. This parameter is reduced when the increase in oxygen flow to the peripheral tissues (cardiac output) does not keep pace with the $\dot{V}O_2$ requirement during increasing work rate exercise. The normal value is about 10 mL/min/W when a 10-watt to 20-watt/min ramp slope is employed, and decreases in cardiac patients, reflecting impaired cardiac function reserve.[12] The index is not affected by the sex and age of subjects.[11] However, it does decrease, even in normal subjects, when the slope of the work rate ramp is steep.

Time Constant of $\dot{V}O_2$

The time constant of the $\dot{V}O_2$ curve at the beginning of exercise represents the cardiac output response when the patient starts to exercise.[13] This reflects the increase in venous return by the muscle pumping effect, heart rate response, and afterload reduction caused by dilatation of peripheral resistance vessels.

Short-Term Exercise Training After Cardiac Surgery Based on *AT*

Determination of Exercise Intensity for Training

A cycle ergometer is our preferred form of training in the early postoperative phase since it has the following advantages over the treadmill (walking exercise): 1) the work rate can be quantified, 2) it is easy to monitor ECG and blood pressure, and 3) it is safer in case of emergencies such as severe arrhythmia, hypotension, or faintness. We prefer a ramp protocol to determine *AT* because it is rapid and does not require great strength by the patient or physical stress. Exercise begins with a 4-minute warm up at 20 watts at 50 rpm, followed by 1-watt incremental loading every 6 seconds.

Figure 4 shows how we determined the work intensity for training at *AT*. Initially, the ramp test was used to determine *AT* (Figure 4, *left panel*); normally a work rate of 10 watts less than the work rate at *AT* in the ramp test is used for training to take into account the time delay of the physiological response to increasing work rate.[14] In pa-

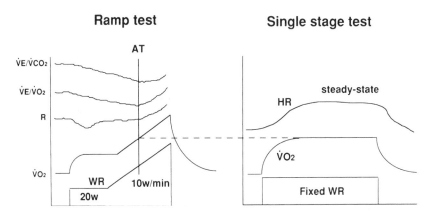

Figure 4. Method to determine the work intensity for training at *AT* level. *AT* was determined by ramp test. The work rate at 10 watts less than the work rate at *AT* in the ramp test gives the $\dot{V}O_2$ at the *AT* (takes into account the time delay of the physiological response to increasing work rate) used for training. In patients with ischemic changes on ECG or hypertension, a fixed work rate at *AT* level was performed to confirm that the exercise training intensity was safe. (R=respiratory exchange ratio, WR=work rate, HR=heart rate.)

tients with ischemic changes on ECG or hypertension, a fixed work rate at the *AT* level was done to confirm that the exercise intensity recommended was safe and was at or below *AT* level (Figure 4, *right panel*). Exercise training was performed based on the heart rate and work rate at *AT* level. It is important not to determine the exercise intensity from heart rate alone since many patients with valvular disease, complicated by atrial fibrillation, and patients with ischemic heart disease will show a suppressed heart rate response.

Training of Patients After Valve Replacement Surgery

In general, exercise capacity transiently decreases after cardiac surgery. Figure 5 shows the time courses of peak $\dot{V}O_2$ and *AT* after mitral valve replacement and/or aortic valve replacement. Both peak $\dot{V}O_2$ and *AT* decreased 1 month after surgery while cardiac output at peak exercise increased. We planned a postoperative training protocol to improve the exercise capacity in valve replacement patients. Training started about 7 days after surgery. Twenty-four patients, most of them admitted to our hospital for mitral valve replacement, entered the study. They were randomly allocated to the control group or training group; two thirds of the patients had atrial fibrillation.

Cardiopulmonary exercise testing (CPX) was done before and 3 weeks after the operation to evaluate the effects of training. The cardiac output was measured every 2 minutes during CPX. In the train-

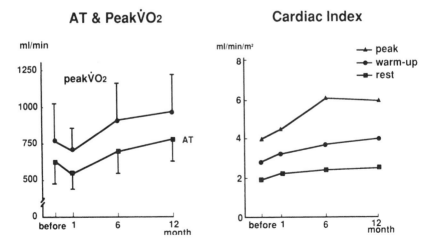

Figure 5. Time course of exercise tolerance (**left**) and cardiac index during exercise test (**right**) before and after valve replacement surgery. Peak $\dot{V}O_2$ and *AT* decreased significantly 1 month after surgery compared with preoperative state while cardiac index had the tendency to increase at rest and during exercise.

ing group, CPX was performed to determine their *AT* a week after the operation, when patients had no fever and could walk at least 200 meters without symptom or changes on ECG. The exercise program consisted of the 30 minutes of training on a cycle ergometer twice daily for 1 week. One week later, the CPX for the new exercise program was done, and patients did the training based on a new prescription for another week. In contrast, the patients in the control group were advised to walk 200 meters three times a day at the onset, and then increase the distance to 500 meters.

Table 1 shows the results of exercise testing before and 3 weeks after the operation for both the control and training group. Exercise time and time to *AT* did not change within the groups. Target heart rate for training, based on the *AT* determined from the ramp exercise protocol, was 100 bpm for the first week and 106 bpm for the second. Peak $\dot{V}O_2$ tended to increase in the training group from 780 ± 178 to 828 ± 163 mL/min while the control group showed a tendency to decrease from 764 ± 270 to 677 ± 160 mL/min. Almost the same changes were noted in the *AT*. No significant differences were found in the *AT* (-91 ± 144 mL/min in control and +17 ± 83 mL/min in training group), and peak $\dot{V}O_2$ (−87 ± 228 mL/min in control and 49 ± 99 mL/min in training group) over the 3-week period in the two groups. $\Delta\dot{V}O_2/\Delta WR$ decreased in the control group, but increased in the training group. The changes in $\Delta\dot{V}O_2/\Delta WR$ in the two groups were significantly different. However, the absolute value of $\Delta\dot{V}O_2/\Delta WR$ even in the training group was still low compared with normal (normal value: 10.0 ± 1.1 mL/min/W[12]). The time constant of $\dot{V}O_2$ for the 20-watt exercise increased for the control, but decreased for the training group (from 47.1 ± 10.3 seconds to 56.2 ± 6.9 seconds in control group; from 53.4 ± 13.5 seconds to 42.0 ± 10.3 seconds in training group, p<0.05). The shortened time constant of $\dot{V}O_2$ suggests an improvement in cardiac output response to exercise.

Table 2 shows the changes in cardiac indices during exercise testing. In the control group, cardiac indices at rest, 20 watts steady state, and peak exercise did not change 3 weeks after the operation compared with preoperative measurements. In contrast, the cardiac index at peak exercise increased in the training group (p<0.01). The lower part of Table 2 shows changes in oxygen delivery, calculated using cardiac output, hemoglobin, and oxygen saturation of arterial blood. Because of the limited volume of autologous blood transfusion, hemoglobin was decreased in both groups to the same extent (from 12.9 ± 1.4 to 11.8 ± 1.7 g/dL in control group, and from 12.6 ± 1.6 to 12.1 ± 1.4 g/dL in training group). There was a tendency for oxygen delivery to decrease during exercise in the control group in which the cardiac

Table 1

Results of Cardiopulmonary Exercise Testing before (pre) and 3 Weeks after Valve Replacement (post) in the Training and Control Groups

	Control Group (n = 14)			Training Group (n = 10)		
	Pre	Post	Post-Pre	Pre	Post	Post-Pre
Exercise time (min)	8.2 ± 2.0	7.6 ± 1.3	−0.6 ± 1.3	8.3 ± 1.7	8.3 ± 1.1	0 ± 1.7
Work rate at AT (W)	48 ± 9	43 ± 9	−5 ± 11	40 ± 27	38 ± 8	−2 ± 25
Peak $\dot{V}O_2$ (mL/min)	764 ± 270	677 ± 160	−87 ± 228	780 ± 178	828 ± 163	49 ± 99
AT (mL/min)	691 ± 143	600 ± 75	−91 ± 144	594 ± 115	611 ± 57	17 ± 83
$\Delta\dot{V}O_2/\Delta WR$ (mL/min/W)	7.2 ± 2.8	5.5 ± 2.3*	−1.7 ± 2.8	6.6 ± 2.4	7.2 ± 2.2*	0.7 ± 1.2†
τ (sec)	47.1 ± 10.3	56.2 ± 6.9*	9.1 ± 7.4	53.4 ± 13.5	42.0 ± 10.3*	−11.4 ± 5.8†

In some patients, AT (7 cases in the control groups and 1 in the training group) and $\Delta\dot{V}O_2/\Delta WR$ (3 cases in the control group) were not determined because of short exercise time, oscillatory ventilation, etc.

*: P < 0.05, **: P < 0.01 before surgery vs. 3 weeks after surgery. +: P < 0.05, ++: p < 0.01 control group vs. training group.

Table 2

Effects of Training on Cardiac Index and Oxygen Delivery During Exercise before (pre) and 3 Weeks after Valve Replacement (post) in the Training and Control Groups

		Control Group (n = 14)			Training Group (n = 10)		
		Pre	Post	Post-Pre	Pre	Post	Post-Pre
Cardiac Index (L/min/m²)	Rest	1.98 ± 0.71	2.29 ± 0.67	0.31 ± 1.59	2.01 ± 0.56	2.21 ± 0.53	0.19 ± 0.47
	20W Steady state	3.20 ± 0.84	3.43 ± 0.86	0.23 ± 0.70	2.87 ± 0.74	3.41 ± 0.71	0.54 ± 0.50
	Peak exercise	4.88 ± 1.42	5.04 ± 1.27	0.16 ± 0.92	4.08 ± 1.27	5.30 ± 1.22**	1.22 ± 0.68
O_2 Delivery (mL/min)	Rest	500 ± 199	506 ± 187	6 ± 141	542 ± 148	564 ± 145	21 ± 111
	20W Steady state	811 ± 261	756 ± 251	−55 ± 194	776 ± 210	879 ± 238	103 ± 126+
	Peak exercise	1258 ± 513	1107 ± 332	−151 ± 341	1118 ± 416	1376 ± 438	258 ± 241++

The O_2 delivery was calculated as followsss: O_2 delivery (mL/min) = Cardiac output (L/min) × Hemoglobin (g/dL) × 1.36 × O_2 saturation of arterial blood (%) ÷ 10

*: $P < 0.05$, **: $P < 0.01$ before surgery vs. 3 weeks after surgery. +: $P < 0.05$, ++: $p < 0.01$ control group vs. training group.

output during exercise did not increase; however, oxygen delivery increased in the training group due to increased cardiac output.

In this study, CPX was performed preoperatively and 3 weeks postoperatively. The results indicate that exercise training prevented a decrease in exercise capacity and increased the cardiac output response after surgery for valve replacement compared to the preoperative state. (Table 2).

Training of Patients After Coronary Artery Bypass Graft Surgery

Thirty patients entered the study 1 week after coronary artery bypass graft surgery. Their mean age was 63.3 ± 7.1 years and mean number of grafts was 2.5 ± 0.8. The patients were randomly divided into two groups: training group and control group. The training protocol was the same as that used for the post-valve replacement surgery patients.

There was no statistical difference in the backgrounds of patients in the control and training groups. Heart rate at rest and at given work rate decreased in both groups after 2 weeks of rehabilitation, but statistical significance was noted only in the training group (77 ± 12 bpm to 74 ± 17 bpm in control group, and 80 ± 14 bpm to 73 ± 12 bpm at rest in training group, 92 ± 13 to 89 ± 15 bpm at 20 watts in control group, and 96 ± 15 bpm to 88 ± 15 at 20 watts in training group). On the other hand, peak heart rate showed a tendency to increase, but it was significant only in the training group (113 ± 19 bpm to 120 ± 25 bpm in control group, and 119 ± 14 bpm to 129 ± 17 bpm in training group).

Exercise time was prolonged in both groups 2 weeks after patients were assigned to either the control or training groups (Table 3). The difference in exercise time was greater in the training group than the control group, but this difference was not significant. Peak $\dot{V}O_2$ increased in both groups, although the training group showed better improvement.

Peak oxygen pulse, which is closely related to stroke volume at peak exercise, increased significantly in both groups. The degree of improvement was greater in the training group (Table 3). Peak cardiac output did not change in the control group (from 10.8 ± 1.7 L/min to 11.3 ± 2.1 L/min). However, it increased from 10.5 ± 1.7 L/min to 12.2 ± 3.4 L/min in the training group.

Figure 6 shows the changes in peak $\dot{V}O_2$, AT, $\Delta\dot{V}O_2/\Delta WR$, and the time constant for $\dot{V}O_2$ (τ) in response to 20-watt constant work rate for the control and training group over the 2-week training program. *AT*

Table 3

Results of Cardiopulmonary Exercise Testing before Training (pre) and 2 Weeks after (post) Coronary Bypass Graft Surgery in the Training and Control Groups

| | Control Group (n = 14) | | | Training Group (n = 10) | | |
	Pre	Post	Post-Pre	Pre	Post	Post-Pre
Exercise time (min)	7.6 ± 2.3	8.8 ± 1.9**	1.2 ± 0.9	7.8 ± 1.3	9.5 ± 1.5**	1.7 ± 0.9
Work rate at AT (W)	52 ± 16	53 ± 17	1 ± 10	56 ± 21	60.1 ± 22**	9 ± 9
Peak $\dot{V}O_2$ (mL/min)	782 ± 202	834 ± 220**	53 ± 58	755 ± 156	878 ± 202*	123 ± 144†
Peak CO (L/min)	10.8 ± 1.7	11.3 ± 2.1	0.6 ± 1.5	10.5 ± 1.7	12.2 ± 3.4	1.7 ± 2.2
Peak O_2 Pulse	6.3 ± 1.7	6.6 ± 2.0*	0.3 ± 0.4	6.1 ± 1.0	6.9 ± 1.8*	0.8 ± 1.0
AT (mL/min)	676 ± 124	634 ± 124*	−42 ± 62	628 ± 92	654 ± 142*	59 ± 84†
$\Delta\dot{V}O_2/\Delta WR$ (mL/min/W)	8.6 ± 3.0	7.7 ± 3.0	−0.3 ± 1.6	8.1 ± 3.4	9.6 ± 3.1**	1.5 ± 1.3††
τ (sec)	46.5 ± 15.7	51.3 ± 12.1	4.80 ± 12.5	50.5 ± 8.4	43.9 ± 10.1**	−6.7 ± 6.6††

*: P < 0.05, **: P < 0.01 before training vs. 2 weeks after training. +: P < 0.05, ++: p < 0.01 control group vs. training group.

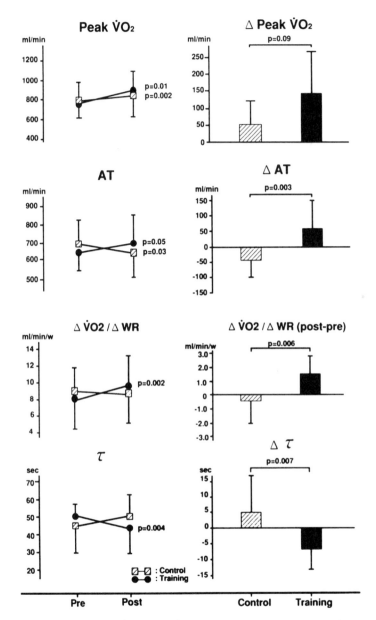

Figure 6. Changes in peak $\dot{V}O_2$, *AT*, $\Delta\dot{V}O_2/\Delta WR$, and time constant of $\dot{V}O_2$ (τ) for 20 watts constant work rate exercise in the training group and the control group after coronary bypass surgery. Peak $\dot{V}O_2$ increased in both groups, though the training group showed a tendency toward better improvement. *AT* increased significantly only in the training group. $\Delta\dot{V}O_2/\Delta WR$ increased in the training group and not in the control group. The differences between the groups were highly significant. The time constant of $\dot{V}O_2$ (τ) was obtained by fitting the $\dot{V}O_2$ curve to the formula; $\dot{V}O_2(t)=(\dot{V}O_2$ at rest $- \dot{V}O_2$ at 20W) $\times$ {1-EXP(t/τ)} + $\dot{V}O_2$ at rest. τ was shortened only within the training group, which indicated that the training improved cardiac output response.

increased significantly from 628 ± 92 mL/min to 654 ± 142 mL/min in the training group, with a decrease from 676 ± 124 to 634 ± 124 in the control group (Table 3); these findings suggest that the non-supervised walking exercise is insufficient to prevent deconditioning after operation. $\Delta\dot{V}O_2/\Delta WR$ also increased in the training group, but not in the control group. The differences between the groups were highly significant (p=0.006). The time constant of $\dot{V}O_2$ (τ) was shortened only in the training group (Table 3).

Interestingly, submaximal parameters depending on cardiac output response to exercise such as $\Delta\dot{V}O_2/\Delta WR$, time constant for $\dot{V}O_2$, and to a lesser extent AT are more sensitive than measurements at peak exercise for the purpose of determining the efficacy of short-term training rehabilitation (Table 3). These findings may reflect the fact that peak $\dot{V}O_2$, and probably AT to some extent, are dependent on muscle volume and function, while the time constant and $\Delta\dot{V}O_2/\Delta WR$ are less dependent on muscle, but depend on the increase in cardiac output. The shortened time constant for $\dot{V}O_2$ at the beginning of exercise after training implies that the cardiac output responded more promptly to the cellular respiratory requirement. This depends on both the contractility of cardiac muscle, and the rapid reduction in afterload caused by dilatation of the resistance vessels.

We conclude that exercise training at the AT level has many advantages in cardiac patients. It allows the circulation, ventilation, and metabolic responses to function at a constant level during exercise. Parameters obtained from cardiopulmonary exercise are useful not only in determining the work intensity for training, but in evaluating the effectiveness of training. Supervised aerobic training increases exercise capacity in patients after cardiac surgery by improving cardiac reserve and possibly in peripheral function.

Summary

Physical training is useful in improving exercise capacity and therefore the quality of life in patients following cardiac surgery (coronary artery bypass graft or valve replacement). There has been no established method to determine exercise intensity for training cardiac patients in the early postoperative stage. We propose that exercise training can be safely done at the AT level and that it is effective. Exercise intensity at AT has many advantages: 1) no development of systemic acidosis, 2) no powerful drive to progressively increase ventilation, 3) no release of excessive catecholamines, and 4) no decrease in LV ejection fraction. These are very important factors in avoiding arrhythmias, excessive ventilation, and left ventricular deterioration due to afterload mismatch in cardiac patients. Moreover, determination of exercise intensity for training in patients with atrial fibrillation can be performed with ease when $\dot{V}O_2$ is used as the index of exercise intensity. In our two recent studies, one following valve replacement, the other after coronary artery bypass graft surgery, indices representing general exercise capacity (peak $\dot{V}O_2$ and AT), cardiac response to exercise (time constant of $\dot{V}O_2$, $\Delta\dot{V}O_2/\Delta WR$), and cardiac output during exercise improved significantly in patients training for 30 minutes at the AT level twice daily for 2 weeks compared with patients who underwent the traditional nonsupervised walking rehabilitation. These results suggest that supervised physical training at the AT level soon after cardiac surgery increases exercise capacity in patients through the improvement in the cardiac response to exercise.

References

1. Degre S, Degre-Coustry C, Hoylarts M: Therapeutic effects of physical training in coronary heart disease. *Cardiology* 62:206–217, 1977.
2. ACSM's guidelines for exercise testing and prescription. *Am Coll Sport Med,* 5th edition. Baltimore: Williams & Wilkins; 151–235, 1995.
3. Wasserman K: The anaerobic threshold: definition, physiological significance and identification. *Adv Cardiol* 35:1–23, 1986.
4. Taniguchi K, Itoh H, Yajima T, Doi M, Niwa A, Marumo F: Predischarge early exercise therapy in patients with acute myocardial infarction on the basis of anaerobic threshold. *Jpn Circ J* 54:1419–1425, 1990.
5. Tanabe K, Osada N, Noda K, et al: Changes in hemodynamics and catecholamines during single-level exercise at the anaerobic threshold and 120% of the anaerobic threshold in normal subjects. *J Cardiol* 24:61–69, 1994.
6. Koike A, Itoh H, Taniguchi K, Hiroe M: Detecting abnormalities in left ventricular function during exercise by respiratory measurement. *Circulation* 80:1737–1746, 1989.
7. Asanoi H, Kameyama T, Ishizaka S, Miyagi K, Sasayama S: Ventriculoarterial coupling during exercise in normal human subjects. *Int J Cardiol* 36:177–186, 1992.
8. Yamaguchi I, Komatsu E, Miyazawa K: Intersubject variability in cardiac output-oxygen uptake relation of men during exercise. *J Appl Physiol* 61:2168–2174, 1986.
9. Kumagai S, Tanaka K, Matsuura Y, Hirikoba K, Asano K: Relationships of the anaerobic threshold with the 5 km, 10 km, and 10-mile races. *Eur J Appl Physiol* 49:13–23, 1982.
10. Matsumura N, Nishijima H, Kojima S, Hashimoto F, Minami M, Yasuda H: Determination of anaerobic threshold for assessment of functional state in patients with chronic heart failure. *Circulation* 68:360–367, 1983.
11. Itoh H, Taniguchi K, Koike A, Doi M: Evaluation of severity of heart failure using ventilatory gas analysis. *Circulation* (suppl II) 81:II31–II37, 1990.
12. Itoh H: Oxygen uptake: work rate relationship in patients with heart disease. *Med Sport Sci* 37:374–380, 1992.
13. De Cort SC, Innes JA, Barstow TJ, Guz A: Cardiac output, oxygen con-

sumption and arteriovenous oxygen difference following a sudden rise in exercise level in humans. *J Physiol* 441:501–512, 1991.

14. Hansen JE, Casaburi R, Cooper DM, Wasserman K: Oxygen uptake as related to work rate increment during cycle ergometer exercise. *Eur J Appl Physiol* 57:140–145, 1988.

17

Use of Exercise Gas Exchange Measurements in Multicenter Drug Studies

Jay N. Cohn, MD; Susan Ziesche, RN
Gary Johnson, MS; Frederick Cobb, MD

Background

Exercise capacity frequently is utilized as an end point in intervention trials in patients with heart failure.[1-7] The duration of exercise on a graded treadmill protocol commonly serves as a guide to efficacy, but peak exercise capacity during a progressive exercise test is subjective at best. Patients may terminate exercise because of complaints of generalized fatigue, leg fatigue, dyspnea, chest pain, or orthopedic disabilities. Determination of whether the test was a suitable maximal test is then left to the attending staff whose aggressiveness in pushing patients to greater exercise capacity also may be an important variable in the duration of time on the treadmill.

Gas exchange measurements during exercise provide a more quantitative assessment of the amount of exercise performed and of the degree of exertion expended.[8] By continuously monitoring oxygen consumption and carbon dioxide production, it is possible to determine when patients have exceeded their anaerobic threshold (*AT*) and are reaching the physiological maximum of exercise capacity.[9] When subjects have not approached this physiological limit, encouragement to continue the protocol is appropriate. Gas exchange studies performed in a single center can easily address equipment calibration and

From Wasserman, K (ed): *Exercise Gas Exchange in Heart Disease.* Armonk, NY: Futura Publishing Company, Inc., © 1996.

staff training to minimize variability. However, in the setting of multi-center trials, the challenge of performing gas exchange measurements in the sequential assessment of exercise capacity raises a number of logistic and scientific issues. We shall therefore utilize the experience in the Vasodilator-Heart Failure Trials (V-HeFT) performed in Veterans Affairs Hospitals to describe the methods employed in these multi-center trials and the benefits that accrued from monitoring gas exchange.

V-HeFT Protocols

V-HeFT I was carried out from 1980 to 1985 in 11 VA Centers[10]; V-HeFT II was carried out from 1986 to 1991 in 13 VA Centers.[11] V-HeFT III was initiated in 1991 and was completed on March 31, 1995. The protocols for these studies differed.

V-HeFT I: Patients with heart failure taking digoxin and diuretic therapy were randomized to receive hydralazine 300 mg plus isosorbide dinitrate 160 mg daily, prazosin 20 mg daily, or matching placebo tablets and capsules. Bicycle exercise was performed twice at baseline and at regular intervals during follow-up. The protocol consisted of exercise beginning at 25 watts with increments of 25 watts at 4-minute intervals. Expired gas was collected utilizing a mixing chamber, and Beckman oxygen and carbon dioxide analyzers. A peak oxygen consumption ($\dot{V}O_2$) less than 25 mL/kg/min was an entrance criterion for this study.

V-HeFT II: Patients taking digoxin and diuretic therapy were randomized to receive the hydralazine-isosorbide dinitrate combination from V-HeFT I or enalapril in a daily dose of 20 mg. Bicycle exercise was carried out beginning at 25 watts for 3 minutes followed by increments of 25 watts at 2-minute intervals. Gas exchange was measured breath-by-breath utilizing a Medical Graphics Corporation 2001 metabolic gas analysis system.

V-HeFT III: Patients receiving diuretic and enalapril with or without digoxin were randomized to receive felodipine 10 mg daily or placebo. Exercise was carried out on a bicycle utilizing a 3-minute unloaded warm-up period followed by a ramp protocol with an increase of 12 watts per minute. Breath-by-breath analysis of gas exchange was carried out utilizing a Medical Graphics Corporation CPX (cardiopulmonary exercise testing) system.

In all three protocols, the criteria for baseline eligibility included a peak $\dot{V}O_2$ less than 25 mL/kg/min, exercise terminated because of dyspnea or fatigue, two tests 2 weeks apart with a peak $\dot{V}O_2$ varying by less than 4 mL/kg/min, and a respiratory exchange ratio increase of greater than 0.1 from the trough and to a value greater than 1.0 at peak.

Quality Control

In order to assure comparability of data from 11 centers in V-HeFT I, 13 centers in V-HeFT II and 4 centers performing gas exchange in V-HeFT III, a number of quality control efforts were carried out. Staff members at each hospital performing the tests were given hands-on experience with the instrumentation at a training session prior to beginning the study. Common equipment was bought for all centers. Each center was instructed to carry out pilot studies on three normal volunteers and three patients with heart failure. Tests results from these pilot studies were forwarded to the office of the study chairman (JNC) where they were reviewed by the study coordinator (SZ). Any deficiencies in the calibration, conduct of the study, or quality of the data were promptly reported to the center. Patients screened for this study were subjected to an exercise test and the data forwarded to the chairman's office for review before the patient could be randomized. Frequent communication between the study coordinator and the local study personnel was an important aspect during the conduct of this study.

In order to maintain calibration of both the bicycle and the gas exchange equipment, three normal volunteers from each center were subjected to a maximal exercise test annually as a biological calibration technique. Stability of the gas exchange measurements from year to year could then be assumed to represent stability of the gas exchange methodology, whereas a change in gas exchange measurements with time might suggest a deficiency in the instrumentation.

Results

Control Subject Calibration

Annual calibrations of the same normal volunteers were carried out at each of the study sites. The results from three representative centers in V-HeFT II are depicted in Figures 1 through 3. In some centers, as exemplified in Figure 1, the mean $\dot{V}O_2$ at each increment in exercise load was quite stable from year to year and approximated 10 mL/W/min. In other centers, as exemplified in Figure 2, a deficiency in the linear response of the system was detected. In this example, an apparent plateau of $\dot{V}O_2$ was noted from about 25 to 70 watts of workload and resulted in an abnormally low slope. This defect was attributed to a poorly calibrated bicycle which was replaced and resulted in appropriate slopes in 1988 and 1989. In one center, depicted in Figure 3, problems with the instrumentation resulted in an abnormally low

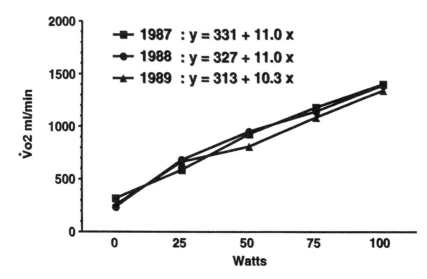

Figure 1. Mean annual gas exchange measurements in three normal volunteers in one center. Equipment functioned well each year.

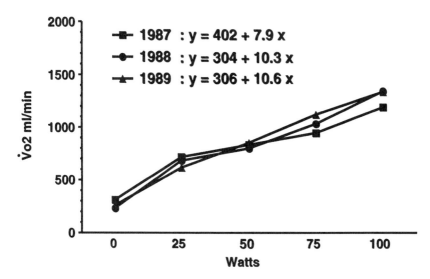

Figure 2. Mean annual gas exchange measurements in three normal volunteers in one center. Plateau in $\dot{V}O_2$ in 1987 was corrected by replacing bicycle ergometer.

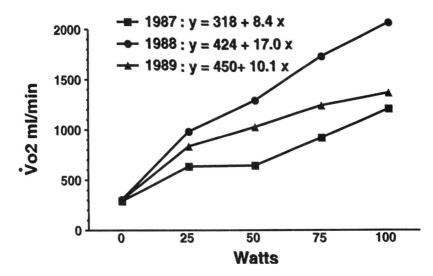

Figure 3. Mean annual gas exchange measurements in three normal volunteers in one center. Instrumentation problems in 1987 and 1988 were apparently corrected in 1989.

slope in 1987 and an abnormally high slope in 1988. The 1989 data are approaching normal functioning of the system. The data from this center, therefore, must be viewed with some caution.

$\dot{V}O_2$ as a Guide to Risk Assessment

Although, as expected, duration of exercise and peak $\dot{V}O_2$ were closely related in V-HeFT, the virtue of having a more precise end point for peak exercise was a valuable addition to exercise duration. As noted in Figure 4, $\dot{V}O_2$ served as a powerful guide to annual mortality rate in V-HeFT I when exercise was associated with a rise of respiratory exchange ratio (RER) by greater than 0.2, but it was not discriminating when exercise did not appear to approach physiological limits.

Effect of Therapy on Peak $\dot{V}O_2$

In V-HeFT I and V-HeFT II, peak $\dot{V}O_2$ was monitored sequentially. There were three treatment arms in V-HeFT I and two treatment arms in V-HeFT II. The smaller size of the treatment arms in V-HeFT I may have contributed to some unexplained variability in the peak $\dot{V}O_2$ measurements made sequentially. Although the hydralazine and isosorbide dinitrate group exhibited increments in peak $\dot{V}O_2$ that were borderline

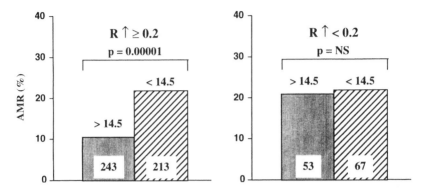

Figure 4. Annual mortality rate (AMR) in V-HeFT in patients whose peak $\dot{V}O_2$ was above the median (>14.5 mL/kg/min) and below the median (<14.5 mL/kg/min). In those who became anaerobic during exercise (R ≠ ≥ 0.2), $\dot{V}O_2$ was a powerful discriminator. In those who did not become anaerobic (R ≠ ≤ 0.2), AMR did not differ between the groups.

significant at 2 months, and highly significant at 12 months over baseline, an inexplicable decrease of peak $\dot{V}O_2$ at 6 months reduced the statistical significance of the overall response in that treatment arm (Figure 5). In contrast, both the placebo and prazosin groups exhibited a progressive decline over time. As noted, because of the modest sample size, only a small number of late measurements were available.

In V-HeFT II, the sample size was considerably larger and resulted in more stability in peak $\dot{V}O_2$ (Figure 6). Hydralazine and isosor-

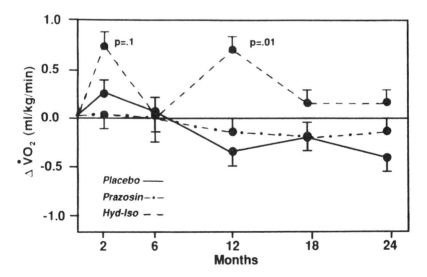

Figure 5. Change in peak $\dot{V}O_2 (\Delta \dot{V}O_2)$ after randomization to three treatment groups in V-HeFT I.

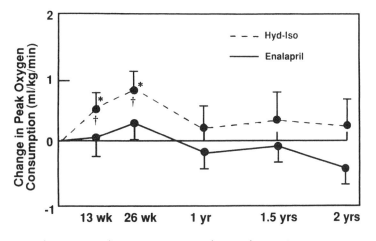

Figure 6. Change in peak O_2 consumption after randomization to two treatment groups in V-HeFT II. *$p < 0.05$ compared to baseline. †$p < 0.05$ compared to enalapril.

bide dinitrate exhibited a significant increment in peak $\dot{V}_{O_2}$ at 3 months and 6 months that was significantly greater than that observed in the enalapril treated group. Peak $\dot{V}_{O_2}$ in the hydralazine-isosorbide dinitrate group was also significantly better at 24 months and 48 months. A gradual decline of peak $\dot{V}_{O_2}$ appeared to emerge in the enalapril treated group.

Of the 804 patients entered in the V-HeFT II, 759 had adequate measurement of peak $\dot{V}_{O_2}$ for inclusion in the baseline database. During the conduct of V-HeFT II, 6098 exercise tests were scheduled per protocol and 4,983 or 81.7% of the scheduled tests were completed. Of the 4,983 tests completed, 4,508 were deemed to be valid. Therefore 90.5% of the tests done achieved the criteria for validity established for this protocol.

Determination of Anaerobic Threshold

In V-HeFT II, breath-by-breath analysis was carried out utilizing Medical Graphics Corporation equipment. Since it was determined prior to initiating this study that gas exchange anaerobic thresholds (ATge) would be assessed in an effort to evaluate the effect of therapy on submaximal exercise performance, graphic records of gas exchange during each exercise test were forwarded to a central reading laboratory (FC) for independent assessment of ATge. Initial attempts to utilize traditional criteria for assessing the ATge were plagued by ventilatory variation that made detection of the ATge questionable in a large proportion of cases. Subsequently, the data diskettes from each center were reassessed on the basis of the V-slope technique described by Beaver et al.[12] Utilizing this technique with a computer program,[13] an ATge could be identified in 58% of the tests. In an additional 16% of the tests, the ATge could be identified manually using this technique. In 25% of the tests, an ATge could not be identified. Examples of the value of measuring ATge are depicted in Figure 7, and the inability to measure ATge in Figure 8, since the

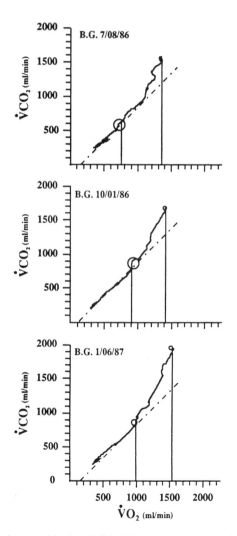

Figure 7. Sequential anaerobic threshold (AT) measurements in the same patient: **upper panel** (7/8/86) shows clear AT and peak $\dot{V}O_2$ (vertical lines); **middle panel** (10/1/86) shows modest improvement; **lower panel** shows further improvement in ATge and peak $\dot{V}O_2$.

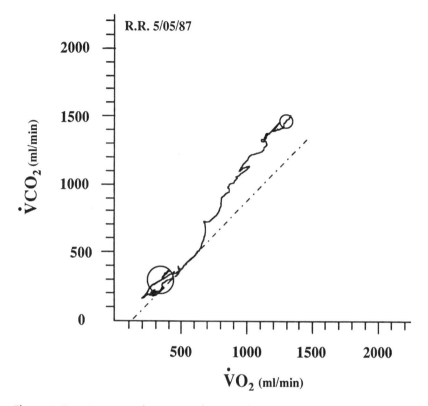

Figure 8. Exercise test in this patient does not demonstrate an identifiable ATge, during exercise. The $\dot{V}CO_2$ inflection occurs at rest due to hyperventilation.

study patient hyperventilated at rest and masked detection of ATge during exercise.

In V-HeFT II, the mean ATge in the two treatment arms was not significantly affected by therapy. In general, the ATge followed the peak $\dot{V}O_2$ exhibiting a slight, but insignificant increase in the hydralazine + isosorbide dinitrate treatment arm, and a gradual decline from baseline in the enalapril treated group.

V-HeFT III

In an effort to utilize a more precise method to identify the *AT* and the peak $\dot{V}O_2$ in patients with heart failure, V-HeFT III was designed utilizing a ramp protocol. An example of ATge measurement in one of the V-HeFT III patients is displayed in Figure 9. As noted in this figure, the *AT* is more clearly defined by the ramp protocol than it was by previous tests utilizing load increments at 2-minute intervals.

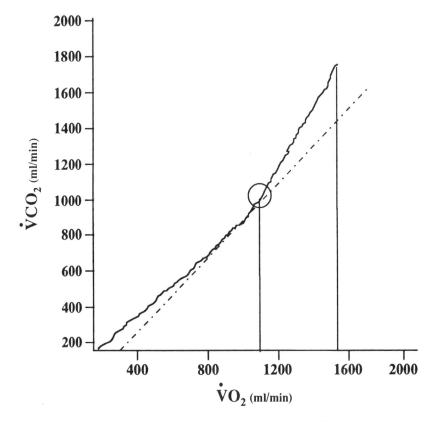

Figure 9. Ramp protocol in a patient in V-HeFT III provides clearer end point for anaerobic threshold and peak $\dot{V}O_2$.

Discussion

The V-HeFT studies have documented the safety of maximal exercise testing in patients with heart failure[14] and have demonstrated the use of gas exchange measurements in a multicenter study. A well-trained staff and common instrumentation that undergoes regular calibration are important factors in the success of such exercise studies carried out in multiple centers. Stability of the staff at the individual centers in V-HeFT was an important factor in the quality of the data. Close communication between the study sites and the chairman's office was vital to the success of the studies. One lesson learned in V-HeFT is the need for more frequent calibration of instrumentation. Nonlinearity of exercise oxygen consumption during increments of workload was apparent in some of the centers and may not have been corrected promptly enough to maintain precision of all of the data collected.

Although it was the initial design in V-HeFT to utilize peak $\dot{V}O_2$ as a guide to drug-induced improvements in exercise tolerance, subsequent experience has led to some controversy regarding the optimal exercise test to evaluate efficacy of an intervention in heart failure. Peak $\dot{V}O_2$ measured during a maximal test may be a poor guide to the comfort with which a patient can carry on his daily activity. Therefore, a submaximal exercise test might be more meaningful than a maximal test in assessing the therapeutic benefit of an intervention. Unfortunately, however, submaximal tests do not lend themselves to precise or quantitative end points.[8] In V-HeFT II, we chose the gas exchange *AT* as a quantitative measure of submaximal exercise capacity; however, difficulties in identifying the *AT* despite a number of additional and newer methods reduced the sensitivity of this technique. Indeed, *AT* did not appear to be more discriminating than peak $\dot{V}O_2$ in assessing the response to the vasodilators utilized in V-HeFT II.[15] A ramp protocol has been substituted in V-HeFT III. Since analysis of that trial is still ongoing, the results of that method in assessing efficacy of the therapeutic interventions are not yet available.

One of the more important lessons gained from V-HeFT is the value of an accurate measurement of peak $\dot{V}O_2$ in risk assessment of the individual. Peak exercise capacity measured by either exercise time or peak $\dot{V}O_2$ is an independent predictor of mortality in patients with heart failure, but the sensitivity of this measurement in V-HeFT may well be importantly related to the availability of gas exchange measurements that allowed staff to prod patients to further exercise when the gas exchange measurements revealed they had not yet surpassed their *AT*. Indeed, peak $\dot{V}O_2$ did not appear to be a discriminator for mortality when exercise was terminated prior to surpassing the *AT*.

Summary

Gas exchange measurements provide an objective end point for peak exercise capacity and a potential objective end point for submaximal exercise capacity in patients with heart failure. Application of gas exchange measurements in a multicenter clinical trial requires well-trained technicians, common instrumentation, regular calibration, and intense supervisory dedication to quality control.

Data from the Vasodilator-Heart Failure Trials (V-HeFT) have confirmed that gas exchange can be satisfactorily performed in a multicenter study and that peak $\dot{V}O_2$ can serve as a powerful predictor of survival. It can also be used to assess clinical efficacy of vasodilator drug therapy, but the sensitivity of this end point was disappointingly small in these multicenter studies. The gas exchange *AT*, which was determined in an attempt to identify a more sensitive guide to drug-induced changes in exercise capacity, did not exhibit a prominent response to therapy, either because the drugs were not adequately effective or because the gas exchange measurement, as performed, was not a sensitive guide to clinical efficacy of therapy. A ramp protocol introduced in V-HeFT III may improve reliability of the measurement.

References

1. Franciosa JA, Goldsmith SR, Cohn JN: Contrasting immediate and long-term effects of isosorbide dinitrate on exercise capacity in congestive heart failure. *Am J Med* 69:559–566, 1980.
2. Colucci WS, Wynne J, Holman RL, Braunwald E: Long-term therapy of heart failure with prazosin: A randomized double blind trial. *Am J Cardiol* 45:337–344, 1980.
3. Massie BM, Kramer B, Haughom F: Acute and long-term effects of vasodilator therapy on resting and exercise hemodynamics and exercise tolerance. *Circulation* 64:1218–1226, 1981.
4. Franciosa JA, Weber KT, Levine B, et al: Hydralazine in long-term treatment of chronic heart failure: lack of difference from placebo. *Am Heart J* 104:587–594, 1982.
5. Leier CV, Huss P, Magorien RD, Unverferth DV: Improved exercise capacity and differing arterial and venous tolerance during chronic isosorbide dinitrate therapy for congestive heart failure. *Circulation* 67:817–822, 1983.
6. Captopril Multicenter Research Group: a placebo-controlled trial of captopril in refractory chronic congestive heart failure. *J Am Coll Cardiol* 2:755–763, 1983.
7. Creager MA, Massie BM, Faxon DP, et al: Acute and long-term effects of enalapril on the cardiovascular response to exercise and exercise tolerance in patients with congestive heart failure. *J Am Coll Cardiol* 6:163–170, 1985.
8. Cohn JN, Rajfer SF: Evaluation of functional capacity in heart failure: a consensus conference. *Heart Failure* 6:169–173, 1990.
9. Wasserman K, McIlroy MB: Detecting the threshold of anaerobic metabolism in cardiac patients during exercise. *Am J Cardiol* 14:844–852, 1964.
10. Cohn JN, Archibald DG, Ziesche S, et al: Effect of vasodilator therapy on mortality in chronic congestive heart failure. *N Engl J Med* 314:1547–1552, 1986.
11. Cohn JN, Johnson G, Ziesche S, et al: A comparison of enalapril with hydralazine-isosorbide dinitrate in the treatment of chronic congestive heart failure. *N Engl J Med* 325:303–310, 1991.
12. Beaver WL, Wasserman K, Whipp BJ: A new method for selecting the anaerobic threshold by gas exchange. *J Appl Physiol* 60:2020–2026, 1986.
13. Dickstein K, Barvik S, Aarsland T, Snapinn S, Millerhagen J: Validation of a computerized technique for detection of the gas exchange anaerobic threshold in cardiac disease. *Am J Cardiol* 66:1363–1367, 1990.
14. Tristani FE, Hughes CV, Archibald DG, Sheldahl LM, Cohn JN, Fletcher R, for the VA Cooperative Study: Safety of graded symptom-limited exercise testing in patients with congestive heart failure. *Circulation* (suppl VI)76:VI-54–VI-58, 1987.
15. Ziesche S, Cobb FR, Cohn JN, Johnson G, Tristani F, for the V-HeFT VA Cooperative Studies Group: Hydralazine and isosorbide dinitrate combination improves exercise tolerance in heart failure: results from V-HeFT I and V-HeFT II. *Circulation* 87:VI-56–VI-64, 1993.

18

Exercise Gas Exchange to Evaluate Cardiac Pacemaker Function

Norbert Treese, MD

Introduction

In normal subjects, maximal exercise capacity is defined by maximal oxygen uptake ($\dot{V}O_2$max). According to Fick's principle, $\dot{V}O_2$max is the product of heart rate, the arteriovenous oxygen content difference, and stroke volume at maximal exercise. At lower work rate, stroke volume increases by the Frank Starling mechanism. At higher work rate, exercise tachycardia is more important[1] and, despite increasing filling pressure, systolic and diastolic volume may decrease.[2]

Exercise capacity is very much dependent on the ability to increase heart rate. An abnormal heart rate response to exercise, therefore, can cause reduced exercise performance and low aerobic capacity.[3,4] The patient's inability to provide an appropriate heart rate increase in response to exercise is considered as chronotropic incompetence. An abnormal heart rate behavior, however, may also be found in patients with a normal peak heart rate with a too-slow heart rate increase at the beginning of exercise, an unstable heart rate during prolonged exercise, or a too-slow decrease at the end of exercise.

Rate-Variable Pacing

The traditional goal of pacemaker therapy is to prevent symptoms associated with excessive bradycardia. Modern cardiac pacing has, in

From Wasserman, K (ed): *Exercise Gas Exchange in Heart Disease.* Armonk, NY: Futura Publishing Company, Inc., © 1996.

addition, attempted not only to maintain atrioventricular synchrony, but also to provide an appropriate heart rate response to exercise. In the absence of normal sinus node function, patients may benefit from pacing systems that simulate physiological heart rate changes during exercise using sensors to provide heart rate variability independent of atrial activity. It has been proposed that rate-variable pacing should normalize the heart rate response to exercise in proportion to the exercise metabolic demand.[5] Therefore, the analysis of respiratory gas exchange during exercise may be of particular importance in patients with sensor-triggered rate-variable pacing.

The usefulness of such pacing systems in selected patients is established. Many studies have demonstrated that single chamber rate-variable pacing is superior to fixed-rate atrial or ventricular pacing.[6-14] In a crossover study, Smedgard et al[14] demonstrated a 7% increase of exercise capacity on the bicycle and a 19% increase during treadmill exercise when activity-triggered pacing was compared with fixed-rate ventricular pacing. Benditt and co-workers[7] found a consistently lower level of perceived exertion during activity-triggered rate-variable single chamber pacing compared to fixed-rate stimulation. In addition, these authors assessed exercise capacity during both pacing modalities using cardiopulmonary exercise testing. During treadmill exercise, rate-responsive pacing provided a 42% increase of heart rate which was related to a 22% increase in aerobic capacity.

Cardiopulmonary Exercise Testing

Rossi et al[11-13] were the first to assess respiratory-controlled pacemaker systems employing the principles of respiratory gas analysis during exercise. According to their findings, rate-variable pacing is of particular value in patients with chronotropic incompetence and heart failure.[13] To achieve a sufficient level of exercise, these patients appear to be dependent on an approriate increase in heart rate as the myocardial contractile reserve and stroke volume capacity are limited. More recently, Kay et al[15] showed that respiratory-controlled pacing improved maximal oxygen uptake by 22% from 13.4 to 16.3 mL/kg/min as compared to fixed-rate pacing.

Our first experience with respiratory gas analysis was based on 17 patients with rate-variable single chamber pacing.[16] Chronotropic incompetence was present in all patients, due to His bundle ablation or high-degree atrioventricular (AV) block.

All patients were exercised sequentially either in a fixed rate of 70 beats per minute (VVI-70 bpm) or in the sensor-triggered pacing mode (VVIR) 4 months to 6 months after pacemaker implantation. Exercise was performed on a bicycle in a semisupine position using a ramp protocol with 10 watts to 20 watts per minute increase in work rate.[17] Respiratory gas exchange was analyzed using a computerized breath-by-breath technique (Medical Graphics Corporation, St. Paul, MN, USA). The anaerobic threshold (*AT*) was determined according to the V-slope method proposed by Beaver et al.[18]

Our findings demonstrated that a 42% increase of heart rate was associated with a 22% increase of $\dot{V}O_2$max from 14.3 to 18.3 mL/kg/min. At the *AT*, $\dot{V}O_2$ increased by 13%. In these patients, a normalized heart rate response appears to delay the onset of anaerobic glycolysis, thus improving aerobic exercise capacity. Similarly, Hatano et al[19] have shown that rate-responsive pacing at a given workload lowered the venous lactate production when compared to fixed-rate pacing, indicating an increase of aerobic capacity.

Oxygen Uptake and Work Rate

Oxygen uptake during exercise is closely related to the level of work that can be performed. Hansen et al[20,21] have studied the slope of $\dot{V}O_2$ as a function of work rate ($\dot{V}O_2$/WR) which is important because it measures the aerobic work efficiency. The authors showed that the $\dot{V}O_2$/WR ratio below the *AT* was constant over a wide range of workloads. During incremental exercise this ratio appears to be predictable for normal subjects,[22] and a reduction in this ratio may indicate cardiovascular dysfunction.[23–25]

Rate-variable pacing in patients with chronic heart failure and chronotropic incompetence may also influence the $\dot{V}O_2$/work-rate ratio. Figure 1 shows a typical example in a patient with advanced chronic heart failure and high-grade AV-block in whom a respiratory-controlled ventricular pacing system was implanted. The $\dot{V}O_2$/work-rate ratio was 9.2 mL/min/W during fixed-rate pacing, and increased to 12.5 mL/min/W during exercise in the rate-variable pacing mode.

The value of the $\dot{V}O_2$/work-rate ratio was studied in 27 patients with chronotropic incompetence who received a respiratory-controlled pacing system (META MV 1202, Teletronics Pacing Systems, Inc., Englewood, CO, USA).[26] At the *AT*, heart rate increased from 75 ± 9 in the VVI mode to 113 ± 21 bpm in the VVIR mode. $\dot{V}O_2$ increased from 9.3 ± 3.4 to 10.9 ± 4.3 mL/kg/min and work rate from 52 ± 20 to 65 ± 24 watts. The $\dot{V}O_2$/work-rate ratio below the *AT* improved from 7.9 ± 2.3 to 10.2 ± 2.4 mL/min/W (Figure 2) and was equal to the mean value for normal subjects (Figure 3). The $\dot{V}O_2$/work-rate ratio appears to be an additional parameter to assess the aerobic capacity in these patients, especially if the *AT* is not attained.

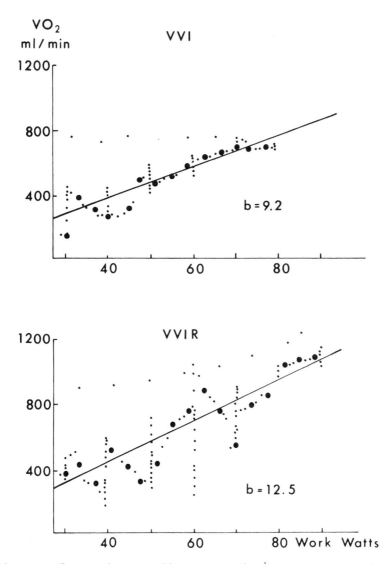

Figure 1. Influence of rate-variable pacing on the $\dot{V}O_2$ (mL/min) to work-rate (W/min) ratio above the oxygen cost of unloaded cycling (y axis intercept) in a patient with heart failure and chronotropic incompetence. The **upper panel** shows the $\dot{V}O_2$/work-rate ratio (b = 9.2) during fixed-rate (heart rate = 70 bpm) pacing (VVI 70), and the **lower panel** shows the results (b = 12.5) during rate-variable pacing (VVIR). The exercise settings were identical during both tests.[39]

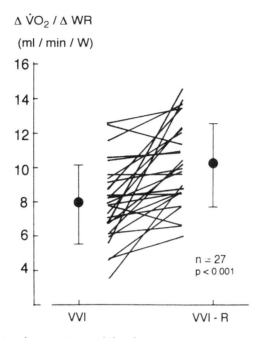

Figure 2. V̇O₂/work-rate ratio, as defined in Figure 1, in 27 patients with a respiratory dependent rate-variable pacemaker during VVI and VVIR pacing.

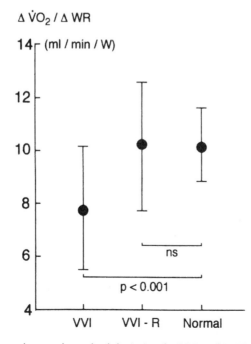

Figure 3. Mean values and standard deviation for VVI and VVIR pacing in 27 patients with a respiratory dependent rate-variable pacemaker, as in Figure 2. These results are compared to values obtained in middle-aged sedentary subjects without overt heart disease.[26]

Cardiopulmonary Exercise Capacity and Long-Term Rate-Variable Pacing

While most studies have demonstrated improved exercise capacity during short-term rate-variable pacing,[7,11,14,16,26] the long-term advantage of this pacing mode is not well established.[27] Therefore, we performed a crossover exercise study in 15 patients with a respiratory-controlled pacemaker (META MV 1202) to compare the rate-variable and fixed-rate pacing mode during short-term and long-term pacing.[28] Four weeks after the pacemaker implantation, the patients were exercised during both VVI and VVIR pacing and randomized to either pacing mode. The test was repeated 10 weeks later. All patients then crossed over to the alternative pacing mode and were reassessed after a further study period of 10 weeks. During short-term assessment, exercise performance was improved with VVIR pacing. A 68% increase in heart rate with an increase in peak $\dot{V}O_2$ from 15.4 ± 4.4 to 17.6 ± 55.5 mL/kg/min and an increase of exercise time from 358 ± 92 to 394 ± 108 seconds was observed. During long-term assessment, however, the improved exercise capacity was not maintained in these patients. Despite a similar increase in heart rate, peak $\dot{V}O_2$ (15.6 ± 5.1 versus 15.9 ± 5.2 mL/kg/min) and exercise time (345 ± 81 versus 342 ± 63 seconds) did not change significantly. The slope of the $\dot{V}O_2$/work-rate ratio normalized during acute VVIR pacing from 7.8 ± 1.9 to 11.0 ± 3.4 mL/min/W and decreased to 9.0 ± 2.1 mL/min/W during chronic VVIR pacing (Figure 4). No change of left ventricular dimensions was observed during echocardiographic examinations at any time during the study.

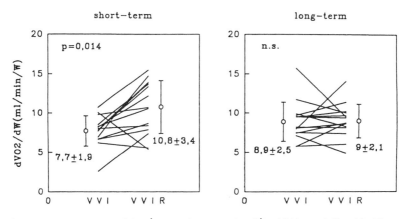

Figure 4. Comparison of the $\dot{V}O_2$ work-rate ratio (d$\dot{V}O_2$/dW), as defined in Figure 1, in 15 patients with a respiratory dependent rate-variable pacemaker during VVI and VVIR pacing during short-term and long-term assessment.[28]

We concluded from these findings that the initial improvement of exercise capacity with rate-variable ventricular pacing is not maintained over time. We hypothesized that not only the peak heart rate, but also the heart rate increase may be an important determinant for exercise performance.

Heart Rate and Oxygen Uptake

Norländer et al[29] reviewed exercise studies in pacemaker patients, and pointed out that the degree of heart rate increase is directly proportional to the patients' exercise capacity regardless of what pacing system has been used. McElroy et al[5] focused on the close relationship between heart rate increase and metabolic demand during exercise and underlined the importance of this relationship for rate-variable pacing. These investigators described a linear relationship between heart rate and $\dot{V}O_2$ in patients with different degrees of heart failure. Individual slopes of this relationship ranged from 2 beats to 6 beats for an increase in $\dot{V}O_2$ of 1 mL/kg/min. A linear relationship was also found between heart rate and minute ventilation, which is not dependent on the patient's functional status. These findings have important implications for rate-variable pacemakers. Ideally an optimally programmed rate-variable pacemaker should reproduce these normal relationships at all levels of exercise.

We analyzed the heart rate response to exercise in relation to the $\dot{V}O_2$ and the minute ventilation in a group of 39 middle-aged sedentary subjects without overt cardiovascular disease.[30] Exercise testing was performed on a bicycle in semisupine position, using a progressively increasing work-rate protocol with a work slope of 20 watts per minute. Linear regression analysis was performed for heart rate as a function of $\dot{V}O_2$ and minute ventilation ($\dot{V}E$). Initially all data from rest to peak exercise were included in the analysis. A linear regression analysis for HR/$\dot{V}O_2$, however, was only found in 16 of 39 subjects and for HR/$\dot{V}E$ in 11 of 39 subjects. Assuming the AT as the breaking point of two linear curves, it could be demonstrated that compared to low-intensity exercise HR appeared to increase more in relation to $\dot{V}O_2$, but less in relation to $\dot{V}E$ near maximal exercise intensity (Figures 5 and 6). In men, the individual slopes for HR/$\dot{V}O_2$ were 2.6 $\pm$ 0.7 below, but 3.22 $\pm$ 1.0 beats/mL/kg above the AT and the slopes for HR/$\dot{V}E$ were 1.6 $\pm$ 0.5 below, but 1.0 $\pm$ 0.44 beats/1 above AT. Similarly, in women the individual slopes for HR/$\dot{V}O_2$ were 3.7 $\pm$ 1.4 below, but 4.3 $\pm$ 1.4 beats/mL/kg above AT and the slopes for HR/$\dot{V}E$ were 2.1 $\pm$ 0.9 below, but 1.3 $\pm$ 0.4 beats/1 above AT.

These findings have been recently confirmed by Lewalter et al.[31] These investigators used a symptom-limited, modified Chronotropic

HR-O$_2$ UPTAKE RELATION

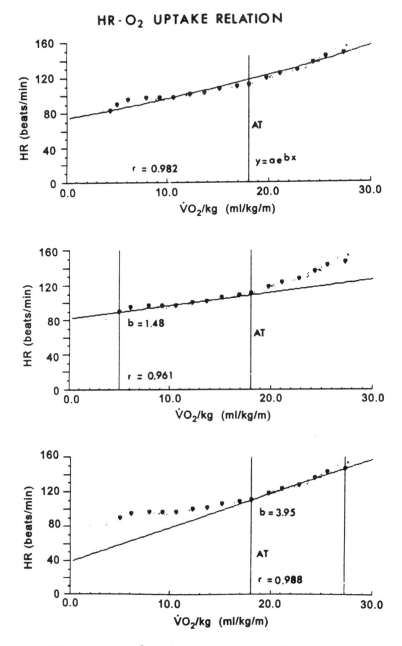

Figure 5. The heart rate to $\dot{V}O_2$ relation in a single healthy subject. Note the exponential relationship with a high correlation coefficient of 0.982 (**upper panel**). The two-phase curve analysis using a linear regression model shows different slopes below (**middle panel**) and above (**lower panel**) the anaerobic threshold (*AT*).[30]

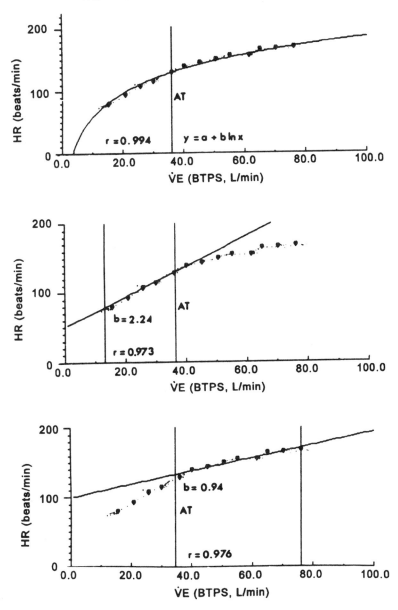

Figure 6. The heart rate to minute ventilation (HR-V̇E) relation in the same healthy subject as in Figure 5. The best fit curve analysis showed a logarithmic relationship with a correlation coefficient of 0.994 (**upper panel**). The two-phase curve analysis using a linear regression model showed different slopes below (**middle panel**) and above (**lower panel**) the anaerobic threshold (*AT*).[30]

Assessment Exercise Protocol (CAEP) as recently proposed by Black-burn et al.[32] For men, an HR/$\dot{V}$E slope of 1.41 ± 0.43 below and 1.05 ± 0.25 beats/L above *AT* was observed. In women, a steeper slope for HR/$\dot{V}$E with 1.78 ± 0.54 and 1.27 ± 0.48 beats/1 respectively was found.

The slopes of the function of heart rate versus $\dot{V}O_2$ and $\dot{V}$E could be used to optimize rate-variable pacing systems. The post hoc analysis of these relationships in our study population with chronic VVIR pacing[28] was 5.0 ± 1.7 beats/mL/kg for HR/$\dot{V}O_2$ and 3.5 ± 1.0 beats/L for HR/$\dot{V}$E. Since these values were steeper than those measured in normal sedentary subjects without overt heart disease, we may have overshot the pacing rate needed for exercise. This "overpacing" might be responsible for the decline in exercise capacity during chronic VVIR pacing.

Kay et al[33] evaluated the heart rate response in rate-variable pacing, using the concept of the heart rate and metabolic reserve as proposed by Wilkoff.[34] The metabolic-chronotropic relation plots normalized heart rate response (percentage heart rate reserve) versus normalized oxygen consumption (percent metabolic reserve) as a linear function. In normal subjects, this response appears to be independent of age, peak aerobic capacity, resting heart rate, and exercise protocol. In Wilkoff's study,[34] however, oxygen consumption was calculated and not directly measured. Therefore, the concept of the metabolic-chronotropic relationship needs to be validated by breath-by-breath analysis of respiratory gas exchange.

Lewalter et al[35] recently described a different method to evaluate the heart rate response in rate-variable pacing using a low-intensity steady state treadmill protocol. During the early phase of dynamic exercise, oxygen consumption was measured and the oxygen deficit calculated. Heart rate was then programmed to minimize this early metabolic deficit.[35] A similar approach quantitating the oxygen deficit during constant levels of submaximal exercise has recently also been used to study rate behavior at onset of exercise in patients with rate-variable pacing.[36]

Chronotropic Incompetence

According to the definition of the American College of Cardiology/American Heart Association, rate-variable pacing is indicated when, during maximal exercise, a heart rate of 100 bpm is not achieved.[37] Age-specific and gender-specific differences, however, are not taken into account. Furthermore, maximal exercise and thus maximal heart rate will not be attained in many patients because of concomitant, noncardiovascular disease, or lack of the patient's willingness to exercise. Another approach defined chronotropic incompetence as one or two standard deviations from age- and protocol-specific deviations from a mean heart rate at every stage of exercise.[38]

We considered the slope of the $HR/\dot{V}O_2$ function to define chronotropic incompetence. In a recent study, we evaluated the impact of the rate-variable pacing mode in 23 patients with dual chamber pacemakers. In a chronic crossover study, dual chamber pacing (DDD) was compared to the dual chamber rate-variable pacing mode (DDDR). Chronotropic incompetence was defined as a slope of $HR/\dot{V}O_2 < 2.0$ beats/mL/kg. According to this definition, 9 patients were classified as chronotropic incompetent with a maximal heart rate below 100 bpm (Table). During chronic assessment of these patients, $\dot{V}O_2$max increased 12.7 $\pm$ 33.1 mL/min/kg in the DDD pacing mode to 15.3 $\pm$ 33.2 mL/kg/min in the DDDR pacing mode and exercise time from 252 $\pm$ 59 to 301 $\pm$ 96 seconds respectively. Quality of life improved significantly in the DDDR pacing mode. By contrast, among the remaining 14 chronotropically competent patients, $\dot{V}O_2$max was higher as compared to the chronotropic incompetent patients, but did not change when chronic DDD pacing was compared with chronic DDDR pacing (17.7 $\pm$ 5.9 versus 16.8 $\pm$ 5.9 mL/kg/min). The exercise time was 407 $\pm$ 159 and 406 $\pm$ 165 seconds respectively (Table). The quality of life, however, deteriorated in these 14 patients with a

	Group A HR/$\dot{V}O_2$ <2b/ml/kg		Group B HR/$\dot{V}O_2$<2b/ml/kg	
Table				
Parameter	DDD	DDDR	DDD	DDDR
HRmax (bpm)	83±13	132±7#	120±21*	130±24
HR-AT (bpm)	77±44	107±15#	101±13*	107±15
$\dot{V}O_2$max (ml/kg/min)	12.7±3.1	15.3±3.2$	17.7±5.9§	16.8±5.9
$\dot{V}O_2$-AT (ml/kg/min)	9.9±2.9	11.6±3.1$	12.3±3.3	12.1±2.9
Wmax (W)	93±22	107±36	140±49§	137±51
W-AT (W)	55±15	66±24	80±28§	78±28
Exercise time (sec)	252±59	301±96$	407±159§	406±165
HR/$\dot{V}O_2$ (b/ml/kg)	1.5±0.4	4.2±0.5#	2.7±0.4*	3.6±1.0
$\dot{V}O_2$/W	8.1±1.0	9.0±0.9$	9.8±2.3§	9.2±2.5

Respiratory gas exchange data in patients with dual chamber pacing during chronic DDD (dual chamber pacing mode) and DDDR (dual chamber rate variable pacing mode) classified according to chronotropic responsiveness into chronotropic competent: n=14 (Group B) and incompetent: n=9 (Group A) patients. HRmax, $\dot{V}O_2$max, Wmax $\simeq$ heart rate, oxygen uptake, and work rate at maximal exercise; HR-AT, $\dot{V}O_2$-AT, W-AT = heart rate, oxygen uptake, and work rate at the anaerobic threshold; HR/$\dot{V}O_2$ − heart rate/$\dot{V}O_2$ slope; $\dot{V}O_2$/W − $\dot{V}O_2$/work rate slope.

Statistical significance (p<0.05) is shown: # - group A, comparison between DDD and DDDR pacing; *= group B comparison between DDD and DDDR pacing; § - DDD pacing, comparison between group A and B; $ - DDDR pacing, comparison between A and B.

significant increase of the symptom score. Holter monitoring showed a significant increase of mean maximal heart rate from 69 ± 7 bpm in the DDD pacing mode to 78 ± 9 bpm in the DDDR pacing mode with no significant incidence of atrial arrhythmias in chronotropic incompetent patients (Table). The maximum heart rate, however, was similar for both pacing modes in the chronotropic competent patients. In these patients, the incidence of atrial arrhythmias increased from median 1.6 under DDD to 4.8 episodes under DDDR pacing, which may account for the decline in the symptom score. The study shows that respiratory gas exchange analysis may identify patients suitable for the rate-variable pacing mode which would benefit patients with chronotropic incompetence.

Summary

Cardiopulmonary exercise testing appears to be of particular value in patients with rate-variable pacing. The influeuce of an appropriate sensor-triggered heart rate response to exercise on the patient's aerobic capacity can be assessed by continuous monitoring of respiratory gas exchange. Changes in the *AT*, as an objective measure of a submaximal exercise level, are most useful for demonstrating the overall benefit of rate-variable pacing in these patients. The $\dot{V}O_2$/work-rate ratio appears to provide additional information. Furthermore, respiratory gas exchange analysis may be useful in evaluating chronotropic responsiveness and in selecting suitable patients for rate-variable pacing. Finally, the close relationship between heart rate and $\dot{V}O_2$ as well as $\dot{V}E$ should play a key role in optimizing pacemaker programming according to the individual metabolic demand.

References

1. Astrand PO, Cuddy TE, Saltin B, Sternberg J: Cardiac output during submaximal and maximal work. *J Appl Physiol* 19:268, 1964.
2. Higginbotham MB, Morris KG, Williams RS, McHale PA, Coleman RE, Cobb FR: Regulation of stroke volume during submaximal and maximal upright exercise in normal man. *Circ Res* 58:281, 1986.
3. Ikkos D, Hanson JS: Response to exercise in congenital complete artrioventricular block. *Circulation* 22:583, 1960.
4. Reybrouck T, Eynde BV, Dumoulin M, Van der Hauwaert LC: Cardiorespiratory response to exercise in congenital complete atrioventricular block. *Am J Cardiol* 64:896, 1989.
5. McElroy P, Janicki JS, Weber KT: Physiologic correlates of the heart rate response to upright isotonic exercise: relevance to rate responsive pacemakers. *J Am Coll Cardiol* 11:94, 1988.
6. Alt E, Hirgstetter C, Heinz M, Blömer H: Rate control of physiologic pacemakers by central venous blood temperature. *Circulation* 73:1206, 1986.

7. Benditt DG, Mianulli M, Fetter J, et al: Single chamber cardiac activity-initiated chronotropic response: evaluation by cardiopulmonary exercise testing. *Circulation* 75:184, 1987.
8. Benditt DG, Milstein S, Buetikkoffer J, Gornick CC, Mianulli M, Fetter J: Sensor-triggered rate variable cardiac pacing: current technologies and clinical implications. *Ann Intern Med* 107:704, 1987.
9. Den Dulk KC, Bouwels L, Lindemann F, Rankin I, Brugada P, Wellens H: The activitrax rate response pacing system. *Am J Cardiol* 61:107, 1988.
10. Rickards AF, Donaldson RM, Thalen TH: The use of QT interval to determine pacing rate: early clinical experience. *PACE* 10:650, 1983.
11. Rossi P, Rognoni G, Orchetta E, Prando MD, Plicchi G, Minella M: Respiration dependent ventricular pacing compared with fixed ventricular and atrioventricular synchronous pacing: aerobic and hemodynamic variables *J Am Coll Cardiol* 6:646, 1986.
12. Rossi P, Prando MD, Ochetta E, Aina F, Rognoni G, Magnami A: Influence of heart rate on anaerobic threshold. *Adv Cardiol* 35:108, 1986.
13. Rossi P, Prando MD, Ochetta E, Rognoni G, Aina F: Rate responsive pacing in patients with left ventricular failure. *Adv Cardiol* 36:115, 1986.
14. Smedgard P, Kristensson BE, Kruse I, Ryden L: Rate-response pacing by means of activity sensing versus single rate ventricular pacing: a double blind crossover study. *PACE* 10:902, 1987.
15. Kay GN, Bubien RS, Epstein AE, Plumb VJ: Rate-modulated cardiac pacing based on transthoracic impedance measurements of minute ventilation: correlates with exercise gas exchange: *J Am Coll Cardiol* 14:1283, 1989.
16. Treese N, Coutinho M, Ophoff N, Rhein S, Pop T, Meyer J: Kardiopulmonale Belastung: Funktionskontrolle für frequenzvariable Schrittmachersysteme. *Z Kardiol* 79:396, 1990.
17. Davis JA, Whipp BJ, Lamarra N, Huntsman DJ, Frank MH, Wasserman K: Effects of ramp slope on measurements of aerobic parameters from ramp exercise test. *Med Sci Sports Exerc* 14:339, 1982.
18. Beaver WL, Wasserman K, Whipp BJ: A new method for detecting the anaerobic threshold by gas exchange. *J Appl Physiol* 60:2020, 1986.
19. Hatano K, Kato R, Hayashi H, Noda S, Sobota I, Murase M: Usefulness of rate response pacing in patients with sick sinus syndrome. *PACE* 12:16, 1989.
20. Hansen JE, Sue DY, Oren A, Wasserman K: Relation of oxygen uptake to work rate in normal men and women with circulatory disorders. *Am J Cardiol* 59:669, 1987.
21. Hansen JE, Casaburi R, Cooper DM, Wasserman K: Oxygen uptake as related to work rate increment during cycle ergometer exercise. *J Appl Physiol* 57:140, 1988.
22. Treese N, Akbulut Ö, Coutinho M, Epperlein S, Meyer J: Halbliegende kardiopulmonale Belastung bei Herzgesunden mittleren Alters. *Z Kardiol* 83: 138, 1994.
23. Itoh H, Tanguchi K, Koike A, Doi M: Evaluation of severity of heart failure using ventilatory gas exchange analysis. *Circulation* (suppl) 81:31, 1990.
24. Koike A, Hiroe M, Adachi H, et al: Anaerobic metabolism as an indicator of aerobic function during exercise in cardiac patients. *J Am Coll Cardiol* 20: 120, 1992.
25. Coutinho M: Spiroergometrische Untersuchungen bei chronischer Herzinsuffizienz (medical thesis). Mainz, Germany, 1990.
26. Epperlein S, Treese N, Stegmeier A, Coutinho M, Meyer J: Der $\dot{V}O_2$-Leistungsindex zur Beurteilung der kardiopulmonalen Leistungsfähigkeit

unter atemminutenvolumen-gesteuerter VVIR Stimulation. *Z Kardiol* 83: 343, 1994.

27. Lipkin D, Boller N, Frenneaux M, et al: Randomized crossover trial of rate responsive activitrax and conventional fixed-rate ventricular pacing. *Br Heart J* 58:613, 1987.

28. Epperlein S, Himmrich E, Herrig I, Zegelman M, Treese N: Akute und chronische kardiopulmonale Leistungsfähigkeit unter atemminutenvolumen-gesteuerter VVIR Stimulation. *Herzschr Elektrophys* 5:73, 1994.

29. Norländer R, Hedman A, Pehrsson SK: Rate-variable pacing and exercise capacity, a comment. *PACE* 12:749, 1989.

30. Treese N, McCarter S, Akbulut O, et al: Ventilation and heart rate response during exercise in normals: relevance for rate variable pacing. *PACE* 17: 1693, 1993.

31. Lewalter T, Jung W, McCarter D, et al: Heart rate during exercise: what is the optimal goal of rate adaptive pacemaker therapy. *Am Heart J* 127:1026, 1994.

32. Blackburn B, Harvey S, Wilkoff B: A chronotropic assessment exercise protocol to assess the need and efficacy of rate responsive pacing (abstr). *Med Sci Sports Exerc* 20:S21, 1988.

33. Kay GN: Quantitation of chronotropic response: comparison of methods for rate modulating permanent pacemakers. *J Am Coll Cardiol* 20:1533, 1992.

34. Wilkoff B, Corey J, Blackburn G: A mathematical model of the cardiac chronotropic response to exercise. *J Electrophysiol* 3:176, 1989.

35. Lewalter T, Jung W, McCarter D, et al: Heart rate and oxygen uptake kinetics: a goal of rate adaptive pacemakers (abstr). *PACE* 16:4, 1993.

36. Dailey SM, Bubien RS, Kay GN: Effect of chronotropic response pattern on oxygen kinetics. *PACE* 17:2307, 1994.

37. Dreifus LS, Fish C, Griffin JC, et al (ed): Guidelines for implantation of cardiac pacemakers and antiarrhythmic devices: a report of the ACC/AHA task force on assessment of diagnostic and therapeutic cardiovascular procedures. *Circulation* 84:455, 1991.

38. Ellestad MH, Wan M: Predictive implications of stress testing: follow-up of 2700 subjects after maximum treadmill stress testing. *Circulation* 51:363, 1975.

39. Treese N, Coutinho M, Stegmeier A, et al: Influence of rate responsive pacing on aerobic capacity in patients with chronotropic incompetence. In: Winter U, Wasserman K, Treese N, Höpp H, eds: *Computerized Cardiopulmonary Exercise Testing*. Darmstadt, Germany: Steinkopff Verlag, 139–146, 1991.

19

Role of Exercise Testing in the Evaluation of Candidates for Cardiac Transplantation

Lynne Warner Stevenson, MD

Prognosis in Advanced Heart Failure

When cardiac transplantation was an experimental therapy for heart failure, candidacy was limited largely to bedridden patients who usually underwent the procedure within a few weeks. As transplantation evolved, medical therapy also evolved to improve quality and length of life without surgery for many heart failure patients. Transplantation continues to be indicated for patients who remain bedridden with heart failure despite tailoring of therapy with vasodilators and diuretics. Among patients who can be rendered ambulatory, however, the current challenge is to distinguish those who will do well without transplantation from those who require early listing in order to survive the long waiting period. As survival after cardiac transplantation has improved to 80% to 85% at 1 year,[1] it is anticipated that ambulatory candidates for transplantation should have a predicted 1-year survival of less than 50% to 60% without transplantation. Many factors which distinguish normal from abnormal circulatory integration for large populations with moderate heart failure have been less useful in advanced heart failure, characterized by more severe cardiac and systemic compromise.

Among patients referred for transplantation, the classic indications of low ejection fraction and Class IV symptoms are no longer adequate to identify patients at unacceptably high risk of poor early

From Wasserman, K (ed): *Exercise Gas Exchange in Heart Disease.* Armonk, NY: Futura Publishing Company, Inc., © 1996.

outcome (Figure 1). Even among patients presenting with both ejection fraction <20% and Class IV symptoms, those responding well to tailored medical therapy since 1990 have a 53% chance of surviving 2 years without death or deterioration necessitating urgent transplantation.[2] Numerous predictors specifically in this population have included neurohormonal markers such as serum sodium and norepinephrine levels, left ventricular size, ventricular filling pressures on maximal therapy, and history of arrhythmias.[3-9]

Although many factors may identify statistically separate increases in risk which contribute to our understanding of heart failure progression and sudden death, the definition and comparison of populations between programs requires an integrative predictor which can be uniformly measured and interpreted. Measurement of exercise capacity assesses both cardiac reserve and integrated physical function, which may each contribute to survival. Cardiopulmonary exercise testing, initially providing a new degree of objectivity in the measurement of peak functional capacity in therapeutic trials in heart failure, was found to predict survival as well.[3,10-14]

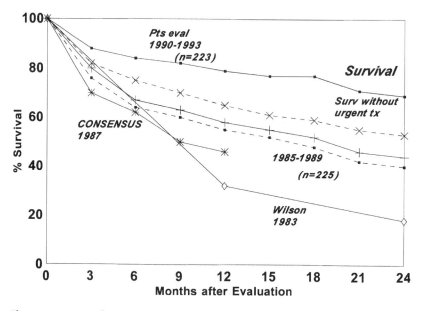

Figure 1. Actuarial **curves** of overall survival on tailored medical therapy and survival without hospitalization for urgent transplantation in 448 patients presenting with Class IV symptoms and subsequently discharged without transplantation. These curves demonstrate improved survival since the series reported by Wilson in 1983,[6] the Consensus trial,[27] and further improvement since 1990. Changes in therapy after 1990 include more aggressive use of angiotensin converting enzyme inhibition for achievement of hemodynamic goals, avoidance of Type I antiarrhythmic agents, and increasing use of amiodarone.

Multivariate analysis in our experience shows peak oxygen consumption ($\dot{V}O_2$) to be an independent variable predicting survival with advanced heart failure in multivariate proportional hazards models including serum sodium, pulmonary capillary wedge pressure on tailored therapy, and left ventricular diastolic dimension.[13] Left ventricular ejection fraction and hemodynamic parameters at the time of referral did not predict survival in patients referred for transplantation. When comparing survival statistics grouped by exercise testing compared to other prognostic factors, it is important to recognize that patients who are bedridden or severely symptomatic at rest have the worst prognosis and generally do not undergo exercise testing, which is of value primarily in the ambulatory population.

Parameters of Exercise Capacity

After the initial work of Mancini,[10] increasing experience has confirmed the value of cardiopulmonary exercise testing specifically in the population of patients evaluated for cardiac transplantation. Testing has been done with both bicycle exercise and treadmill exercise. Although bicycle exercise is not as familiar to most patients as walking, actual workload is easier to quantify without concern regarding upper body support, and debilitated patients may feel less fear of falling than with treadmill exercise. Previous studies in normal populations suggest that peak $\dot{V}O_2$ may be 5% to 10% higher with treadmill exercise. Although it has not been systematically assessed, there is theoretical reason to believe that the recruitment of additional muscle groups during treadmill exercise may have even greater influence on the peak $\dot{V}O_2$ in heart failure, because addition of arm exercise to leg exercise causes a larger increase in peak $\dot{V}O_2$ in heart failure patients than in normal patients. The testing protocol in most centers begins with a period of zero or low level work to allow familiarity with the mouthpiece and exercise equipment. A major benefit of the real time display of $\dot{V}O_2$ and carbon dioxide release is the ability to assess the level of patient effort and urge them past the point at which the respiratory quotient (R) exceeds one. Although this, in general, occurs slightly after the anaerobic or lactate threshold is detectable, it provides a practical guide to reliable exercise testing in this population. As the majority of patients do not achieve limiting symptoms until after several minutes of anaerobic metabolism, a final R value of no more than 1.0 suggests that both effort and peak $\dot{V}O_2$ were submaximal. Most patients will achieve an R value of at least 1.1, and many will achieve 1.3 or higher. Comparison of serial tests in the same patient should include comparison of peak respiratory quotients.

Peak $\dot{V}O_2$ divided by patient weight in kilograms has been the most widely studied parameter of exercise performance in this population. Cohn demonstrated peak $\dot{V}O_2$ less than 15 mL/kg/min to be associated with poorer survival in mild–moderate heart failure.[3] Jessup-Likoff showed peak $\dot{V}O_2$ less than 13 to identify increased risk in more severe heart failure.[11] Slazchic in a small series suggested peak $\dot{V}O_2$ less than 10 to be associated with high mortality.[12] Mancini demonstrated the importance of peak $\dot{V}O_2$ measured at the time of initial transplant evaluation.[10] While 14 mL/kg/min on treadmill testing was the initial recommendation for a threshold regarding need for transplantation, their patients with peak $\dot{V}O_2$ of less than 10 mL/kg/min had the worst prognosis. Further work from that group in 272 patients supported the use of 14 mL/kg/min. Our experience with over 300 ambulatory patients performing bicycle exercise after referral for transplantation[13] reflected a 2-year survival of 57% without urgent transplantation in patients with peak $\dot{V}O_2$ less than 10 mL/kg/min, 70% with peak $\dot{V}O_2$ 10 to 16 mL/kg/min (Figure 2). Patients with peak $\dot{V}O_2 > 16$ mL/kg/min had a 1-year survival without urgent transplantation of 89%, at 2 years 84%. The Stanford experience suggested a threshold value of 12 mL/kg/min.[14] Synthesis of these reports indicates three broad groups divided according to exercise capacity. A very high-risk group can be identified with peak $\dot{V}O_2$ less than 10 to 12 mL/kg/min. Varying estimates of survival in this population may reflect variable exclusion of patients with congestive symptoms at rest. On the other hand, patients with peak $\dot{V}O_2$ over 16 to 18 mL/kg/min appear to have a 2-year prognosis at least as good as that after cardiac transplantation. Estimation of prognosis for patients in the middle range of peak $\dot{V}O_2$ may require use of other information, including that obtained from serial exercise testing.

Peak $\dot{V}O_2$ can also be expressed as a percentage of predicted maximal capacity using the Wasserman et al equation[15] which includes gender, age, and nonobese weight,[15] or the Astrand equation which includes gender and age.[16] This in theory would aid comparison of the relative limitation between the young male patient and the elderly female patient, for example. In multivariate analysis of our population using the proportional hazards model, percent of predicted peak $\dot{V}O_2$ is essentially interchangeable with peak $\dot{V}O_2$ per kilogram. For calculating actuarial survival, percent of predicted peak consumption has not improved distinction between survivors and nonsurvivors beyond that provided by peak mL/kg/min in our experience or that of Mancini, although it was found helpful by another group.[17] This parameter seemed to divide our 320 patients into two rather than three groups (Figure 3). Those with greater than 50% of predicted peak capacity have a 1-year survival of approximately 90%, 2-year survival of approximately 83%.

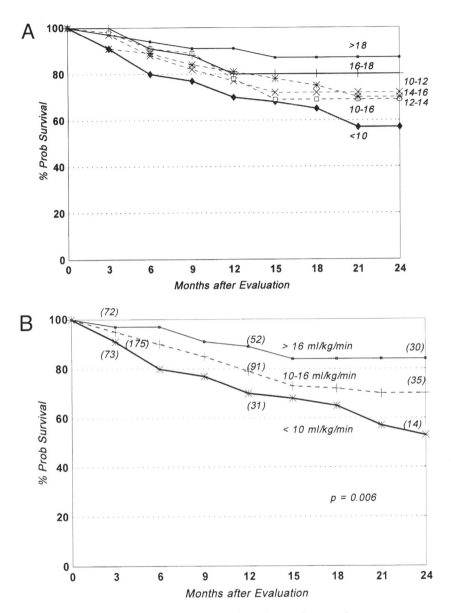

Figure 2. Actuarial **curves** of survival without hospitalization for urgent transplantation, analyzed for 320 patients undergoing cardiopulmonary exercise testing during intial evaluation for transplantation. Both death and urgent transplantation were considered end points of medical therapy, with patients censored at time of elective transplantation. **A**) Division of patients in increments of 2 mL/kg/min peak oxygen consumption ($\dot{V}O_2$): 73 patients < 10 mL/kg/min, 67 patients 10–12, 62 patients 12–14, 46 patients 14–16, 37 patients 16–18, and 35 patients over 18 mL/kg/min. **B**) Division of patients into three groups suggested by the results in A. The test was performed after a 6-minute warm up at 20 watts, followed by a 5- to 10-minute rest period and symptom limited bicycle exercise at a ramping interval of 15 W/min. Significance for prediction of outcome by Mantel-Cox, p = 0.006.

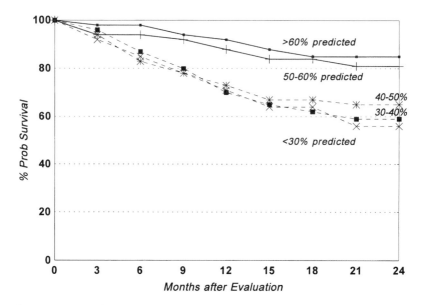

Figure 3. Actuarial **curves** of survival without urgent transplantation for the same patients as in Figure 2, classified according to the peak oxygen consumption ($\dot{V}O_2$) expressed in relationship to maximal values predicted by the Wasserman et al formula[15] according to age, gender, and lean body mass. This calculation appears to divide the population into 2 major groups, those achieving less than 50% of predicted values (38 patients less than 30%, 72 patients 30% to 40%, and 85 patients 40% to 50%), and those achieving ≥ 50% of predicted values (68 patients 50% to 60%. 57 patients > 60%).

Other parameters of exercise capacity may be determined. In our population of patients referred for transplantation, it was possible to compare the results of peak $\dot{V}O_2$, anaerobic threshold (AT), peak watts, and double product of peak blood pressure times peak heart rate in 300 patients. In 180 patients, the 6-minute walk test could also be compared to all of the above peak exercise measurements. Multivariate analysis for prediction of survival or survival without urgent transplant shows AT to be essentially interchangeable with peak $\dot{V}O_2$. Double product and 6-minute walk distance were not significant univariate predictors of survival in the proportional hazards model, so they were not entered into multivariate analysis.

Further analysis of peak watts achieved did identify the small group of patients (10%) achieving less than 40 watts to be at higher risk, with only 53% likelihood of surviving 2 years without urgent transplantation. Those patients (28%) achieving over 100 watts had 83% likelihood of surviving 2 years without urgent transplantation. The majority of the patients achieved between 40 and 100 peak watts

Table 1

Peak Watts Achieved During Incremental Exercise Encouraged
Beyond Respiratory Quotient = 1

| | | Predicted Survival Without Urgent Transplant | |
Watts	# Patients	1 Year	2 Years
≤40	32	70%	53%
40–60	47	73	66
60–80	72	81	70
80–100	70	79	71
>100	86	88	83

and had intermediate survival (Table 1). It is critical to recognize that the peak watts achieved during cardiopulmonary exercise testing are more reflective of true peak capacity than workload achieved during standard cardiac workload testing, due to the on-line availability of the respiratory quotient, which guides the degree of encouragement during the test. Without this information, it is difficult to assess the degree to which exercise is limited by oxygen delivery and utilization. The double product at peak exercise did not distinguish at all between survivors and nonsurvivors (Table 2).

The 6-minute walk test is easily performed without formal exercise equipment. The distance covered is shorter in patients with higher classes of heart failure symptoms.[18] Patients with severe symptoms at rest or minimal exertion will have very low peak $\dot{V}O_2$ and short 6-minute distance, while patients who are extremely fit will have high peak $\dot{V}O_2$ and long 6-minute distance. For 2-year survival, 6-minute walk distance provides only modest information (Figure 4). In most

Table 2

Double Product Achieved During Incremental Exercise

| | | Predicted Survival Without Urgent Transplant | |
Double Product	# Patients	1 Year	2 Years
<12k	34	85%	75%
12–16k	81	72	64
16–20k	82	79	71
20–24k	56	88	81
>24k	32	86	77

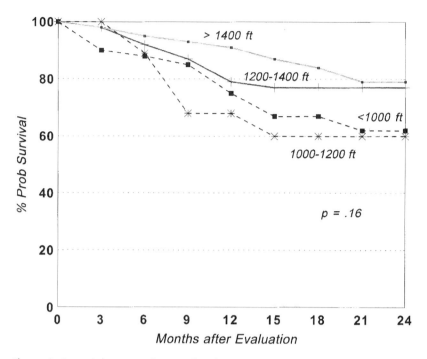

Figure 4. Actuarial **curves** of survival without urgent transplantation for 241 patients undergoing the 6-minute walk test during evaluation for transplantation. The distance walked during the 6 minutes was measured along inside corridors with two right-angle turns and no reversal of direction required for 2000 feet. Trend statistic for prediction of outcome, p = 0.16.

patients, however, factors such as stride length and habit may be more important determinants of 6-minute walk distance than aerobic capacity. In the important range of peak $\dot{V}O_2$ between 10 and 20 mL/kg/min, the correlation coefficient with 6-minute walk distance was only 0.25 in one study of 240 patients.[19] That study suggested that the ability to remain below the *AT* for 6 minutes of low-level exercise did not predict well the distance walked.

As mentioned above, the apparent predictive value of exercise testing may be further enhanced by inclusion of patients with obvious severe symptoms of heart failure at rest or with minimal exertion. As these patients can usually be identified by physical examination and history, the clinical value of exercise testing is less for them than for the ambulatory patient who appears compensated. As in exercise testing for other cardiac diagnoses, survival is significantly worse for these patients who do not perform testing due either to physician concern or patient reluctance (Figure 5).

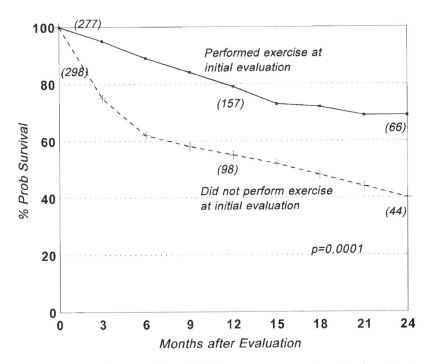

Figure 5. Actuarial **curves** of survival without urgent transplantation for patients completing cardiopulmonary exercise test during evaluation between 1988 and 1993. During this time, protocol included exercise testing of all ambulatory patients except those with resting symptoms of heart failure, severe angina, or recurrent ventricular arrhythmias, or patient refusal or failure to appear as scheduled.

Functional Capacity with Heart Failure and Transplantation

In addition to improving survival, cardiac transplantation is expected to improve functional capacity and quality of life. Some patients do not wish to undergo the rigors of transplantation to improve survival unless major improvement in functional capacity is also anticipated. To assess the potential for improvement requires quantification of the exercise capacity after transplantation.

Although the left ventricular ejection fraction is within normal limits in most patients after transplantation, multiple factors limit peak cardiac output.[20] Denervation reduces peak heart rate, although contractility does increase with exercise. Decreased compliance may limit ventricular filling despite high venous return. The ravages of rejection and transplant coronary artery disease further diminish cardiac reserve. Hypertension can also impair cardiac performance after transplantation. Peripheral factors such as persistent muscle deconditioning and the effects of corticosteroid therapy may limit oxygen utilization by the exercising muscles. Obesity frequently compromises exercise. Studies of peak $\dot{V}O_2$ after transplantation have demonstrated average values between 14 and 22 mL/kg/min, usually between 50% and 70% of predicted normal values.[21-23] Patients with stable heart failure achieve similar levels of peak $\dot{V}O_2$, and are often indistinguishable from heart transplant patients in terms also of *AT* and peak oxygen pulse (Table 3). Interestingly, ventilatory equivalents for carbon dioxide also remain higher than normal after transplantation, suggesting some reduction of ventilatory efficiency. When patients are studied serially before and after transplantation, those with severe initial impairment in peak $\dot{V}O_2$ generally show improvement after transplantation, in one study increasing during the first year after transplantation by 4.5 mL/kg/min from an initial level of 11 mL/kg/min.[23]

Table 3

Quality of Life Factors in Survivors* of Cardiac Transplantation or Sustained Medical Therapy for Stable Heart Failure

	Cardiac Transplantation	Sustained Medical Therapy
Initial ejection fraction, %	15 ± 3	15 ± 3
Late ejection fraction, %*	62 ± 7	22 ± 9
Peak $\dot{V}O_2$, mL/kg/min	17 ± 9	19 ± 4
Predicted peak O_2, %	60 ± 14	62 ± 9
Anaerobic threshold (mL O_2)	820 ± 270	960 ± 330
Peak heart rate, beats/min	137 ± 18	145 ± 20
Peak O_2 pulse, mL/beat	10 ± 2	10 ± 2
$\dot{V}E/\dot{V}CO_2$ at peak ex	43 ± 6	37 ± 9**
6-minute walk, ft	1460 ± 180	1430 ± 190
Adjustment to illness†	47 ± 11	52 ± 8
Anxiety‡	9 ± 4	7 ± 4
Depression‡	14 ± 8	12 ± 7

*Testing at 14 ± 6 months.

**p < 0.05

$\dot{V}E/\dot{V}CO_2$ = ventilatory equivalents for carbon dioxide

†From psychological adjustment to illness scae (PAIS) total score possible 0–138, high scores represent greater impairment.

‡From multiple affective adjective checklist.

(Adapted from Reference 21.)

Indications for Transplantation

Peak $\dot{V}O_2$ provides information to allow prediction of improvement in both survival and functional capacity after cardiac transplantation. While the survival benefits may be largest for patients with initial peak $\dot{V}O_2$ below 10 to 12 mL/kg/min, functional capacity benefits may be expected for patients with peak $\dot{V}O_2$ below 14 to 15 mL/kg/min. Although normalization of peak $\dot{V}O_2$ values to predicted values for age and gender may not significantly improve the prognostic value of the test, it does clarify the relative limitation. A 24-year-old man with a peak $\dot{V}O_2$ of 16 mL/kg/min may experience greater limitation before and better functional capacity after transplantation than a 63-year-old woman with the same initial peak $\dot{V}O_2$.

Peak $\dot{V}O_2$ has become a critical component of the evaluation for transplantation in an ambulatory patient (Table 4). While ejection fraction below 20% and history of severe symptoms of heart failure are no longer adequate indications of the severity of current compromise, measurement of peak $\dot{V}O_2$ quantifies both risk and functional limitation.[24]

Table 4

Bethesda Conference
Selection Criteria for Benefits from Transplantation

I. Accepted Indications for Transplantation
    1. Peak $\dot{V}O_2$ < 10 mL/kg/min with achievement of anaerobic metabolism.
    2. Severe ischemia consistently limiting routine activity not amenable to bypass surgery or angioplasty.
    3. Recurrent symptomatic ventricular arrhythmias refractory to all accepted therapeutic modalites.
II. Probable Indications for Cardiac Transplantation
    1. Peak $\dot{V}O_2$ < 14 mg/kg/min and major limitation of the patient's daily activities.
    2. Recurrent unstable ischemia not amenable to bypass or angioplasty.
    3. Instability of fluid balance/renal function not due to patient noncompliance with regimen of weight monitoring, flexible use of diuretic drugs and salt restriction.
III. Inadequate Indications for Transplantation
    1. Ejection fraction
    2. History functional class III or IV symptoms of heart failure.
    3. Previous ventricular arrhythmias
    4. Peak $\dot{V}O_2$ > 15 m/kg/min without other indications.

(Adapted from Reference 24.)

Role of Exercise Testing in Reevaluation of Candidates Awaiting Transplantation

There are currently twice as many patients listed for transplantation each month as actually undergo the procedure. The average waiting time for an ambulatory patient now exceeds 500 days and will lengthen further.[25] Patients who do not die or deteriorate to require hospitalization for urgent transplantation may demonstrate progressive improvement under the intense medical supervision provided during the waiting period. Although it has been recognized that ambulatory patients surviving to undergo transplantation may have proven themselves to have a good intermediate prognosis without transplantation, the process of reevaluating and removing a patient from the transplant waiting list is emotionally charged. A patient and his family whose lives have focused on the imminent drama of transplantation are understandably reluctant to return the symbolic beeper. The medical staff are intimidated by the continued risks of sudden death or deterioration, even when these risks have declined to equal the risks of death from infection or rejection after transplantation. The use of objective criteria may facilitate reevaluation of the ambulatory waiting list population.

The combination of clinical criteria for stability and improved exercise capacity was tested for reevaluation of waiting candidates.[26] In a study of 107 ambulatory patients listed with an initial peak $\dot{V}O_2$ of < 14mL/kg/min, 68 had neither undergone transplantation, deteriorated to require continued hospitalization, nor died before reevaluation could be performed. While on the list, all patients were supervised on a regimen of vasodilator and diuretic therapy tailored to hemodynamic goals and evaluated for management of ventricular arrhythmias. At an average of 6 months after initial listing, these patients underwent repeat exercise testing and clinical evaluation (Table 5). Of the 68 patients reexercised, 38 showed major improvement, defined as an increase in peak $\dot{V}O_2$ by at least 2 mL/kg/min to at least 12 mL/kg/min (Figure 6 and Table 6)., Of the 38 patients with exercise improvement, 7 had evidence of clinical instability and remained on the list. The other 31 patients were removed from the active waiting list, after an average improvement of 5 mL/kg/min in peak $\dot{V}O_2$. Over the next 2 years after reevaluation, their survival was 92%, and only 5 patients were relisted for transplantation.

Examining the changes occurring in exercise capacity reveals that the increases in peak $\dot{V}O_2$ were accompanied by commensurate changes in the *AT* without increases in the respiratory quotient at peak exercise, confirming that the changes measured were most likely due to true increase in aerobic capacity rather than intensification of effort.

Table 5

Assessment of Clinical Stability

Clinical Criteria
1. Stable fluid balance without orthopnea, elevated jugular venous pressures, or other evidence of congestion on the flexible diuretic regimen.
2. Stable blood pressure with systolic at least 80 mmHg.
3. Stable serum sodium and renal function.
4. Absence of symptomatic ventricular arrhythmias.
5. Absence of frequent angina.
6. Absence of severe drug side effects.
7. Stable or improving activity level without dyspnea during self-care or 1 block exertion.

Exercise Criteria (if initial peak $\dot{V}O_2 < 14$ mL/kg/min)
1. Improvement in peak $\dot{V}O_2$ of $\geqslant 2$ mL/kg/min.
2. Peak $\dot{V}O_2 \geqslant 12$ mL/kg/min.

(Adapted from Reference 26.)

Table 6

Changes in Exercise Performance after Acceptance as Transplant Candidates

| | No Major Improvement | Major Improvement $n = 38$ | |
		Remained On List	Taken Off List
Number of patients	30	7	31
Increased peak $\dot{V}O_2$	0.7 ± 3	(by def) **4 ± 3**[t]	**5 ± 3**[t]
Change in R at peak ex	−.04 ± .10	.02 ± .04	−.03 ± .17
Increased AT	.05 ± 1.7*	**2.3 ± 1.5**	**2.7 ± 2.0****
Increased peak watts	6 ± 22*	**30 ± 15**	28 ± 28
Change in resting HR	−1 ± 13	−3 ± 11	**−11 ± 20**
Increased peak HR	2 ± 21	13±18	−1 ± 25
Increased exercise HR reserve	3 ± 21	**16 ± 16**	10 ± 2.5
Increased O_2 pulse	0.3 ± 2.0*	0.7 ± 1.2	**2.5 ± 2.4****
Change in peak SBP	4 ± 25	−5 ± 6	**15 ± 25****

[t]Boldface italic type indicates significant change from baseline.

*Significant difference between patients with no improvement and patients with major improvement.

**Significant difference between improved patients taken off the list and all others.

AT = anaerobic threshold, HR = heart rate, R = respiratory quotient, SBP = systolic blood pressure, $\dot{V}O2$ = oxygen uptake

All values expressed ± standard deviations.

(Adapted from Reference 26.)

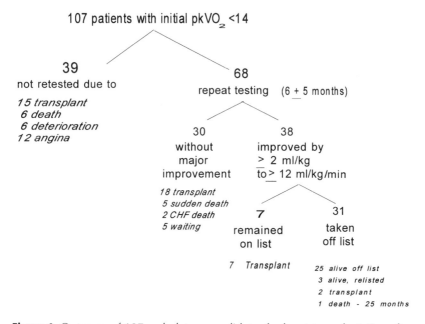

Figure 6. Outcome of 107 ambulatory candidates for heart transplantation after initiation of periodic reevaluation including cardiopulmonary exercise testing. Patients with major improvement in exercise performance who remained on the list failed to meet all criteria for clinical stability as listed in Table 5. (Adapted from Reference 26.)

Although there was only a small group of patients whose unstable clinical picture continued to warrant transplantation despite improved exercise performance, those patients had no significant increase in peak oxygen pulse compared to the patients who were able to leave the transplant list (Table 6). The increase in exercise capacity was accompanied in both groups by an increase in heart rate reserve (heart rate at peak exercise-heart rate at rest), but this resulted in the unstable group from an increase in peak heart rate, while the stable group had a decrease in resting heart rate. Also different in the improved patients was the increase in peak systolic blood pressure, which may reflect either increased central blood flow or improved ability to vasoconstrict nonexercising vascular beds.

Summary

The increasing complexity of heart failure mandates thoughtful initial and serial evaluation of each patient in order to select and assess available therapies. Identification of the candidate for transplantation must be guided by the expected improvements in survival and functional capacity. The peak $\dot{V}O_2$ measured during symptom-limited incremental exercise testing identifies groups of ambulatory patients with low, average, and high risk of death or deterioration to require urgent transplantation within the next 1 to 2 years. In addition, the measured functional capacity can be compared to that described after transplantation to determine the degree of improvement the patient can expect. Peak $\dot{V}O_2$ is a major criterion in the accepted indications for transplantation. Recent work indicates that improvement in peak $\dot{V}O_2$ should also be a major criterion in the reevaluation of ambulatory candidates awaiting transplantation, up to 30% of whom may demonstrate sufficient improvement to leave the active waiting list. As waiting lists lengthen, systematic evaluation and reevaluation of eligible candidates should increase their overall survival, both by increasing the duration of functional time prior to transplantation, and by distributing the donor hearts expeditiously to those candidates least likely to survive without them.

References

1. Hosenpud JD, Novock RJ, Breen TJ, Daily OP: The registry of the international society for heart and lung transplantation: eleventh official report—1994. *J Heart Lung Trans* 13(4):561–570, 1994.
2. Stevenson LW, Fonarow GC, Steimle AE, et al: Survival without transplantation despite ejection fraction < 20% and class IV symptoms. *J of Heart and Lung* 90(1) Part II:S32, 1994.
3. Cohn J, Johnson G, Shabetai R, et al: Ejection fraction, peak exercise oxygen consumption, cardiothoracic ratio, ventricular arrhythmias, and plasma norepinephrine as determinants of prognosis in heart failure. *Circulation* 87: VI-5–VI-6, 1993.
4. Lee W, Packer M: Prognostic importance of serum sodium concentration and its modification by converting-enzyme inhibition in patients with severe chronic heart failure. *Circulation* 73: 257–267, 1986.
5. Franciosa J, Wilen M, Ziesche S, Cohn J: Survival in men with severe left ventricular failure due to either coronary artery disease or idiopathic dilated cardiomyopathy. *Am J Cardiol* 51: 831–836, 1983.
6. Wilson J, Schwartz JS, Sutton MSJ, et al: Prognosis in severe heart failure: relation to hemodynamic measurements and ventricular ectopic activity. *J Am Coll Cardiol* 2: 403–410, 1983.
7. Lee TH, Hamilton MA, Stevenson LW, et al: Impact of left ventricular cavity size on survival in advanced heart failure. *Am J Cardiol* 72:672–676, 1993.
8. Stevenson LW, Tillisch JH, Hamilton M, et al: Importance of hemodynamic response to therapy in predicting survival with ejection fraction ≤ 20% secondary to ischemic or non-ischemic dilated cardiomyopathy. *Am J Cardiol* 66:1348–1354, 1990.
9. Stevenson WG, Stevenson LW, Middlekauff HR, Saxon LA: Sudden death prevention in patients with advanced left ventricular dysfunction. *Circulation* 88:2953–2961, 1993.

10. Mancini D, Eisen H, Kussmaul W, Mull R, Edmunds L, Wilson J: Value of peak exercise oxygen consumption for optimal timing of cardiac transplantation of ambulatory patients with heart failure. *Circulation* 83: 778–786, 1991.

11. Jessup-Likoff M, Chandler S, Kay H: Clinical determinants of mortality in chronic CHF secondary to idiopathic dilated or ischemic cardiomyopathy. *Am J Cardiol* 59(6):634–638, 1987.

12. Slazchic J, Massie B, Kramer B, Topic N, Tuban J: Correlates and prognostic implication of exercise capacity in chronic congestive heart failure. *Am J Cardiol* 55:1037–1042, 1985.

13. Stevenson L, Steimle A, Chelimsky-Fallick C, et al: Outcomes predicted by peak oxygen consumption during evaluation of 333 patients with advanced heart failure. *Circulation* 88: 94A, 1993.

14. Haywood GA, Rickenbacher PR, Trindade PT, Vagelos RH, Oyer P, Fowler MB: Deaths in patients awaiting heart transplantation: the need to identify high risk category two patients. *Circulation* 90: I-360, 1994.

15. Wasserman K, Hansen J, Sue D, Whipp B: *Principles of Exercise Testing and Interpretation*. Philadelphia: Lea and Febiger; 72–86, 1986.

16. Astrand P: Human physical fitness with special reference to sex and age. *Physiol Rev* (suppl 2) 36:307–335, 1956.

17. Stelken AM, Younis LT, Jennison SH, et al: Improved risk stratification of ambulatory congestive heart failure patients using age and gender adjusted percent predicted peak exercise oxygen uptake (abstr). *J Am Coll Cardiol* 23:400A, 1994.

18. Lipkin DP, Scriven AJ, Crake T, Poole-Wilson PA: Six-minute walking test for assessing exercise capacity in chronic heart failure. *Br Med J* 292: 653–655, 1986.

19. Stevenson LW, Lucas C, Hamilton MA, Fonarow GC, Creaser J, Janovsky V: Six-minute walk compared to peak and low-level aerobic capacity in 302 patients with heart failure. *J Am Coll Cardiol* 1995. In press.

20. Stevenson LW, Miller L: Cardiac Transplantation as Therapy for Heart Failure. *Current Problems in Cardiology*. 16;4:219–305, 1991.

21. Stevenson LW, Sietsema K, Tillisch JH, et al: Exercise capacity for survivors of cardiac transplantation or sustained medical therapy for stable heart failure. *Circulation* 81:78–85, 1990.

22. Kavanagh T, Yacoub MH, Mertner DJ, Kennedy J, Campbell RB, Sawyer P: Cardiorespiratory responses to exercise training after orthotopic cardiac transplantation. *Circulation* 77:162–171, 1988.

23. Hauptman PJ, Givertz M, Kartashov AI, et al: Predictive value of functional capacity before and after cardiac transplantation. *Circulation* 90:I-153, 1994.

24. Mudge G, Goldstein S, Addonizio L, et al: 24th Bethesda Conference: Cardiac Transplantation. Task Force 3: Recipient Guidelines/Prioritization. *J Am Coll Cardiol* 22:21–31, 1993.

25. Stevenson LW, Warner SL, Steimle AE, et al: The impending crisis awaiting cardiac transplantation: modeling a solution based on selection. *Circulation* 89:450–457, 1994.

26. Stevenson LW, Steimle AE, Fonarow G, et al: Improvement in exercise capacity of candidates awaiting heart transplantation. *J Am Coll Cardiol* 25:163–170, 1995.

27. The Consensus Trial Study Group. Effects of enalapril on mortality in severe congestive heart failure. *N Engl J Med* 316:1429–1435, 1987.

20

The Role of Cardiopulmonary Exercise Testing for Preoperative Evaluation of the Elderly

Paul Older, MB
Adrian Hall, MB

Introduction

Major abdominal surgery in elderly patients is associated with high mortality.[1] A paper in 1980 quoted a 9% mortality for colon resections.[2] A mortality of 18% for all patients over 80 years for abdominal surgery was reported at the 1994 Royal Australasian College of Surgeons Scientific Meeting (O'Rourke MGE, personal communication 1994). We reported an overall mortality of 7% following invasive hemodynamic measurements made at rest to assess risk.[3]

Comparison of mortality between studies of elderly surgical patients is very difficult. Review of the literature from 1984 to 1993 shows a variation of 1.4% to 11.3%[4–8] in reported mortality. Selection or exclusion criteria for surgery were not made clear in these reports. Low mortality can reflect either good surgery and perioperative care or good selection. The selection process could bias results: being too selective, using subjective criteria of cardiopulmonary function, could deny surgery to potential survivors, while failure to assess risk adequately may shorten the life of the patient.

The precise cause of postoperative death may be difficult to de-

From Wasserman, K (ed): *Exercise Gas Exchange in Heart Disease.* Armonk, NY: Futura Publishing Company, Inc., © 1996.

termine. Often death is ascribed to sepsis. Sepsis or Systemic Inflammatory Response Syndrome (SIRS)[9] places increased demands on oxygen delivery that may not be met if the cardiac output is unable to increase sufficiently. We have found that these patients often have an oxygen consumption ($\dot{V}O_2$) of 220 mL/min/m2 or greater. These patients die from cardiac failure when oxygen delivery is insufficient to meet the oxygen requirement of the organs of the body. Thus, reduced cardiovascular reserve is the pivotal cause of death. Since age is associated with deteriorating cardiac function, the age of the patient to undergo surgery is of concern. The problem with using age to assess the risk of dying from surgery, however, is highlighted by a recent study comparing 116 patients over 80 years to 622 patients under 80 years having elective abdominal aortic aneurysms resected. The difference in mortality was not significantly different (3% and 2% respectively).[10]

The trend in any individual is for cardiac function to decrease

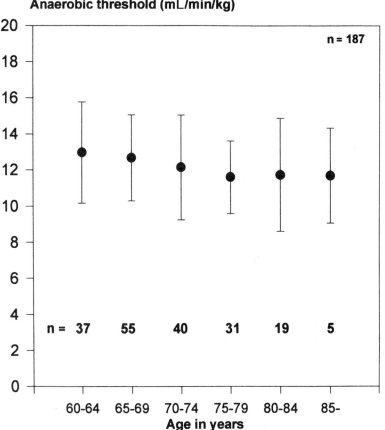

Figure. Comparison of anaerobic threshold (mean and standard deviation) with age for 187 elderly surgical patients.

with age. In fact, cardiac, pulmonary, renal, and immune systems all deteriorate with age and this compromises patients' ability to respond to the increased needs of surgery, trauma, or sepsis. Greenburg et al[11] state that "if senescence alters the ability of the elderly person to respond to stress and trauma, complete preoperative assessment is required to minimize potential difficulties."

Wasserman has pointed out that we all age at different rates, thus chronological age is not the same as physiological age.[12] Our study showed that age is an unreliable indicator of cardiovascular function as measured by anaerobic threshold (AT) (Figure).[13] It is not appropriate to use age alone as a selection criteria for major surgery.

Cardiac Dysfunction as a Cause of Death

Dunlop et al showed that the severity of illness was a much better predictor of outcome than age in elderly patients.[14] Goldman et al showed in 1977 that cardiac failure and arrhythmias were potent causes of perioperative mortality and morbidity and had predictive value.[15] In 1980, an invasive study of 148 elderly surgical patients, preoperatively, showed a 23% incidence of serious cardiopulmonary abnormalities which placed them at high risk of postoperative mortality.[2] We reported that studies performed at rest would not reflect the patient's physiological state post-surgery, and that exercise studies might be a better technique for evaluating the ability of the cardiopulmonary system to respond to stress.[3]

Major surgery is associated with high postoperative $\dot{V}O_2$ and cardiac output requirement.[3,16] We believe that postoperative mortality is high in elderly patients because cardiac reserve is reduced. As a result of cardiac failure, the increased postoperative oxygen demand cannot be met. The only options for raising $\dot{V}O_2$ in postoperative patients are to increase oxygen extraction ratio (OER) and/or to increase oxygen delivery. While increases in OER to 35% are common in surgical cases, we find that an OER above 40% usually results in an increasing blood lactate. This will ultimately lead to a further increase in $\dot{V}O_2$ secondary to Cori cycle conversion of lactate to glucose in the liver. The postoperative use of inotropic drugs to augment cardiac output is widely accepted and it has been shown that this approach reduces mortality.[17]

Use of Cardiopulmonary Exercise Testing to Evaluate Cardiac Function

Cardiac failure is the common denominator in many postoperative deaths. We use cardiopulmonary exercise testing (CPX) to quantify cardiac failure as well as identifying ischemia and arrhythmia. We measure

AT using the technique described by Beaver et al[18] and the classification system of Weber and Janicki to define the grade of the cardiac failure.[19] In our study,[13] we found that postoperative cardiovascular deaths were virtually confined to patients with an AT of less than 11 mL/min/kg (p = 0.001) (Table 1). We also found that an AT of less than 11 mL/min/kg associated with angina or ECG evidence of ischemia during exercise resulted in approximately 40% mortality following defined major surgery in patients over 60 years of age (Table 2). By comparison, myocardial ischemia (ST depression >1mm) with lesser degrees of cardiac failure (AT ≥ 11 mL/min/kg) did not appear to be a major risk factor. Cardiac failure, defined as an AT < 11 mL/min/kg, appeared to be as good an indicator of mortality as evidence of ischemia alone. Elderly patients who exhibited neither cardiac failure nor ischemia based on exercise testing criteria had a mortality of less than 1%, even for major surgery.

Table 1

Postoperative Death Rate as Related to Preoperative Assessment of Anaerobic Threshold (AT)

AT (mL/min/kg)	number	CVS deaths*	percentage mortality
<11	55	10	18
≥11	132	1	0.8
totals	187	11	(p < 0.001)

*CVS = cardiovascular system
(Reproduced with permission from Reference 13.)

Table 2

Postoperative Death Rate as Related to Preoperative Assessment of Anaerobic Threshold (AT) and Exercise ECG Evidence of Ischaemia

AT (mL/min/kg)	number	number with ischemia	CVS deaths	percentage mortality
<11	55	19	8	42
≥11	132	25	1	4
totals	187	44	9	(p < 0.01)

(Reproduced with permission from Reference 13.)

The "Surgical Anaerobic Threshold"

It is our hypothesis that if myocardial ischemia develops at or above the *AT*, it is less likely to develop in the postoperative period. This introduces the concept of a "surgical anaerobic threshold." This is similar to the exercise *AT* in that it is the point at which oxygen delivery is not adequate to support organ metabolism aerobically. This is the metabolic rate at which lactic acidosis develops.

We find that cardiac output, postoperatively, is less than peak cardiac output of preoperative CPX. If myocardial ischemia occurs at relatively high levels of exercise (high cardiac output), the patient is unlikely to reach that level of cardiac demand postoperatively, as compared to the patient who develops ischemia at a low metabolic rate.

The Relationship of Ischemia to Anaerobic Threshold

We studied 214 elderly elective surgical patients by CPX testing. The study concentrated on those patients who developed ischemia or arrhythmia during CPX testing, ischemia being defined as more than 1 mm horizontal depression on continuous 12 lead ECG monitoring (Mortara ELI-100XR, Mortara Instruments, Milwaukee WI). A cardiologist blinded to the CPX study reported every ECG. The relationship between ischemia, arrhythmia, *AT,* and postoperative cardiac events was examined.

Fifty-two out of the 214 patients (24.3%) had myocardial ischemia as defined by ECG criteria compared to 44 out of 187 patients (23.5%) in our initial study[13] (Table 2). There appear to be two patterns of evolution of ST depression: one in which myocardial ischemia occurs very early in exercise, becoming positive within 2 minutes of commencement, and another where ischemia occurs late, i.e., around or above the *AT*. Ischemia may be the cause of the poor cardiac performance in some instances or the result of increased cardiac demand in others. On this basis, we examined the relationship between the time of onset of the ischemia and the *AT*. We found that in those patients in whom myocardial ischemia developed at reduced work rates, the *AT* was usually reduced. The average *AT* for the patients who developed ischemia at low work rates was 10.4 mL/min/kg (SD = 1.74: n = 21). In those patients who developed ischemia at higher work rates, the *AT* averaged 13.9 mL/min/kg (SD = 2.28: n = 31). These groups are significantly different for *AT* by Student's "t" test (p = 0.05). This supports our hypothesis that those patients in whom ischemia develops early in exercise are at higher risk than those in whom it develops late. Thus, patients with early ischemia and low AT are more likely to reach their "surgical AT" postoperatively, and manifest ischemia and cardiac failure. We have found an extremely high mortality rate associated with the combination of low AT and myocardial ischemia.[13]

Conveying the Preoperative Data to Our Colleagues

The whole thrust of our work since 1985 has been to identify patients at risk following major surgery. The logical extension of this work is to evolve a preoperative system which allows anaesthetists and surgeons to easily appreciate operative risk. This would also provide our patients with better information on which to base their consent for treatment.

Ideally the system selected should be based not only on cardiovascular function, but also on the function of other organs which are critically important during the operative and postoperative periods; for example, preexisting pulmonary disease and renal disease are relevant.

The important concept is that perioperative cardiac mortality is an issue of oxygen demand versus oxygen supply. Minor surgery has a much lower oxygen demand than major surgery and therefore a lesser demand on cardiac reserve. A patient having an operation for excision of a bunion is not at the same risk as if he were subjected to an abdominoperineal resection of a rectal tumor. Therefore, we need to know both the cardiovascular status of the patient and the "oxygen demand stress" of the procedure. It follows that any risk assessment must include the planned surgery in the evaluation. We therefore suggest a classification system quite different from the 30-year-old American Society of Anesthesiologists (ASA) Classification.[20]

Proposed Grading of Preoperative Risk

Our classification uses an alphanumeric system. The first digit describes the extent of cardiac failure based on CPX data; the letters A, B, C or D indicate the Weber and Janicki grade.[19] The letter E is used to indicate an emergency procedure and implies that the Weber and Janicki classification is not known.

The second digit, a number $1–3$, indicates the likely extent of the surgical stress response in terms of $\dot{V}O_2$. The number 1 indicates a minor procedure, 2 an intermediate procedure, and 3 a major procedure.

This is based on the average oxygen consumption of 170 mL/min/m^2 observed following major surgery.[3,21] Resting oxygen consumption of the elderly is approximately 110 mL/min/m^2.[3]

Following the first two alphanumerics, a letter or series of letters indicate organ system dysfunction; for example, if the patient has myocardial ischemia, the letter *I* follows the first two alphanumerics. As we have pointed out, the ischemia may have major or minor significance. Therefore, we suggest the use of an uppercase *I* to suggest high significance of the ischemia, or a lowercase *i* if ischemia is of less significance. Cardiac arrhythmias are treated in the same manner with *A* or *a*.

Other organ system dysfunction may influence outcome or postoperative problems. An uppercase *P* implies major pulmonary dysfunction; for example, the presence of severe restrictive or obstructive disease associated with marked elevation in the ventilatory equivalent for oxygen ($\dot{V}E/\dot{V}O_2$) at AT (>35). A lowercase p denotes less significant pulmonary disease.

Uppercase *R* signifies creatinine clearance less than 30 mL/min, or lowercase *r* indicates a lesser degree of renal impairment.

The classification is presented as an alphanumeric series (Table 3). Thus *A1p,* indicates a patient with excellent cardiovascular function (*A*) and insignificant pulmonary disease (*p*) scheduled for a minor procedure (*1*). Alternatively, *B3IR* describes a patient with mild cardiac failure (*B*), significant ischemia (*I*), and severe renal disease (*R*) scheduled for a major procedure (*3*).

Nonoperative Mortality

In our studies, there has always been a group of patients whose operation was cancelled or postponed. In our latest analysis, 10 patients from a group of 118 were not operated on because they were felt to be at high risk for mortality. Six of these are still alive 6 months to 23 months after original presentation. Of the patients who died, three died of cardiovascular disease and one from the original disease. In contrast, of the 108 who had the operation, 3.7% died over the same period.

What is the Significance of Supraventricular Arrhythmia During Cardiopulmonary Exercise Testing?

In our series of 214 patients, there were five patients who developed a supraventricular tachycardia (SVT) during exercise testing. Three of these patients developed significant ST depression during SVT. The ST depression did not exist in the absence of the SVT. We classified these as a rate-dependent ischemia. The same patients de-

Table 3

Proposed Grading of Operative Risk Based on Cardiopulmonary Reserve, Magnitude of Surgery and Functional Status of Heart, Lungs and Kidneys

degree of cardiac failure A–E	postoperative $\dot{V}O_2$ (mL/min/M2) 1–3	organ system dysfunction P, p, A, a, I, i, R, r	
Weber & Janicki grade A, B, C, D (from Ref. 19) 'E' denotes emergency or unknown	1 = $\dot{V}O_2 < 120$ 2 = $120 < \dot{V}O_2 < 150$ 3 = $\dot{V}O_2 > 150$	'P' - $\dot{V}E/\dot{V}O_2 > 35$ 'A' - SVT 'I' - early ischemia 'R' - cr.cl* < 30mL/min	'p' - $28 < \dot{V}E/\dot{V}O_2 < 35$ 'a' - other arrhythmia 'i' - late ischemia 'r' - 30 < cr.cl < 70

*cr.cl = creatinine clearance

veloped supraventricular arrhythmias in the ICU despite preoperative digitalization.

Are the Newer Endoscopic Procedures Less "Stressful"?

Quantification of the oxygen demand stress of surgical procedures has increasing relevance as laparoscopic surgery becomes more prevalent. If the laparoscopic procedure results in a lower postoperative oxygen demand than conventional surgery, then the procedure could be offered to patients with a lower cardiac reserve.

Making the Best Use of Intensive Care Unit/High Dependency Unit Resources

Our indication for admission to the intensive care unit (ICU) or the high dependency unit (HDU) for elderly patients scheduled for major surgery remains unaltered since 1989. Patients with an AT of less than 11 mL/min/kg ($C3$ or worse) are electively admitted to the ICU preoperatively where they are invasively monitored by pulmonary artery catheters. Filling pressures are optimized with appropriate fluid therapy, renal function is estimated via creatinine clearance, and all preoperative surgical and anaesthetic orders are implemented. This policy has the additional benefit of identifying those patients with extremely high values for pulmonary vascular resistance, a known mortality risk factor.[22] It also reduces anaesthetic time in that all "lines" are in place and X-rays are performed prior to anaesthesia. Patients who have an $AT \geq$ 11 mL/min/kg, but exhibit either myocardial ischemia or significant arrhythmia are admitted to HDU postoperatively for cardiovascular system (CVS) monitoring ($A3$ or $B3$ with I or A). We also admit patients to HDU postoperatively if they have significantly disturbed pulmonary function or a $\dot{V}E/\dot{V}O_2$ at AT of >35 during CPX testing. All patients scheduled for major vascular surgery (resection of abdominal aortic aneurysm, distal vascular grafting) are routinely admitted to the ICU regardless of the results of CPX testing. Finally, the very few patients (<4% in our series) who could not successfully perform CPX are invasively monitored preoperatively in the ICU.

We have examined the ICU bed utilization in our hospital over the period of a decade, from 1983 to 1993. Before CPX was available, approximately 450 ICU bed-days were occupied for each 100 elderly patients undergoing major abdominal surgery. Patients who deteriorated on the ward were admitted to the ICU as emergencies, and they had a stay of 10 days or more associated with a high mortality rate.

Since we started to evaluate patients by CPX testing, approximately 40% of patients were managed postoperatively on the wards,

50% were admitted to the ICU preoperatively, and 10% were electively admitted to the HDU postoperatively. Of the last 450 elderly patients evaluated by CPX testing, no patient identified as at low risk was admitted to ICU from the wards as an emergency. The average duration of stay was 4.8 days for patients electively admitted to the ICU.

Only 220 bed-days were occupied for each 100 patients who went to surgery, and this includes the day of preoperative admission. Mortality rate has been reduced to less than 5% from >12%.

Summary

Mortality remains high in elderly patients undergoing major abdominal surgery. While chronological age is a poor guide to physiological status, senescence is associated with a deterioration in cardiopulmonary, renal, and immune function. The importance of both cardiac failure and ischemia in the operative patient has long been recognized. We believe that the reduction in cardiopulmonary reserve is the pivotal factor in mortality following major surgery. Postoperatively, there is a large increase in oxygen demand which requires an increase in cardiac output. We used CPX testing to relate the cardiopulmonary reserve to postoperative mortality. The degree of cardiac failure assessed by CPX testing is an important predictor of mortality. Early onset exercise-induced cardiac ischemia is associated with a low *AT* and this is also an important predictor of mortality.

We found that the patient's ability to transport oxygen during exercise can reasonably predict operative risk when the oxygen demand stress of surgery is taken into account. Outcome is influenced by ventricular function, ischemia, arrhythmia, and impaired pulmonary and renal function. We propose a system for grading operative risk which includes evidence of these abnormalities within the framework of cardiopulmonary function based on CPX testing.

Acknowledgments: The authors would like to acknowledge the continuing support and assistance of Dr. R.E.R. Smith, Director of Department of Anaesthesia at the Western Hospital, and all members of the Division of Anaesthesia and Intensive Care. We also would thank Dr. R. Newman for his assistance with interpretation of exercise ECG's. We are indebted to our biomedical engineers, Rodney Hone and John Menagh, who calibrated the metabolic cart on each and every occasion it was used.

References

1. Buck N, Devlin HB, Lunn JN: *The report of a confidential enquiry into perioperative deaths.* London: The Nuffield Provincial Hospital Trust and the Kings Fund, 1987.
2. Del Guercio LRM, Cohn JD: Monitoring operative risk in the elderly. *JAMA* 243:1350–1355, 1980.

3. Older PO, Smith RER: Experience with the preoperative invasive mea-surement of haemodynamic, respiratory and renal function in 100 elderly patients scheduled for major abdominal surgery. *Anaesth Intens Care* 16: 389–395, 1988.
4. Barlow AP, Zarifa Z, Shillito RG, Crumplin MK, Edwards E, McCarthy JM: Surgery in a geriatric population. *Ann R Coll Surg Engl* 71:110–114, 1989.
5. Vivi AA, Lopes A, Cavalcanti S de F, Rossi BM, Marques LA: Surgical treatment of colon and rectum adenocarcinoma in elderly patients. *J Surg Oncol* 51:203–206, 1992.
6. Williams JH, Collin J: Surgical care of patients over eighty: a predictable crisis at hand. *Br J Surg* 75:371–373, 1988.
7. Rorbaek-Madsen M, Dupont G, Kristensen K, Holm T, Sorensen J, Dahger H: General surgery in patients aged 80 years and older. *Br J Surg* 79: 1216–1218, 1992.
8. Scott A, Baillie CT, Sutton GL, Smith A, Bowyer RC: Audit of 200 consec-utive aortic aneurysm repairs carried out by a single surgeon in a district hospital: results of surgery and factors affecting outcome. *Ann R Coll Surg Engl* 74:205–210, 1992.
9. American College of Chest Physicians/Society of Critical Care Medicine Con-sensus Conference: Definitions for sepsis and organ failure and guidelines for the use of innovative therapies in sepsis. *Crit Care Med* 20:864–874, 1992.
10. Paty PS, Lloyd WE, Chang BB, Darling RC, Leather RP, Shah DM: Aortic replacement for abdominal aortic aneurysm in elderly patients. *Am J Surg* 166:191–193, 1993.
11. Greenburg AG, Saik RP, Pridham D: Influence of age on mortality of colon surgery. *Am J Surg* 150:65–70, 1985.
12. Wasserman K: Preoperative evaluation of cardiovascular reserve in the el-derly. Editorial. *Chest* 104:663–664, 1993.
13. Older PO, Smith RER, Courtney P, Hone R: Preoperative evaluation of car-diac failure and ischemia in elderly patients by cardiopulmonary exercise testing. *Chest* 104:701–704, 1993.
14. Dunlop WE, Rosenblood L, Lawrason L, Birdsall L, Rusnak CH: Effects of age and severity of illness on outcome and length of stay in geriatric sur-gical patients. *Am J Surg* 165:577–580, 1993.
15. Goldman L, Caldera DL, Nussbaum SR, et al: Multifactorial index of cardiac risk in noncardiac surgical procedures. *N Engl J Med* 297:845–850, 1977.
16. Bland RD, Shoemaker WC: Common physiologic patterns in general sur-gical patients: haemodynamic and oxygen transport changes during and after operation in patients with and without associated medical problems. *Surg Clin North Am* 65: 793–833, 1985.
17. Boyd O, Grounds RM, Bennett ED: A randomised clinical trial of the effect of deliberate perioperative increase of oxygen delivery on mortality in high risk surgical patients. *JAMA* 270:2699–2707, 1993.
18. Beaver WL, Wasserman K, Whipp BJ: A new mthod of detecting anaero-bic threshold by gas exchange. *J Appl Physiol* 60:2020–2027, 1986.
19. Weber KT, Janicki JS: *Cardiopulmonary exercise (CPX) testing.* Philadelphia: WB Saunders Co, 153, 1986.
20. New classification of physical status. *Anesthesiology* 24:111, 1963.
21. Shoemaker WC, Appel PL, Kram HB, Waxman K, Lee T-S: Prospective trial of supranormal values of survivors as therapeutic goals in high risk surgical patients. *Chest* 94:1176–1186, 1988.
22. Shoemaker WC: Pathophysiology, monitoring, outcome prediction, and therapy of shock states. *Crit Care Clinics* 3:307–357, 1987.

Index

Adenosine diphosphate, 1
  peripheral arterial disease and, 201
Adenosine triphosphate, 1–2
Aerobic glycolysis, 168
Age
  maximal oxygen consumption and
    hemodynamic variables in, 52
  slope of minute ventilation *versus*
    carbon dioxide production and,
    128
  surgical mortality and, 288–289
  ventilatory response to exercise in
    heart failure and, 136
Aging of heart, 48–52
Alveolar hypoperfusion, dyspnea
  and, 103–104
Alveolar ventilation, at rest and
  during exercise, 150
Alveolar-capillary gas diffusion
  capacity, exercise hyperpnea
  and, 130
Anaerobic glycolysis, 168
Anaerobic threshold, 12, 23, 24
  after coronary artery bypass graft,
    240, 241
  after transplantation, 280
  after valve replacement surgery,
    237
  age and, 288–289
  in drug trials, 251–253
  in evaluation of physical training
    following cardiac surgery,
    231–233
  exercise intensity at, 230
  postoperative cardiovascular
    deaths and, 290
  in precardiac transplantation
    evaluation, 276
  rate-variable pacing and, 259
  relationship to myocardial
    ischemia, 291–292

short-term exercise training after
  cardiac surgery and, 234–242
systolic dysfunction and, 56–61
ventilatory response to exercise in
  heart failure and, 136
Anatomic dead space ventilation,
  100, 101
Angiotensin-converting enzyme
  inhibitors, 100
Ankle, swollen, 84
Arterial blood gases
  added external dead space and,
    148, 149
  changes during exercise in heart
    failure, 87, 125–143
Arterial carbon dioxide tension
  added external dead space and,
    148, 149
  exercise hyperpnea and, 97
  ventilatory response to exercise in
    heart failure and, 87, 137
Arteriovenous oxygen difference
  cardiovascular aging and, 50
  in diastolic heart failure, 44
  leg, 211
  in transplant recipient, 47
Ascites, 84
AT; *see* Anaerobic threshold
ATP; *see* Adenosine triphosphate
Atrophy, skeletal muscle, 218–219
Augmented ventilation, 145–156
  exercise testing with face mask
    using cycle ergometer and, 147
  influence of added external dead
    space on arterial blood gas
    tension during exercise testing,
    148, 149
  mechanical dead space and,
    152–154
  physiological dead space and, 154,
    155

Augmented ventilation (*Continued*)
  at rest and during exercise,
    145–146
  role of lactic acidosis, 148–152

Beta-adrenergic stimulation, post-
  exercise oxygen consumption
  and, 64–65
Bethesda Conference Selection
  Criteria for Benefits from
  Transplantation, 281
Bicarbonate
  critical capillary oxygen partial
    pressure and, 165–166
  exercise and, 5
  inadequate blood supply and, 6
  levels during exercise, 113–114
  ventilatory response to exercise in
    heart failure and, 137
Bicycle exercise test
  in chronic heart failure, 20
  in precardiac transplantation
    evaluation, 273
  rate-variable pacing and, 258
  in Vasodilator-Heart Failure Trial,
    246
Blood flow
  cardiovascular coupling of
    external to cellular respiration
    and, 4–6, 7
  heart failure and, 89, 210–212
Blood lactate
  fitness and, 6–8
  inadequate blood supply and, 6
  response during graded bicycle
    exercise, 24
Bohr equation, 135
Borg scale of dyspnea, 95–96
Breath-by-breath technology, 19–20
Breathing pattern, exercise hyperpnea in heart failure and, 130
Breathlessness, 85
Bronchial hyperresponsiveness,
  96–97
Bruce protocol, 20

CAEP; *see* Chronotropic Assessment
  Exercise Protocol
Calf muscle volume, 219, 220
Capillary blood volume, dyspnea
  and, 101–102

Capillary oxygen partial pressure,
  157–177
  exercise capacity and, 191
  factors limiting exercise in heart
    failure and, 173–176
  femoral vein blood sampling for,
    161–164, 176–178
  lactate increase during exercise
    and, 164–165
  lactate increase in heart disease
    and, 171–173, 174
  lactic acidosis facilitation of
    oxyhemoglobin dissociation
    and, 165–169
  lactic acidosis interaction with
    muscle respiration and, 178–
    179
  respiratory adaptation to heavy
    work and, 169–171
  theory of, 159–160
Carbon dioxide production
  cardiovascular coupling of
    external to cellular respiration
    and, 9, 10
  to determine ventilatory threshold,
    28, 29
  during exercise in cardiac patient,
    114–117
  in heart failure, 86
  minute ventilation in exercise and,
    125–129
  post-exercise, 66–67
Carbon monoxide, effects of acute
  reduction in oxygen transport
  and, 110
Carboxyhemoglobin, effects of acute
  reduction in oxygen transport
  and, 110–113
Cardiac asthma, 96–97
Cardiac index
  after valve replacement surgery,
    235, 238
  cardiovascular aging and, 50
  in diastolic heart failure, 44
  in transplant recipient, 47
  ventilatory response to exercise in
    heart failure and, 136
Cardiac output, 40
  anaerobic threshold and, 232
  in hypertrophic cardiomyopathy,
    44

peak exercise oxygen consumption and, 213
surgical mortality and, 289
in systolic dysfunction, 57–59
in transplant recipient, 46
Cardiac pacemaker, 257–270
cardiopulmonary exercise capacity and long-term rate-variable pacing, 262–263
cardiopulmonary exercise testing and, 258–259
chronotropic incompetence, 266–268
heart rate and oxygen uptake, 263–266
oxygen uptake and work rate, 259–261
rate-variable pacing, 257–258
Cardiac reserve, in systolic dysfunction, 57
Cardiac surgery, 229–244
determination of exercise intensity for physical training following, 229–231, 232
evaluation of exercise training following, 231–234
training based on anaerobic threshold, 234–242
Cardiac transplantation, 271–286
cardiac pressure and volume following, 46–48
exercise testing reevaluation before, 282–284
functional capacity with heart failure and, 279–280
indications for, 181
maximal oxygen consumption and hemodynamic variables in, 52
parameters of exercise capacity before, 273–279
prognosis in advanced heart failure and, 271–273
Cardiomyopathy
hypertrophic, 43–45
left ventricular pressure volume relationship in, 42
peak exercise performance in, 198
Cardiopulmonary exercise testing
after coronary artery bypass graft, 239–242

after valve replacement surgery, 235–239
before cardiac transplantation, 271–286
in chronic heart failure, 17–38
with face mask using cycle ergometer, 147
pacemaker function and, 258–259
peripheral and central oxygen extraction in, 183–196
in peripheral arterial disease, 201–202
in preoperative evaluation of elderly, 287–297
supraventricular arrhythmia during, 293–295
in systolic dysfunction, 55–62
Cardiovascular coupling of external to cellular respiration, 1–15
exercise lactic acidosis and, 6–8
muscle bioenergetics in, 1–2, 3
myocardial ischemia and, 10–12
oxygen consumption and carbon dioxide production in, 9, 10
oxygen consumption and work rate in, 2–4, 5
peripheral blood flow requirements during exercise and, 4–6, 7
peripheral vascular disease and, 13
pulmonary vascular disease and, 13–14
Cardiovascular disease, 71–81
coupling of external to cellular respiration in, 9–14
determinants of oxygen deficit in, 71–72
ejection fraction and maximal oxygen uptake in, 40
exercise lactic acidosis and, 6–8
factors affecting gas exchange dynamics in, 74–76
femoral vein oxygen partial pressure and lactate increase in, 171–173, 174
functional capacity and, 117–121
oxygen consumption dynamics in, 72–74, 76–78
peak exercise performance in, 198

Cardiovascular disease (*Continued*)
potential significance and application of oxygen consumption measurements, 78
Carnitine, peripheral arterial disease and, 200–201
Catecholamines, elevation in heart failure, 66
Cell redox state, 166–169
Chronic heart failure, 17–38
augmented ventilation in, 145–146
blood flow changes in, 210–212
cause of symptoms, 84–85
exercise hyperpnea in, 125, 129–134
exercise response in cardiac index and wedge pressure, 59
exercise response in mixed venous lactate concentration, 61
exercise response in stroke volume, 60
exercise training in, 221–222
femoral vein oxygen partial pressure and lactate increase in, 171–173, 174
indications for exercise testing in, 31–33
maximal aerobic capacity in, 23
methodology of exercise testing, 19–22
oxygen consumption for constant work rate exercise in, 77
parameters of exercise capacity in, 22–31
peak exercise performance in, 198
peripheral and central oxygen extraction in, 183–196
rationale for exercise testing, 17–19
skeletal muscle changes in, 212–221
ventilatory and arterial blood gas changes during exercise in, 125–143
Chronotropic Assessment Exercise Protocol, 263–266
Chronotropic incompetence
oxygen uptake and work rate, 259–261
pacemaker function and, 266–268

Circulatory failure
exertional dyspnea and, 61–62
systolic pump function and, 56
Citrate synthetase, 217
Claudication
exercise training in, 202–205
pathophysiology of, 198–201
Constant-load exercise testing, 202, 203–204
Coronary artery bypass graft, exercise testing after, 239–242
Coronary artery disease, peak exercise performance in, 198
Creatine phosphate, post-exercise oxygen consumption and, 65–66
Critical capillary oxygen partial pressure, 157–177
exercise capacity and, 191
factors limiting exercise in heart failure and, 173–176
femoral vein blood sampling for, 161–164, 176–178
lactate increase during exercise and, 164–165
lactate increase in heart disease and, 171–173, 174
lactic acidosis facilitation of oxyhemoglobin dissociation and, 165–169
lactic acidosis interaction with muscle respiration and, 178–179
respiratory adaptation to heavy work and, 169–171
theory of, 159–160
Cycle ergometer, 147
in short-term exercise training after cardiac surgery, 234–235
Cytokines, heart failure and, 88, 90

Dead space, 145–156
arterial blood gas tension during exercise testing and, 148, 149
augmented ventilation at rest and during exercise, 145–146
exercise testing with face mask using cycle ergometer and, 147
lactic acidosis and augmented ventilation, 148–152
mechanical, 152–154
physiological, 154, 155
ventilatory efficiency and, 100–101

ventilatory response to exercise in heart failure and, 130–132, 137, 138
Denervation, peripheral arterial disease and, 199
Depression after transplantation, 280
Desaturation in heart failure, 86
Diastolic dysfunction, 39–54
    cardiac transplantation and, 46–48
    cardiovascular aging and, 48–52
    etiology and hemodynamic consequences of, 41–42
    in hypertrophic cardiomyopathy, 43–45
Diastolic volume index
    cardiovascular aging and, 51
    in diastolic heart failure, 45
    in transplant recipient, 48
Diffusion abnormality, 101–102
Diffusive membrane, 101–102
Digoxin, Vasodilator-Heart Failure Trial and, 246
Dilated cardiomyopathy
    left ventricular pressure volume relationship in, 42
    maximal oxygen consumption and hemodynamic variables in, 52
Diuretic therapy, Vasodilator-Heart Failure Trial and, 246
Drug studies, 245–256
    anaerobic threshold determination and, 251–253
    control subject calibration in, 247–249
    discussion of, 254–255
    oxygen consumption as risk assessment guide, 249, 250
    peak oxygen consumption and, 249–251
    quality control in, 247
    V-HeFT III protocol in, 253–254
    V-HeFT protocols in, 246
Dual chamber pacing, 267–268
Dual chamber rate-variable pacing, 267–268
Dynamic endurance, 218
Dyspnea, 95–107
    abnormal diffusive membrane in, 101–102
    alveolar hypoperfusion and, 103–104

awareness and measurement of, 95–96
    cardiac asthma and, 96–97
    exercise hyperpnea and, 97
    exercise performance and, 98–99
    reversibility of reduction of ventilatory efficiency and, 99–101
    in systolic dysfunction, 61–62
    ventilatory efficiency and, 97–98

Ejection fraction
    after transplantation, 280
    cardiovascular aging and, 51
    in diastolic heart failure, 45
    maximal oxygen uptake in heart disease and, 40
    in transplant recipient, 46, 47
Elderly, cardiopulmonary exercise testing in preoperative evaluation of, 287–297
Enalapril, Vasodilator-Heart Failure Trial and, 246
End-capillary oxygen partial pressure, 160–171
    femoral vein blood determination of, 161–164
    lactate increase during exercise and, 164–165
    lactic acidosis facilitation of oxyhemoglobin dissociation and, 165–169
    lactic acidosis in respiratory adaptation to heavy work and, 169–171
Excess post-exercise oxygen consumption, 64–65
Exercise
    anaerobic threshold and, 230–231
    augmented ventilation in, 145–146
    femoral vein oxygen partial pressure and lactate increase during, 164–165
    following cardiac surgery, 229–244
    heart failure symptoms during, 85
    lactate levels during, 113–114
    leg venous oxygen partial pressure at peak, 189, 190
    muscle bioenergetics in, 1–2, 3
    peripheral blood flow requirement during, 4–6, 7

Exercise (*Continued*)
  in precardiac transplantation
    evaluation, 283
  ventilatory response as related to
    functional capacity, 109–123
  ventilatory response to, 126–129
Exercise capacity, 257
  cardiac transplantation and,
    273–279
  critical capillary oxygen partial
    pressure and, 191
  in drug studies, 245
  long-term rate-variable pacing
    and, 262–263
Exercise hyperpnea, 97, 125–143
  alveolar hypoperfusion and,
    103–104
  arterial blood gas changes in heart
    failure and, 132–133
  assessment of, 126–129
  clinical meaning of, 138–139
  diffusion abnormalities and,
    101–102
  hemodynamics, functional
    capacity, and arterial blood
    gases and, 134–138
  increased dead space in, 145–146
  increased pulmonary dead space
    and, 130–132
  metabolic acidosis and, 133
  non-carbon dioxide, non-pH
    dependent mechanisms in,
    133–134
  peripheral and central oxygen
    extraction and, 183–196
  peripheral determinants of,
    209–227
  pulmonary pressures and, 129–
    130
  ventilatory efficiency and, 97–98
  ventilatory response as related to
    functional capacity, 109–123
Exercise testing; *see*
    Cardiopulmonary exercise
    testing
Exercise tolerance
  after valve replacement surgery,
    235
  in chronic heart failure, 22–31
  diastolic dysfunction and, 39

oxygen delivery and, 185–187
ventilatory efficiency and, 98–99
Exercise training
  after cardiac surgery, 229–244
  in chronic heart failure, 221–222
  in peripheral arterial disease,
    202–205

Face mask, 147
Fatigue
  in chronic heart failure, 18–19
  post-exercise in heart failure, 68–69
Femoral vein blood sampling,
    161–164, 176–178
Femoral vein oxygen partial
    pressure, 160–173
  in chronic heart failure, 211
  determination of, 161–164
  lactate increase during exercise
    and, 164–165
  lactate increase in heart disease
    and, 171–173, 174
  lactic acidosis facilitation of
    oxyhemoglobin dissociation
    and, 165–169
  lactic acidosis in respiratory
    adaptation to heavy work and,
    169–171
Fick equation, 39
Fick relationship, 72
Fitness, exercise lactic acidosis and,
    6–8
Fluid retention, 84
Functional capacity, 109–123
  carbon dioxide production during
    exercise and, 114–117
  cardiovascular disease and,
    117–121
  changes in lactate and bicarbonate
    levels during exercise, 113–114
  effects of reduction in oxygen
    transport on ventilatory control,
    109–113
  transplantation and, 279–280
  ventilatory response to exercise
    and, 117–121

Gas exchange ratio, 121
Glycolysis, 168, 217
Graded maximal exercise test, 20

Heart disease; *see* Cardiovascular disease
Heart failure, 83–93
    augmented ventilation in, 146
    cardiac transplantation for, 271–273
    cause of symptoms, 84–85
    chronic; *see* Chronic heart failure
    critical capillary oxygen partial pressure and, 173–176
    defined, 55–56
    dyspnea in, 95–107
    exercise arterial blood gas changes in, 132–133
    exercise hyperpnea in, 125, 129–134
    gas exchange during recovery from exercise in, 63–70
    skeletal muscle and, 87–89
    systolic dysfunction and, 55–62
    ventilation in, 86–87
Heart rate
    after transplantation, 47, 280
    cardiovascular aging and, 50
    chronotropic incompetence and, 266–267
    in diastolic heart failure, 44
    exercise capacity and, 257
    pacemaker function and, 263–266
    ventilatory response to exercise in heart failure and, 136
Hemodynamics
    diastolic dysfunction and, 41–42
    in peripheral arterial disease, 198–199
    ventilatory response to exercise in heart failure and, 134–138
Hexokinase, 217
High dependency unit, 295–296
Hydralazine, Vasodilator-Heart Failure Trial and, 246
3-Hydroxyacyl-CoA dehydrogenase, 217
Hypertrophic cardiomyopathy, 43–45, 52

Intensive care unit, 295–296
Isokinetic endurance, peal oxygen consumption and, 219
Isosorbide dinitrate, Vasodilator-Heart Failure Trial and, 246

Kinetics of recovery of oxygen consumption, 31

Lactate
    critical capillary oxygen partial pressure and, 164–165, 171–173, 174
    effects of acute reduction in oxygen transport and, 110–112
    exercise and, 5, 113–114
    peripheral arterial disease and, 200
    post-exercise carbon dioxide production and, 67
    pyruvate and, 158
Lactic acidosis
    augmented ventilation and, 148–152
    cardiovascular coupling of external to cellular respiration and, 6–8
    exercise hyperpnea and, 97
    facilitation of oxyhemoglobin dissociation, 165–169
    inadequate blood supply and, 6
    interaction with muscle respiration, 178–179
    oxygen consumption and carbon dioxide production kinetics in, 9, 10
    respiratory adaptation to heavy work and, 169–171
Lactic acidosis threshold, 12, 23–24, 25
    cardiovascular disease and, 75
    effects of acute reduction in oxygen transport and, 110–113
    glycolysis and, 168
Left ventricular ejection fraction
    anaerobic threshold and, 232
    relation to oxygen consumption in chronic heart failure, 18
    ventilatory response to exercise in heart failure and, 136
Left ventricular filling abnormalities
    cardiovascular aging and, 48–52
    hemodynamic consequences of, 41–42
Left ventricular pressure volume loop, 41–42
Leg arteriovenous oxygen difference, 211

Leg vascular resistance, 211
Leg venous oxygen partial pressure at peak exercise, 189, 190, 191
Long-term rate-variable pacing, 262–263
Lung, chronic heart failure and, 84–85

Maximal exercise cardiac index, 61
Maximal oxygen uptake, 22–23
  during bicycle exercise in chronic heart failure, 26
  cardiovascular aging and, 50
  ejection fraction in heart disease and, 40
  in hypertrophic cardiomyopathy, 43–44
  rate-variable pacing and, 258
  systolic dysfunction and, 56–61
Mean arterial pressure, 136
Mechanical dead space
  augmented ventilation and, 152–154
  at rest and during exercise, 150
Mechanoreceptors, 134
Metabolic acidosis, 114, 133
Metabolism, peripheral arterial disease and, 199–201
Metaboreceptors, 134
Methoxamine, 96–97
Minute ventilation
  after transplantation, 280
  to determine ventilatory threshold, 28, 29
  heart rate relation to, 265–266
  peak exercise, 126
  post-exercise, 67, 68
Mitochondrial redox state, 166–169
Mitral valve stenosis, 73
Mixed venous lactate concentration, 61
Modified Naughton treadmill protocol
  in chronic heart failure, 20
  in systolic dysfunction, 57
Mortality following surgery, 287–297
  cardiac dysfunction and, 289
  cardiac transplantation and, 271–273
  exercise testing to evaluate cardiac function and, 289–292

intensive care unit and high dependency unit resources and, 295–296
  proposed grading of preoperative risk, 292–295
Muscle
  cardiovascular coupling of external to cellular respiration and, 1–2, 3
  increased ventilation in heart failure and, 83–93
  peripheral arterial disease and, 199–201
Muscle hypothesis for origin of symptoms in heart failure, 89–90
Muscle oxidative enzymes
  heart failure and, 88, 216–217
  peripheral arterial disease and, 200–201
Myocardial ischemia
  anaerobic threshold and, 291–292
  cardiovascular coupling of external to cellular respiration and, 10–12
  postoperative cardiovascular deaths and, 290
Myophosphorylase deficiency, 171

Naughton treadmill protocol
  in chronic heart failure, 20
  in systolic dysfunction, 57
New York Heart Association classification
  in chronic heart failure, 31–32
  in dyspnea, 95–96
  ventilatory response to exercise in heart failure and, 136
Norepinephrine, anaerobic threshold and, 230–231

Oxygen consumption
  after transplantation, 46, 280
  during bicycle exercise test, 22
  bicycle *versus* treadmill exercise, 20, 21
  carbon dioxide production and, 116–117
  cardiovascular coupling of external to cellular respiration and, 2–4, 5, 9, 10

cardiovascular disease and, 72–74, 76–78

chronotropic incompetence and, 267

to determine ventilatory threshold, 29

in drug trials, 249, 250

effects of acute reduction in oxygen transport and, 110–113

heart rate and pacemaker function, 263–266

increase for work rates with and without lactic acidosis, 169–171

measurement of, 184–185

muscle bioenergetics and, 1–2, 3

oxygen extraction ratio and, 187–188

post-exercise gas exchange and, 64–66, 72, 73

relation to left ventricular ejection fraction, 18

in systemic inflammatory response syndrome, 288

Oxygen consumption time constant

after coronary artery bypass graft, 240, 241

after valve replacement surgery, 237

in evaluation of physical training following cardiac surgery, 233–234

post-exercise in heart failure, 68

Oxygen consumption/work-rate ratio, 29–31

after coronary artery bypass graft, 240, 241

after valve replacement surgery, 237

cardiovascular disease and, 9–14, 75

in evaluation of physical training following cardiac surgery, 233

pacemaker function and, 259–261

Oxygen debt, 64, 65

Oxygen deficit, 64, 65, 71–72

Oxygen delivery

after valve replacement surgery, 238

exercise tolerance and, 185–187

measurement of, 184–185

peak oxygen uptake coupling and, 192

Oxygen extraction

exercise tolerance in chronic heart failure and, 192–193

leg venous oxygen partial pressure at peak exercise in, 189, 190

limitations of study, 193–194

measurement of, 184–185

peak oxygen consumption and peak oxygen delivery coupling in, 192

physiological basis of exercise capacity and critical capillary oxygen partial pressure in, 191

relation of oxygen delivery and exercise tolerance in, 185–187

relation of oxygen extraction ratio and oxygen consumption in, 187–188

severity of chronic heart failure and, 185, 186

study design in, 184

surgery and, 289

test results in, 189–191

Oxygen partial pressure

added external dead space and, 148, 149

exercise capacity and, 191

exercise-induced changes in heart failure and, 132

femoral vein lactate and, 174

leg venous, 189, 190

ventilatory response to exercise in heart failure and, 87, 137

Oxygen pulse response

after coronary artery bypass graft, 240

in chronic heart failure, 28–29

in evaluation of physical training following cardiac surgery, 233

Oxygen transport

effects of acute reduction, 109–113

normal, 18, 19

peak oxygen consumption in chronic heart failure and, 192–193

Oxygen uptake; see Oxygen consumption

Oxyhemoglobin dissociation, lactic acidosis facilitation of, 165–169

Oxyhemoglobin saturation
   during exercise, 167
   femoral venous oxygen partial
      pressure and, 161–164

Pacemaker function, 257–270
   cardiopulmonary exercise capacity
      and long-term rate-variable
      pacing, 262–263
   cardiopulmonary exercise testing
      and, 258–259
   chronotropic incompetence,
      266–268
   heart rate and oxygen uptake,
      263–266
   oxygen uptake and work rate,
      259–261
   rate-variable pacing, 257–258
PAD; see Peripheral arterial disease
Peak carbon dioxide production
   after coronary artery bypass graft,
      240
   after transplantation, 280
   ventilatory response to exercise in
      heart failure and, 136
Peak exercise performance, 198, 202
Peak oxygen consumption
   after coronary artery bypass graft,
      240, 241
   after transplantation, 280
   after valve replacement surgery,
      237
   age and, 128
   during bicycle exercise in chronic
      heart failure, 26
   chronic heart failure prognosis
      and, 33
   in drug trials, 249–251, 255
   in evaluation of physical training
      following cardiac surgery,
      231–233
   isokinetic endurance and, 219
   leg venous oxygen partial pressure
      at peak exercise and, 189, 190
   muscle mass and, 88
   peak oxygen delivery coupling
      and, 192
   in peripheral arterial disease, 202
   in precardiac transplantation
      evaluation, 274–276, 281

ventilatory response to exercise in
   heart failure and, 136
Peripheral and central oxygen
   extraction, 183–196
   exercise tolerance in chronic heart
      failure and, 192–193
   leg venous oxygen partial pressure
      at peak exercise in, 189, 190
   limitations of study, 193–194
   measurement of, 184–185
   peak oxygen consumption and
      peak oxygen delivery coupling
      in, 192
   physiological basis of exercise
      capacity and critical capillary
      oxygen partial pressure in, 191
   relation of oxygen delivery and
      exercise tolerance in, 185–187
   relation of oxygen extraction ratio
      and oxygen consumption in,
      187–188
   severity of chronic heart failure
      and, 185, 186
   study design in, 184
   test results in, 189–191
Peripheral arterial disease, 197–208
   exercise testing and performance
      in, 201–202
   hemodynamic changes in, 198–
      199
   muscle histology, function, and
      metabolism in, 199–201
Peripheral determinants of exercise
   intolerance, 209–227
   blood flow changes in, 210–212
   exercise training and, 221–222
   skeletal muscle changes in,
      212–221
Peripheral resistance, heart failure
   and, 88–89
Peripheral vascular disease, 13
pH
   anaerobic threshold and, 230
   at rest and during exercise, 150
   ventilatory response to exercise in
      heart failure and, 87, 137
Phosphate, muscle bioenergetics and,
   1–2
Phosphocreatine, 1–2
Phosphofructokinase deficiency, 171

Physiologic dead space, 154, 155
    at rest and during exercise, 150
    ventilatory efficiency and, 100, 101
Physiologic dead space to tidal
        volume ratio, 130–132, 137, 138
Plasma potassium, 134
Post-exercise gas exchange, 63–70
    in healthy subject, 64–67
    in heart failure, 67–69
Prazosin, Vasodilator-Heart Failure
        Trial and, 246
Preoperative evaluation of elderly,
        287–297
    cardiac dysfunction as cause of
        death in, 289
    exercise testing to evaluate cardiac
        function in, 289–292
    intensive care unit and high
        dependency unit resources and,
        295–296
    proposed grading of preoperative
        risk, 292–295
Pulmonary artery pressure,
        ventilatory efficiency and,
        103–104
Pulmonary capillary wedge pressure
    in chronic heart failure, 213
    in diastolic heart failure, 45
Pulmonary pressures, 129–130
Pulmonary vascular disease, 13–14
Pulmonary wedge pressure
    in diastolic heart failure, 45
    in transplant recipient, 48
    ventilatory efficiency and, 103–
        104
    ventilatory response to exercise in
        heart failure and, 136
Pyruvate, lactate and, 158

Quality of life after transplantation,
        279–280

Ramp protocol
    in chronic heart failure, 21
    in short-term exercise training
        after cardiac surgery, 234–235
    in V-HeFT III, 253–254
Rate-variable pacing, 257–258
    exercise capacity and, 262–263
    heart rate and oxygen uptake,
        263–266

oxygen uptake and work rate,
        259–261
Respiratory adaptation to heavy
        work, 169–171
Respiratory exchange ratio to
        determine ventilatory threshold,
        28, 29
Respiratory gas analysis
    in chronic heart failure, 32
    rate-variable pacing and, 258
Respiratory muscles
    exercise hyperpnea and, 139
    ventilatory efficiency and, 99
Right atrial pressure, ventilatory
        response to exercise and, 136
Roughton and Forster formula,
        101–102

Single leg blood flow, 211, 213
Single leg oxygen consumption, 211
6-minute walk test, 277–278
Skeletal muscle
    chronic heart failure and, 84,
        87–89, 212–221
    peripheral arterial disease and, 199
    ventilatory response to exercise in
        heart failure and, 134
Slope of minute ventilation *versus*
        carbon dioxide production
    in chronic heart disease, 125–129,
        136, 137
    post-exercise, 66–67
Slow-twitch type I fibers, 215–216
Static endurance, 218
Stenosis, claudication and, 199
Stroke volume
    anaerobic threshold and, 232
    cardiovascular aging and, 51
    in diastolic heart failure, 44
    exercise response in chronic
        cardiac failure and, 60
    in transplant recipient, 47
Succinate dehydrogenase, 217
Supraventricular arrhythmia during
        exercise testing, 293–295
Surgical anaerobic threshold, 291
Swollen ankle, 84
Systemic inflammatory response
        syndrome, 288
Systolic dysfunction, 55–62
    exertional dyspnea in, 61–62

Systolic dysfunction (*Continued*)
  heart failure defined in, 55–56
  maximal oxygen uptake, anaerobic
    threshold, and severity of, 56–61
Systolic volume index
  cardiovascular aging and, 51
  in diastolic heart failure, 45
  in transplant recipient, 48

Tidal volume
  exercise hyperpnea in heart failure
    and, 130–132
  respiratory frequency at rest and
    during exercise and, 152
Time constant of oxygen
    consumption
  after coronary artery bypass graft,
    240, 241
  after valve replacement surgery,
    237
  in evaluation of physical training
    following cardiac surgery,
    233–234
  post-exercise in heart failure, 68
Total ventilation, dead space and,
    153
Treadmill exercise
  in chronic heart failure, 20
  in peripheral arterial disease,
    201–202, 203–205
  in precardiac transplantation
    evaluation, 273
  rate-variable pacing and, 258
  in systolic dysfunction, 56–57

Valve replacement surgery, exercise
    training after, 235–239
Vasodilator-Heart Failure Trials, 246,
    253–254
Ventilation
  carbon dioxide production and,
    114–117
  effects of acute reduction in
    oxygen transport, 109–113
  in heart failure, 86–87
Ventilation/perfusion mismatch,
    increased physiologic dead
    space and, 146
Ventilation/perfusion ratio, at rest
    and during exercise, 155

Ventilatory efficiency
  alveolar hypoperfusion and,
    103–104
  diffusion abnormalities and, 102
  exercise hyperpnea and, 97–98
  exercise performance and, 98–99
  reversibility of reduction, 99–101
Ventilatory equivalent for carbon
    dioxide
  functional capacity and, 118, 120
  at rest and during exercise, 151
Ventilatory equivalent for oxygen,
    118, 120
Ventilatory equivalents *vs.* time
    curve, 28, 29
Ventilatory response to exercise in
    heart failure, 109–143
  arterial blood gas changes in heart
    failure and, 132–133
  assessment of, 126–129
  carbon dioxide production during
    exercise and, 114–117
  changes in lactate and bicarbonate
    levels during exercise, 113–114
  clinical meaning of, 138–139
  effects of reduction in oxygen
    transport on ventilatory control,
    109–113
  functional capacity and, 117–121,
    134–138
  hemodynamics and arterial blood
    gases and, 134–138
  increased dead space in, 145–156
  increased pulmonary dead space
    and, 130–132
  metabolic acidosis and, 133
  non-carbon dioxide, non-pH
    dependent mechanisms in,
    133–134
  pulmonary pressures and, 129–130
  transplantation and, 279–280
Ventilatory threshold
  in chronic heart failure, 24–26, 27
  determination of, 28, 30
V-HeFT protocols, 246
V-slope method, 29

Walking
  oxygen consumption in mitral
    valve stenosis and, 73

in precardiac transplantation
evaluation, 277–278
Weber and Janicki grade, 292, 294
Wedge pressure, 59
Work rate
after coronary artery bypass graft,
240
after valve replacement surgery, 237

carbon dioxide production and,
117
cardiovascular coupling of
external to cellular respiration
and, 2–4, 5
effects of acute reduction in
oxygen transport and, 110
pacemaker function and, 259–261